The Washington Manual™ Cardiology Subspecialty Consult

W9-AWM-418

The Washington Manual™ Cardiology Subspecialty Consult

Faculty Advisors
Jane Chen, M.D., F.A.C.C.
Assistant Professor of Medicine
Division of Cardiology, Arrhythmia Service
Washington University School of Medicine
St. Louis, Missouri

Keith Mankowitz, M.D., F.A.C.C.
Assistant Professor of Medicine
Division of Cardiology
Washington University School of Medicine
St. Louis, Missouri

The Washington Manual™ Cardiology Subspecialty Consult

Editor
Peter A. Crawford, M.D., Ph.D.
Postdoctoral Fellow
Department of Internal Medicine
Division of Cardiology
Department of Molecular Biology and
Pharmacology
Washington University School of Medicine
Barnes-Jewish Hospital
St. Louis, Missouri

Series Editor
Tammy L. Lin, M.D.
Adjunct Assistant Professor of Medicine
Washington University School of Medicine
St. Louis, Missouri

Series Advisor
Daniel M. Goodenberger, M.D.
Professor of Medicine
Washington University School of Medicine
Chief, Division of Medical Education
Director, Internal Medicine Residency
Program
Barnes-Jewish Hospital
St. Louis, Missouri

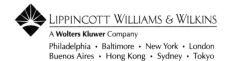
LIPPINCOTT WILLIAMS & WILKINS
A **Wolters Kluwer** Company
Philadelphia · Baltimore · New York · London
Buenos Aires · Hong Kong · Sydney · Tokyo

Acquisitions Editors: Danette Somers and James Ryan
Developmental Editors: Scott Marinaro and Keith Donnellan
Supervising Editors: Allison Risko and Mary Ann McLaughlin
Production Editor: Erica Broennle Nelson, Silverchair Science + Communications
Manufacturing Manager: Colin Warnock
Cover Designer: QT Design
Compositor: Silverchair Science + Communications
Printer: RR Donnelley

©2004 by Department of Medicine, Washington University School of Medicine

Printed in the USA

Library of Congress Cataloging-in-Publication Data

The Washington manual cardiology subspecialty consult / editor, Peter A. Crawford.
    p. ; cm. -- (Washington manual subspecialty consult series)
  Includes bibliographical references and index.
  ISBN 0-7817-4370-2
  1. Cardiology--Handbooks, manuals, etc. 2. Heart--Diseases--Handbooks, manuals, etc.
I. Title: Cardiology subspecialty consult. II. Crawford, Peter A. (Peter Alan), 1969- III. Series.
  [DNLM: 1. Cardiovascular Diseases--Handbooks. 2. Cardiology--methods--Handbooks. WG 39 W319 2003]
  RC669.15.W37 2003
  616.1'2--dc21

                                    2003047695

---

10 9 8 7 6 5 4 3 2 1

Contents

Contributing Authors

Ryan G. Aleong, M.D.

Cardiology Fellow
Department of Cardiology
University of Pittsburgh
Medical Center
Pittsburgh, Pennsylvania

Michael O. Barry, M.D.

Clinical Instructor of Medicine
Department of Internal Medicine
Washington University School of
Medicine
Barnes-Jewish Hospital
St. Louis, Missouri

Douglas R. Bree, M.D.

Cardiology Fellow
Department of Internal Medicine
Washington University School of
Medicine
Barnes-Jewish Hospital
St. Louis, Missouri

Peter A. Crawford, M.D., Ph.D.

Postdoctoral Fellow
Department of Internal Medicine,
Division of Cardiology
Department of Molecular Biology and
Pharmacology
Washington University School of
Medicine
Barnes-Jewish Hospital
St. Louis, Missouri

Richard G. Garmany, M.D.

Cardiology Fellow
Department of Internal Medicine
Washington University School of
Medicine
Barnes-Jewish Hospital
St. Louis, Missouri

Michael E. Lazarus, M.D.

Instructor of Medicine
Internal Medicine Division of
Hospital Medicine
Washington University School of
Medicine
Barnes-Jewish Hospital
St. Louis, Missouri

Christopher R. Leach, M.D.

Cardiology Fellow
Department of Internal Medicine
Division of Cardiology
Washington University School of
Medicine
Barnes-Jewish Hospital
St. Louis, Missouri

Martin S. Maron, M.D.

Cardiology Fellow
Division of Cardiology
Tufts University School of Medicine
New England Medical Center
Boston, Massachusetts

Tuan D. Nguyen, M.D.

Fellow in Cardiology
Department of Cardiovascular
Medicine
Texas Heart Institute
St. Luke's Episcopal Hospital
Houston, Texas

Michael J. Riley, M.D.

Cardiology Fellow
Department of Cardiovascular
Medicine
Cleveland Clinic Heart Center
Cleveland, Ohio

J. Mauricio Sánchez, M.D.

Cardiology Fellow
Department of Medicine
Washington University School of
Medicine
Barnes-Jewish Hospital
St. Louis, Missouri

Navinder S. Sawhney, M.D.

Instructor in Medicine
Department of Medicine
Washington University School of
Medicine
Barnes-Jewish Hospital
St. Louis, Missouri

Adam B. Stein, M.D.

Cardiology Fellow
Department of Internal Medicine
Division of Cardiology
University of Louisville School of
Medicine
Louisville, Kentucky

Alan Zajarias, M.D.

Cardiology Fellow
Department of Internal Medicine
Washington University School of
Medicine
Barnes-Jewish Hospital
St. Louis, Missouri

Chairman's Note

Medical knowledge is increasing at an exponential rate, and physicians are being bombarded with new facts at a pace that many find overwhelming. The Washington Manual™ Subspecialty Consult Series was developed in this context for interns, residents, medical students, and other practitioners in need of readily accessible practical clinical information. They therefore meet an important unmet need in an era of information overload.

I would like to acknowledge the authors who have contributed to these books. In particular, Tammy L. Lin, M.D., Series Editor, provided energetic and inspired leadership, and Daniel M. Goodenberger, M.D., Series Advisor, Chief of the Division of Medical Education in the Department of Medicine at Washington University, is a continual source of sage advice. The efforts and outstanding skill of the lead authors are evident in the quality of the final product. I am confident that this series will meet its desired goal of providing practical knowledge that can be directly applied to improving patient care.

Kenneth S. Polonsky, M.D.
Adolphus Busch Professor
Chairman, Department of Medicine
Washington University School of Medicine
St. Louis, Missouri

Series Preface

The Washington Manual™ Subspecialty Consult Series is designed to provide quick access to the essential information needed to evaluate a patient on a subspecialty consult service. Each manual includes the most updated and useful information on commonly encountered symptoms or diseases and highlights the practical information you need to gather before formulating a plan. Special efforts have been made to organize the information so that these guides will be valuable and trusted companions for medical students, residents, and fellows. They cover everything from questions to ask during the initial consult to issues in subsequent management.

One of the strengths of this series is that it is written by residents and fellows who know how busy a consult service can be, who know what information will be most helpful, and can detail a practical approach to patient care. Each volume is written to provide enough information for you to evaluate a patient until more in-depth reading can be done on a particular topic. Throughout the series, key references are noted, difficult management situations are addressed, and appropriate practice guidelines are included. Another strength of this series is that it was written in concert. All of the guides were designed to work together.

The most important strength of this series is the collection of authors, faculty advisors, and especially lead authors assembled to write this series. In addition, we received incredible commitment and support from our chairman, Kenneth S. Polonsky, M.D. As a result, the extraordinary depth of talent and genuine interest in teaching others at Washington University is showcased in this series. Although there has always been house staff involvement in editing The Washington Manual™ series, it came to our attention that many of them also wanted to be involved in writing and making decisions about what to convey to fellow colleagues. Remarkably, many of the lead authors became junior subspecialty fellows while writing their guides. Their desire to pass on what they were learning, while trying to balance multiple responsibilities, is a testament to their dedication and skills as clinicians, teachers, and leaders.

We hope this series fulfills the need for essential and practical knowledge for those learning the art of consultation in a particular subspecialty and for those just passing through it.

Tammy L. Lin, M.D., Series Editor
Daniel M. Goodenberger, M.D.,
Series Advisor

Preface

Handbooks covering cardiovascular topics reign in abundance. Physicians and physicians-in-training have no difficulty finding a pocket-sized text that comprehensively covers the fundamentals of cardiovascular medicine, physiology, imaging, electrocardiography, and/or cardiovascular pharmacotherapy.

Why, then, did we venture to add another ship to the armada? The overall content of our handbook is not particularly unique, nor should it be. However, three primary reasons explain our undertaking and render our text very useful to you.

First, the style in which the material is presented places this text among the best companions to the practicing internist, resident physician on the cardiology service or consult rotation, junior or senior medical student on the cardiology service, or motivated freshman or sophomore medical student interested in cardiology. This handbook's curriculum was devised and edited by a cardiology fellow, written by motivated residents, and reviewed by attending cardiologists. Material is presented with a singular intention: to convey concepts of pathophysiology, diagnosis, and management in a pragmatic manner. However, because the practice of cardiology today is—more so than any other field in medicine—a product of rapidly evolving, evidence-based medicine, the practical approach is clearly supported by relevant clinical investigations. This blend of focused, practical content in an academic backdrop enhances our handbook and reflects the tradition of patient care at Washington University of St. Louis and Barnes-Jewish Hospital.

For example, readers will find descriptions at many locations within the text—"classes" of indications for a particular diagnostic study or therapeutic intervention. These classes have been diligently described by the American College of Cardiology and the American Heart Association for almost all cardiovascular conditions (see http://www.ahajournals.org/misc/sci-stmts_topicindex.shtml for a complete listing); the guidelines derive from clinical scientific trials. These classes are summarized as follows:

Class I: Conditions for which there is evidence and/or general agreement that the procedure or treatment is useful and effective.

Class II: Conditions for which there is conflicting evidence and/or a divergence of opinion about the usefulness/efficacy of a procedure or treatment.

Class IIa: The weight of evidence or opinion is in favor of the procedure or treatment.

Class IIb: Usefulness/efficacy is less well established by evidence or opinion.

Class III: Conditions for which there is evidence and/or general agreement that the procedure or treatment is not useful/effective and in some cases can be harmful.

The second reason we believe our handbook is most useful is the unique format. The text is divided into three parts, each with its own set of chapters. The topics addressed in Part I, Common Presentations in Cardiology (chest pain, dyspnea, syncope, cardiac emergencies), may be the only substantive information you have before seeing a new patient. Many pathophysiologic processes are discussed, because a given presentation can be due to multiple (including noncardiac) mechanisms of disease. Diagnostic means for distinguishing those presentations are highlighted, as are the assessment and management of cardiac emergencies. It is important for readers to be familiar with the information in these chapters so that you, as a diagnostician, do not become biased toward a certain diagnosis before others are eliminated. Part II, Cardiovascular Disease Entities, covers the most common disease processes in cardiovascular medicine, providing important aspects of epidemiology, pathophysiology, appropriate history and physical exams, diagnostic testing, and management. Part III, Testing and Procedures in Cardiology, reviews diagnostic testing, procedures, and assessment and management of noncardiac surgical patients. Readers will find partial overlap in the content between Parts I and II, as well as between Parts II and III. This is intentional. Although redundancy is limited in the text, we believe a modest amount of repetition is useful. Repetition allows one to gain different perspectives on a given topic, which in turn increases the likelihood of solidifying one's knowledge, and it improves access to information. Cross-references to appropriate chapters make these relationships convenient.

Although this text contains detailed descriptions of the appropriate care of the patient with a cardiovascular emergency (balancing terseness and comprehensiveness more effectively than any other handbook), there is no section on ACLS protocols, as these are widely available through hardcopy or electronic sources (e.g., Tarascon Pharmacopeia and ePocrates for the Palm). Furthermore, although a brief outline of salient tips is provided in Chapter 1, Approach to the Cardiovascular Patient and Basic Electrocardiography, we have not provided a detailed text on ECG reading. We refer you to *Chou's Electrocardiography*

in Clinical Practice (an unabridged format) or O'Keefe et al., *The ECG Criteria and ACLS Handbook* (Physicians Press), both excellent texts on ECG criteria. Each chapter in this text highlights relevant electrocardiographic manifestations of disease and demonstrates them where appropriate.

The third reason this text is useful is accessibility. In addition to hardcopy, the text will also be available in personal digital assistant (PDA) format, allowing even faster cross-referencing within the book. Therefore, this handbook, whether used as a hardcopy or a PDA, is indispensable on the wards (a) when first learning about a new patient before your workup, (b) after you've performed your history and physical exam to help you focus your thoughts on diagnosis and management, and (c) in subsequent management of the patient after your attending has made his or her initial recommendations.

Despite the strengths of our text, it is in no way a substitute for reading the primary literature, reviews written in peer-reviewed journals, and unabridged textbooks. The information presented here is your guide to information, but it is nowhere near a complete authority. We recommend strongly further reading of the texts, articles, and Web sites referred by this handbook. We encourage you to share your thoughts and questions with us, as well as with your attending cardiologists or cardiology fellows, as the exchange of knowledge and ideas will never become mundane.

P.A.C.

Key to Abbreviations

ACC/AHA	American College of Cardiology/American Heart Association
ACE	angiotensin-converting enzyme
ACLS	advanced cardiac life support
ACS	acute coronary syndrome
AF	atrial fibrillation
AFl	atrial flutter
AI	aortic insufficiency
ANA	antinuclear antibody
ARDS	acute respiratory distress syndrome
AS	aortic stenosis
ASA	aspirin
AV	atrioventricular
AVM	arteriovenous malformation
BCLS	basic cardiac life support
BP	blood pressure
bpm	beats per minute
BUN	blood urea nitrogen
CABG	coronary artery bypass grafting
CAD	coronary artery disease
cAMP	cyclic adenosine 3',5'-monophosphate
CBC	complete blood count
CHF	congestive heart failure
CMV	cytomegalovirus
CNS	central nervous system
COPD	chronic obstructive pulmonary disease
CPR	cardiopulmonary resuscitation
CRP	C-reactive protein
CT	computed tomography
ECG	electrocardiogram
EEG	electroencephalogram
ER	emergency room
ESR	erythrocyte sedimentation rate
FDA	U.S. Food and Drug Administration
FEV_1	forced expiratory volume in 1 second
GI	gastrointestinal
HCM	hypertrophic cardiomyopathy
Hct	hematocrit
HDL	high-density lipoprotein
HIV	human immunodeficiency virus
HTN	hypertension
ICP	intracranial pressure
ICU	intensive care unit
INR	international normalized ratio
LDL	low-density lipoprotein
LMWH	low-molecular-weight heparin

LV	left ventricle
LVH	left ventricular hypertrophy
MI	myocardial infarction
MRI	magnetic resonance imaging
MVP	mitral valve prolapse
NPO	nothing by mouth (nil per os)
NSAIDs	nonsteroidal antiinflammatory drugs
NSR	normal sinus rhythm
(N)STEMI	(non) ST-segment elevation myocardial infarction
NSVT	nonsustained ventricular tachycardia
NTG	nitroglycerin
NYHA	New York Heart Association
OR	operating room
PET	positron-emission tomography
PPD	purified protein derivative
PT	prothrombin time
PTT	partial thromboplastin time
RFA	radiofrequency ablation
RV	right ventricle
SLE	systemic lupus erythematosus
SPECT	single-proton emission computed tomography
SVT	supraventricular tachycardia
TB	tuberculosis
TEE	transesophageal echocardiogram
TIA	transient ischemic attack
TSH	thyroid-stimulating hormone
UA	urinalysis
U/S	ultrasound
$\dot{V}/\dot{Q}$	ventilation/perfusion
VF	ventricular flutter
VSD	ventricular septal defect
VT	ventricular tachycardia
WBC	white blood cell

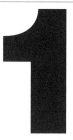

Approach to the Cardiovascular Patient and Basic Electrocardiography

Peter A. Crawford

APPROACH TO THE CARDIOVASCULAR PATIENT

Taking care of patients with cardiovascular problems is among the most rewarding pursuits in medicine. Rarely will you have the opportunity to integrate essential physiology with the most rapidly developing techniques, evidence-based medicine, and cutting-edge molecular pharmacotherapeutics *and* be able to make a significant difference for your patient.

So, you are on the cardiology service, or perhaps you have a patient who may have a cardiovascular problem. Where do you begin? An incredible abundance of literature in cardiovascular medicine continues to accumulate; it far exceeds one individual's personal hard-drive's data space. How in the world do you apply it? Remember that even in the face of the most rapidly evolving field, fundamental **principles** and **concepts** guide your caregiving. The history and physical exam remain the cornerstones of evaluation. First, let's take a look at the kind of patients you're likely to find on your service.

The most common **presentations** for patients admitted to the cardiology service, in descending order of frequency, are

1. Chest discomfort
2. Dyspnea
3. Syncope
4. Lower extremity/diffuse edema
5. Palpitation

The most common reasons for **consultation** by general medicine and surgical services include (in no particular order of frequency)

1. Atrial fibrillation
2. Positive troponin I
3. Positive stress test
4. History of (or significant risk factors for) CAD in the preop patient
5. Chest pain
6. New-onset heart failure
7. Tachycardia, not otherwise specified
8. Bradycardia, not otherwise specified
9. Abnormal ECG, not otherwise specified
10. Abnormal echocardiogram, not otherwise specified (including vegetation or mass)
11. Pulmonary embolism
12. Evaluation for/management of pericardial effusion

Other presentations and reasons for consult exist, but this list covers >90% of the reasons you will be asked to see a patient, whether by the ER physician, house staff from another service, admitting office secretary, or nurse or secretary for the consulting physician. The assessment and management of these presentations are thoroughly discussed elsewhere in this manual.

Approach the patient systematically. There are several general **critical questions** applicable to all cardiology patients that you, as the consulted physician or physician to whom this patient is going to be admitted, should learn as quickly as possible:

1. Why am I being asked to see the patient?
2. What is the patient's primary problem? (often distinct from #1)
3. What are his or her approximate vital signs right now?
4. Where is the patient right now (home, clinic, patient testing, ER, ward, OR, holding area, ICU)?
5. How long has the problem been present?
6. What is the patient's mental status?
7. What does the ECG show?

To answers these questions, formulate the following **critical parameters** in your mind:

1. What diagnostic study, procedure, or medicinal intervention is appropriate for this patient?
2. When does he or she need it?
3. Where does this patient need to be physically located now (e.g., floor, ICU) to best receive his or her care?

After you have asked these critical questions and formulated the patient's critical parameters, you are ready to begin your workup and management. Obviously, the amount of time you have to execute this process, as well as the history and physical exam, will vary and depends on the answers to the critical questions above. Your ability to determine the three critical parameters will develop with knowledge and experience. Of note, **patients with (a) unstable vital signs (including tachypnea), (b) poor mental status (i.e., a change from baseline), (c) refractory chest discomfort with a high suspicion of ischemia, or (d) newly diagnosed aortic dissection (any anatomic location) should be triaged to an ICU for appropriate management.**

Not infrequently, your caller won't be able to answer your critical questions. **Do not punish the patient (by not seeing him or her) because of the caller's lack of knowledge.** Sometimes, as in the case of a nurse or secretary, it is not his or her job to have the answers to those questions. It is incumbent on **you** to assess the patient.

This guidebook takes you through the assessment and management of the aforementioned chief complaints and reasons for consult. Chapters in Part I highlight the incorporation of a broad differential diagnosis into histories and physical exams while also explaining how to apply expedient and appropriate care. Chapters in Part II discuss, from a disease-entity perspective, details of epidemiology, pathophysiology, appropriate history and physical exam, diagnostic testing, and management. Finally, chapters in Part III serve as a reference for diagnostic testing procedures.

ELECTROCARDIOGRAPHY

This manual provides you with the tools to approach the cardiology patient. The ECG is second to the history and physical exam in the hierarchy of patient assessment. As mentioned in the preface, this text does not provide a complete guide to ECG reading, which can be found elsewhere. However, the ECG is discussed and presented in the manual where appropriate. In addition, there are a few tenets of ECG reading that warrant mentioning here.

A systematic approach to ECG reading is taught in medical school and should be used whether you are a first-year medical student or senior cardiology attending. The following order can be used as a guideline:

1. **Verify the patient's name.**
2. The **scales** should be evaluated before reading the ECG proper (indicated in the upper left-hand corner of the page and/or the bottom of the page). Many a cardiology fellow has been thwarted in the middle of the night because the scale on the ECG is not at standard, and he or she did not detect this immediately. This is particularly an issue on surgical services, where ECGs are performed less frequently.
   a. The standard voltage scale is 10 mm/mV (0.1 mV/little vertical box). Half standard (5 mm/mV) will underrepresent amplitudes, and double standard (20 mm/mV) will overrepresent them.
   b. The standard for chart speed is 25 mm/sec (0.2 sec/big box—five little boxes).

Alterations of this will generate **apparent** interval lengthening (and heart rate decrease) if chart speed is increased or shortening if it is decreased.

The rhythm strips at the bottom of a standard ECG provide 10 secs of data.

3. **Rate** can be determined in multiple ways. Heart rate equals
   a. 300/(number of large boxes in the RR interval) (if the chart speed is 25 mm/sec)
   b. 1500/(number of small boxes in RR interval) (if the chart speed is 25 mm/sec)
   c. The number of QRS complexes counted over a period of three hash marks at the bottom of the ECG × 10 (each hash-marked interval is 3 secs, two intervals is 6 secs, × ten is 60 secs)

      Memorizing the pattern 300, 150, 100, 75, 60, 50, etc., is a derivation of equation (a), in which the number of large boxes between RR intervals allows you to count down in this series.

4. **Rhythm** can be very easy or difficult to assess. First, look to see if there is a P wave associated with each QRS complex and a QRS complex associated with each P wave. Exclude premature ventricular contractions from underlying rhythm assessment. If a rhythm other than that which consists of a P wave in front of each QRS complex is present, then count the P waves and QRS complexes. If the number of P waves exceeds QRS complexes, then AV block exists. If the number of QRS complexes is greater than the number of P waves, then AV dissociation exists. If the number of P waves equals the number of QRS complexes, AV block or AV dissociation can still exist, depending on the relationship between them. Second, look at the P wave morphology in leads II, III (inferior), and V_1. If the rhythm is sinus, the P wave is upright in the inferior leads. If this is not true, an ectopic atrial rhythm may exist, in which atrial automaticity is determined outside the sinus node. This can yield a rhythm that is regular, with P waves and QRS complexes, but is not "normal sinus."

   Examine also for "buried" P waves, which are those that may be hidden in the QRS or T. This is particularly important in tachycardias. You will not infrequently encounter ECGs in which the differential diagnosis is supraventricular tachycardia, atrial flutter, atrial tachycardia, sinus tachycardia, accelerated junctional rhythm, and even VT. **Beware in particular of heart rates of approximately 150 bpm that look like sinus tachycardia.** In this case, particularly in older patients, have a high suspicion for 2:1 atrial flutter (with half of the F waves buried) (see Chap. 11, Atrial Fibrillation; Chap. 14, Bradycardia and Permanent Pacemakers; and Chap. 15, Tachyarrhythmias, Sudden Cardiac Death, and Implantable Cardioverter-Defibrillators).

5. **Axis**, which is the vector sum of the major QRS deflection and thus the major direction of the heart's depolarization in the chest cavity, is usually easy to determine. Two methods are useful:
   a. If the net QRS deflection is positive in limb leads I (whose positive pole is at 0 degrees in the frontal plane) and aVF (whose positive pole is at $^+$90 degrees), the axis is normal (0–90 degrees, lower **anatomic** left quadrant of the Cartesian plane). If the net deflection is positive in I and negative in aVF, the axis is leftward (0–$^-$90 degrees, upper left quadrant). If the QRS deflection is negative in I and positive in aVF, the axis is rightward ($^+$90–180 degrees, lower right quadrant). Finally, if the QRS deflection is negative in both I and aVF, the axis is extreme rightward ($^-$90–180 degrees, upper right quadrant).
   b. A more exact determination of the axis can be made by the following: The lead whose net QRS amplitude is isoelectric is exactly perpendicular to the axis, in degrees. I (0 degrees for positive pole/180 degrees for negative pole) is perpendicular to aVF ($^+$90 degrees for positive/$^-$90 for negative); II (60 degrees for positive/$^-$120 degrees for negative) is perpendicular to aVL ($^-$30 degrees for positive/$^+$150 degrees for negative); III ($^+$120 degrees for positive/$^-$60 degrees for negative) is perpendicular to aVR ($^-$150 degrees for positive/$^+$30 degrees for negative). The decision to use the negative or positive pole for the appropriate perpendicular axis lead is determined by the net voltages in I and aVF. *For example*, if the QRS is isoelectric in III, then the axis (aVR) is $^-$150 degrees (extreme right) if the QRS is negative in I and aVF; however, it is normal ($^+$30 degrees) if the QRS is positive in I and aVF.

6. **Ischemic changes**, such as ST depression, ST elevation (semantically, convex ST elevation is an **injury** pattern, rather than an ischemic pattern), T wave inversion, and Q waves (sign of prior infarct), should be carefully assessed and noted. Remember that ST elevation is not always caused by acute CAD (pericarditis, normal variant early repolarization, ventricular aneurysm, etc.); ST depression similarly can also be due to LVH, digitalis effect, Wolff-Parkinson-White (WPW) syndrome, electrolyte abnormalities, etc.; T wave inversion is even less specific for ischemia; and Q waves can also be caused by HCM, as well as other cardiomyopathies. Thus, these changes should be carefully sought and noted. Further reading and experience will allow you to discriminate among the different etiologies for these changes. This manual and the referred ECG references (see Suggested Reading) will assist you with details.

7. **Intervals** should be carefully assessed. An **interval** includes the wave mentioned in its name; a **segment** is the region between the named waves, **not** including the waves.

   a. A long **PR interval** (>200 msecs) suggests AV block; a short PR interval (<120 msecs) may be seen in WPW. Of note, a given PR interval is usually **normal** in type II second-degree AV block in those cycles in which P waves are conducted through to generate QRSs; the PR interval in type I second-degree AV block (Wenckebach) gradually lengthens until a QRS is dropped.

   b. The **QRS interval duration** can be lengthened (>120 msecs) by a variety of conditions such as bundle-branch block, MI, LVH, WPW, drugs (antiarrhythmics, tricyclic antidepressants), and others.

   c. The **QT interval** is important to assess, as its lengthening is associated with a higher risk of a potentially lethal rhythm, torsades de pointes. The corrected QT interval, or **QTc**, is used as a standard. It is defined as

   $$QTc = \frac{QT \ (msec)}{\sqrt{RR \ \text{interval (sec)}}}$$

   A QTc >450 msecs is considered prolonged and warrants evaluation. The most common causes for a long QTc are drugs (antiarrhythmics, antibiotics, etc.), hypocalcemia, hypomagnesemia, hypokalemia, and congenital disorders (see Chap. 15, Tachyarrhythmias, Sudden Cardiac Death, and Implantable Cardioverter-Defibrillators). The most common cause for a short QTc is **hypercalcemia.**

8. **Classic patterns** will become familiar as you gain experience, but you should try to acquire a database of gestalt patterns that immediately trigger your memory. Such patterns do not exempt clinicians from a systematic evaluation of ECGs but help increase awareness of particular issues. Some classic examples:

   a. **LVH** carries formal criteria such as Cornell and Romhilt-Estes. Nevertheless, your suspicion for LVH should be raised on an ECG with high-amplitude voltage and lead you to suspect that your patient may have a history of poorly controlled HTN or HCM.

   b. **Wellens' waves, or very deep** T wave inversions across the precordial leads, should signify a differential diagnosis that includes a critical proximal left anterior descending artery lesion; a CNS catastrophe, such as subarachnoid hemorrhage; or (much less likely) the apical variant of HCM (Fig. 1-1).

   c. **Pre-excitation** (the delta wave), as seen in WPW, should jump out immediately on the ECG. **AF in a patient with WPW** should become immediately recognizable and easy to distinguish from VT (see Chap. 15, Tachyarrhythmias, Sudden Cardiac Death, and Implantable Cardioverter-Defibrillators).

   d. **Digoxin effect** is characterized by downsloping ST depressions, particularly in the precordial leads.

   e. The **Brugada ECG,** which is associated with a syndrome of polymorphic VT and sudden cardiac death in patients with structurally normal hearts, shows coved ST elevation and an incomplete right bundle-branch block in leads V_1-V_3 (see Chap. 15, Tachyarrhythmias, Sudden Cardiac Death, and Implantable Cardioverter-Defibrillators).

   f. **Osborne waves.** J waves are inscribed between the end of the QRS and early ST segment in the setting of profound hypothermia.

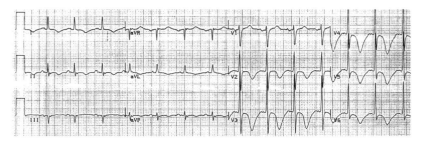

FIG. 1-1. Wellens' deep T wave inversions.

KEY POINTS TO REMEMBER

• Patients presenting to a hospital with known or presumed cardiovascular problems need to be evaluated expeditiously to ensure appropriate triage and management.
• Second to history and physical, the ECG is a key component in the evaluation of the cardiovascular patient.
• ECG reading should always be performed in a systematic fashion; otherwise, the likelihood of errors in interpretation goes dramatically up.

REFERENCES AND SUGGESTED READINGS

ePocrates for the Palm (www.epocrates.com)

O'Keefe J, Hammill S, Freed M, et al. *The ECG criteria and ACLS handbook*. Royal Oak, MI: Physicians Press, 1998.

Surawicz B, Knilans T. *Chou's electrocardiography in clinical practice*, 5th ed. Philadelphia: WB Saunders, 2002.

Tarascon pocket pharmacopeia. Loma Linda, CA: Tarascon Publishing, 2002.

Common Presentations in Cardiology

2

Chest Pain

Michael J. Riley

INTRODUCTION

Each year, millions of patients in the United States visit ERs and medical offices with a chief complaint of "chest pain." Every physician at one time or another is confronted with this problem, and having a basic approach to chest pain is extremely important for health care providers, regardless of specialty.

Despite the unremitting frequency with which it occurs, chest pain remains a challenging problem, not only because of the ominous connotation the phrase carries (i.e., heart attack), but also because of the vast number of disorders—both cardiac and noncardiac—that can underlie this complaint. A systematic approach to history, physical exam, and lab and other testing helps ensure that patients with chest pain are evaluated and treated appropriately.

The differential diagnosis of chest pain is extensive (Table 2-1), but historical features, along with physical exam, usually lead to the diagnosis.

PRESENTATION

History

General

Despite the eruption in technologies used to diagnose heart disease, the most useful and reliable diagnostic tool remains a thorough history. History, when done completely and systematically, helps the physician differentiate between truly active CAD and the myriad other causes of chest pain. Additionally, in the setting of a true ACS, it allows the clinician to gauge more accurately the degree and severity of cardiac ischemia (e.g., unstable angina vs acute MI). When taking a history, the examiner should elicit many specific details, including the quality of the pain; location of pain and pattern of radiation, if any; precipitating, aggravating, and mitigating factors; time course and nature/pattern of recurrence; and associated symptoms. Question all patients complaining of chest pain about risk factors for CAD.

Quality

Because "chest pain" can take on a variety of different connotations, it is important to ask the patient to elaborate on the exact nature and quality of pain. First, **realize that the patient may deny frank "pain,"** per se, instead complaining of chest discomfort, heaviness, pressure, or burning sensation, or may use various other descriptors. The patient may complain of "an elephant standing on my chest" or "a vice gripping my chest." All of these specific complaints may signify active underlying CAD. Certain types of patients—e.g., those with diabetes mellitus—may not complain of or experience chest pain in the setting of active myocardial ischemia. It is also useful to have the patient gauge his or her pain in terms of severity. A 0–10 scale is widely used, but the examiner must remember that tolerance for pain can vary markedly among individuals. If the patient has documented CAD and has suffered an ACS in the past, one

TABLE 2-1. DIFFERENTIAL DIAGNOSIS OF CHEST PAIN

1. Angina pectoris/MI
2. Other cardiovascular causes
   a. Likely ischemic in origin
      (1) Aortic stenosis
      (2) Hypertrophic cardiomyopathy (HCM)
      (3) Severe systemic HTN
      (4) Severe right ventricular HTN
      (5) Aortic regurgitation
      (6) Severe anemia/hypoxia
   b. Nonischemic in origin
      (1) Aortic dissection
      (2) Pericarditis
      (3) Mitral valve prolapse
3. GI
   a. Esophageal spasm
   b. Esophageal reflux
   c. Esophageal rupture
   d. Peptic ulcer disease
4. Psychogenic
   a. Anxiety
   b. Depression
   c. Cardiac psychosis
   d. Self-gain
5. Neuromusculoskeletal
   a. Thoracic outlet syndrome
   b. Degenerative joint disease of cervical/thoracic spine
   c. Costochondritis (Tietze's syndrome)
   d. Herpes zoster
   e. Chest wall pain and tenderness
6. Pulmonary
   a. Pulmonary embolus with or without pulmonary infarction
   b. Pneumothorax
   c. Pneumonia with pleural involvement
7. Pleurisy

From Fuster V, Alexander RW, O'Rourke RA, eds. *Hurst's the heart*, 10th ed. New York: McGraw-Hill, 2000.

should ask about similarity between this pain episode and that experienced with previous anginal attack or acute MI. Pain described as "lancinating," "knifelike," "sharp," or "stabbing" is less typical for myocardial ischemia, suggesting instead pericarditis or a musculoskeletal problem (e.g., Tietze's syndrome). Pain that is pleuritic (increasing with inspiration) is more typical of pneumonia or acute pulmonary embolism with possible pulmonary infarction.

Location and Radiation

The location and pattern of radiation, if any, can provide important clues to the underlying disease process. Pain due to myocardial ischemia is typically difficult to characterize (i.e., the pain tends to be diffuse and generalized across the chest). Thus, if pain can be localized to a small, specific area (e.g., by pointing with one finger) on the chest, it is less likely to be due to true angina. Chest pain may be limited to a certain dermatomal distribution, as in early herpes zoster. The pattern of radiation is also helpful in narrowing the diagnosis. *Classically, chest pain due to cardiac ischemia radiates from the chest to the left shoulder and down the ulnar aspect of the left arm and hand*. Alternatively, it may radiate to the epigastrium, across the chest, to the right shoulder (less common), to the neck or jaw, and to the back (usually between the scapulae). Acute pericarditis, however, may follow the same pattern. For patients with pain radiating to the back, other etiologies, such as aortic dissection, expanding thoracic aortic aneurysm, ruptured peptic ulcer, or pancreatitis, should be considered. Also note that pain isolated to areas, such as the neck or jaw, epigastrium, or shoulder, may be an anginal equivalent despite the absence of frank chest pain. Pain localized to areas above the neck or below the umbilicus is unlikely to reflect myocardial ischemia.

Modifying Factors

Examiners should also inquire about any factors, circumstances, or interventions that may aggravate or mitigate the chest pain. Typically, chest pain due to angina is precipitated and/or exacerbated by exertion and relieved by rest or NTG. Other situations, such as emotional upset, anxiety, or cold exposure, may also precipitate angina. Response to NTG is important to ascertain, as a positive response increases the likelihood that the pain is due to symptomatic CAD. Remember, however, that other conditions, particularly esophageal spasm, are also frequently relieved with nitrates. Pain that changes in intensity with changing body position is less likely to be angina and more likely to be due to another condition, such as pericarditis (which often abates after leaning forward) or musculoskeletal problems. Pain worsened by touching the chest suggests costochondritis of other musculoskeletal disorders or herpes zoster. Pain from a GI problem, such as esophagitis, esophageal spasm, or gastroesophageal reflux disease, typically changes in intensity after meals or when lying supine. It is often relieved not only by nitrates but also by milk and antacids.

Duration, Frequency, and Timing of Recurrence

The duration of episodes of chest pain and the frequency and timing with which they recur can provide useful information for narrowing the differential diagnosis. Typically, angina pectoris is crescendo/decrescendo in nature and lasts a few minutes, on average. It usually recurs in a fairly predictable manner with consistent levels of exertion (e.g., "pain after walking two blocks" or "climbing three flights of stairs"). Pain similar to a patient's usual anginal symptoms but occurring with less exertion, recurring more frequently, or at rest should alert the examiner to the possibility of unstable angina. If pain lasts >30 mins, it could signal either unstable angina or acute MI or may be due to such noncardiac conditions as aortic dissection, costochondritis, or psychogenic pain syndrome. Variant (Prinzmetal's) angina due to coronary vasospasm can occur in any pattern, or none at all, and often occurs at rest. Pain that lasts only seconds or that recurs several times in a short period is less likely due to cardiac ischemia, as is pain that endures for many hours.

Associated Symptoms

Often, the presence of specific associated symptoms serves as an important clue to the underlying disorder. Chest pain from cardiac ischemia is classically accompanied by one or more of the following symptoms: shortness of breath, nausea, vomiting, diaphoresis (with this, more than any other co-complaint, serving as a red flag for a serious problem—i.e., acute MI, aortic dissection), palpitations, lightheadedness, and dizziness. Pain due to various GI disorders is often accompanied by nausea and/or vomiting, but in contrast to angina, dysphagia and a bitter taste are often also present. Pain from a pulmonary embolism or spontaneous pneumothorax is often pleuritic and has associated shortness of breath. The presence of hemoptysis can point to a lung tumor or pulmonary embolism with pulmonary infarction. Fever or chills may indicate an underlying pneumonia or other infectious process. Mood changes may point to a psychogenic cause. It is vital to inquire about these various features when eliciting history.

Cardiac Risk Factors
Everyone evaluated with a chief complaint of chest pain should be screened for known risk factors for CAD. The number of risk factors present will help determine the probability that chest pain is due to symptomatic CAD. These risk factors include

- **Smoking.** The risk of CAD is dose related—i.e., the greater the number of cigarettes consumed, the more likely that CAD is present. Studies have shown that patients who smoke ≥ 1 pack of cigarettes or more/day have at least double the risk for CAD of nonsmokers.
- **HTN.** This also includes isolated systolic HTN (a common comorbidity in older adults).
- **Hyperlipidemia.** This includes high LDL, low HDL, and various other dyslipoproteinemias.
- **Diabetes mellitus.** The presence of diabetes independently increases the risk of CAD by four- to fivefold compared to nondiabetic patients. It also increases the risk for asymptomatic ischemia.
- **Family history of early CAD.** Risk increases if CAD developed in male relatives <55 yrs or female relatives <60 yrs.
- **Obesity/deconditioning.**
- **Postmenopausal state.**
- High-sensitivity C-reative protein has been shown to be an independent risk factor.

Physical Exam

After taking a thorough history, the clinician should be able to narrow the differential diagnosis for chest pain considerably. The physical exam then serves as a tool for further narrowing the list, confirming or supporting suspicions, and occasionally uncovering problems not suspected based to history alone. Like history taking, the physical exam should be thorough, as well as focused and systematic.

Vital Signs
Vital signs are usually nonspecific but can occasionally point to certain diagnoses. Is the patient febrile? Hypertensive? Are BPs equivalent in all bilateral extremities (sometimes unequal in aortic dissection)? Hypotensive (as in tension pneumothorax or cardiac tamponade)? Tachypneic (as with pulmonary embolism)? Tachycardic (as with underlying arrhythmia)? Is pulsus paradoxus present (suggesting large pericardial effusion with tamponade)?

General Appearance
One should get an immediate sense of the patient's degree of distress, as this may call for immediate intervention. Is the patient clenching his or her chest? Cold or clammy? Diaphoretic? Is the patient's breathing labored or is he or she speaking full sentences comfortably?

HEENT/Neck
The presence of arcus senilis may alert the examiner to the presence of occult hyperlipidemia. Does the patient have jugular venous distention? Are there carotid bruits present (since the presence of stenosis in any vascular bed predicts probable CAD)?

Lungs/Chest
Can pain be reproduced with palpation along the sternum or chest wall? Are there abnormal breath sounds present (e.g., unilateral reduction in breath sounds in pneumothorax and pleural effusion; rales in congestive heart failure, possibly complicating an ACS; egophony suggests consolidation as in pneumonia; wheezing as in asthma vs "cardiac asthma," which occurs with elevated left-sided filling pressures)? A "PA (pulmonary artery) tap" is suggestive of pulmonary HTN, as is a loud P_2, right-sided S_4 or S_3.

Cardiovascular

Pay particular attention to the rate, presence of murmurs, rubs, S_3 or S_4, and position of point of maximal impulse. Are these findings new, or have they been described previously?

Abdomen

Is there tenderness to palpation? If so, where? Guarding or rebound? Are bowel sounds present? Organomegaly?

Extremities

Is edema present? Is it equal bilaterally (as in heart failure) or asymmetric (as is sometimes seen with deep vein thrombosis, suggesting pulmonary embolism as the possible cause of chest pain)? Is clubbing or cyanosis present? Are pulses unequal or reduced (peripheral vascular disease)?

Skin

Is there erythema or are there vesicles on the chest wall in a dermatomal distribution (herpes zoster)?

Neurologic Considerations

What is the patient's mood/affect? Are there any focal deficits (e.g., asymmetric weakness, sensory deficits, or mental status changes sometimes seen as a complication of acute aortic dissection)?

MANAGEMENT

Lab Studies and Diagnostic Tests

Routine Labs

Routine labs include measurements of blood counts, electrolytes, liver function tests, and amylase/lipase (if pancreatitis or other GI process is suspected).

Cardiac Enzymes

Cardiac-specific troponin assays are the preferred test for cardiac injury. A patient with a presentation suggestive of symptomatic CAD should be ruled out for MI with two successive measurements of serum troponin I or T, 12 hrs apart. Troponin I does not become elevated in MI for 4–6 hrs after the initial ischemic insult. Myoglobin is usually elevated early in MI, but it has poor specificity.

ECG

ECG is the most important test to obtain in patients presenting with chest pain. When possible, it should be compared to a previous (baseline) ECG to look for acute changes. Much valuable information can be found here, including presence or absence of ST-segment abnormalities (elevation, depression), other changes suggesting possible ischemia (e.g., T wave abnormalities), pathologic Q waves (suggesting old infarction), arrhythmia, evidence of hypertrophy (HTN vs HCM), and low-voltage or electrical alternans (as in pericardial effusion). If evidence of acute ischemia is found on ECG, consider whether the patient meets criteria for thrombolytic administration or urgent revascularization. This should be obtained quickly in the evaluation process and repeated serially, especially if a patient's complaints or clinical picture change.

Chest X-Ray

Chest x-ray also provides much useful information, such as possible cardiomegaly, pulmonary edema, pleural effusion or other findings consistent with heart failure, infiltrates or masses, and pneumothorax. A widened mediastinum suggests the possibility of aortic dissection but has poor sensitivity and specificity.

Other Studies

Various other studies may be performed based on clinical suspicion (e.g., ABG measurement and $\dot{V}/\dot{Q}$ lung scanning if acute pulmonary embolism suspected; chest CT, TEE, or MRI for aortic dissection; spiral CT for pulmonary embolism).

Focused Therapy

If symptomatic CAD is suspected based on history, physical exam, and ECG and other findings, therapy should be tailored to the specific ACS (see Chap. 6, Stable Angina; Chap. 7, Acute Coronary Syndromes: Unstable Angina/Non–ST-Segment Elevation Myocardial Infarction; and Chap. 8, Acute ST-Segment Elevation Myocardial Infarction, which discuss the assessment and management of these clinical entities in detail).

KEY POINTS TO REMEMBER

- The etiologies for chest pain are broad and need to be considered in every patient. History and physical exam are critically important.
- Chest pain is often not described as "pain" by a presenting patient. Seek other adjectives in your histories.
- The most important immediate causes to rule out with history, physical, ECG, and diagnostic testing are ACS/acute MI, aortic dissection/dissecting aortic aneurysm, and pulmonary embolism.

REFERENCES AND SUGGESTED READINGS

Braunwald E, Antman EM, Beasley JW, et al. ACC/AHA guidelines for management of patients with unstable angina: a report of the American College of Cardiology/American Heart Association Task Force on Practice Guidelines (Committee on the Management of Patients with Unstable Angina). *J Am Coll Cardiol* 2000;36:970–1062.

Braunwald E. Examination of the patient/the history. In: Braunwald E, Zipes DP, Libby P, eds. *Heart disease: a textbook of cardiovascular medicine*. Philadelphia: WB Saunders, 2001.

Ryan TJ, Antman EM, Brooks NH, et al. 1999 update: ACC/AHA Guidelines for the Management of Patients with Acute Myocardial Infarction: a report of the American College of Cardiology/American Heart Association Task Force on Practice Guidelines (Committee on Management of Acute Myocardial Infarction). *J Am Coll Cardiol* 1999;34(3):890–911.

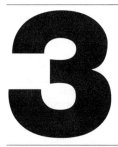

Evaluation of the Patient with Dyspnea

Adam B. Stein

INTRODUCTION

Much of what cardiologists do is see people who are acutely or chronically short of breath. The range of possible causes and, therefore, appropriate treatments is extremely long, but you can rapidly focus your range of options based on a patient's history and physical exam.

Dyspnea is an uncomfortable and abnormal awareness of breathing. It results from a complex interrelation between ventilatory requirements (the amount of ventilation necessary to support the body), ventilatory capacity (the ability to breath), and the ventilatory effort needed to meet these requirements. Analogous to pain, dyspnea is a sensory modality that involves the activation of sensory receptors, transmission of sensations to the CNS, integration and processing of sensations, and, finally, interpretation of these inputs. The sensory components in the processing of dyspnea include

- Respiratory chemoreceptors in the periphery (carotid bodies sensitive to PO_2) and central chemoreceptors (sensitive to pH and PCO_2)
- Lung and thoracic cage receptors
- Central motor command efforts
- Vascular mechanoreceptors
- CNS integration and interpretation sites

Although the exact neurophysiologic causes of dyspnea are difficult to pinpoint, it is often thought to result from the awareness of discrepancies between sensory input from the lungs and chest wall during respiratory activity and the expected perceptions based on motor command.

PRESENTATION

History and Physical Exam

A comprehensive history and physical exam are of utmost importance in diagnosing the cause of dyspnea.

One must inquire about **timing, place, and position** at onset of symptoms; **precipitating** factors; **ameliorating or aggravating** factors; **associated conditions**; and **alterations in overall health status.**

- Intermittent dyspnea suggests a reversible process [e.g., congestive heart failure (CHF), asthma, pulmonary embolism].
- Acuity of symptoms guides the differential diagnosis and determines how rapidly a diagnosis must be made.
- Nocturnal dyspnea suggests CHF, gastroesophageal reflux disorder, or asthma.
- **Orthopnea** (difficulty breathing in the recumbent position, usually relieved with sitting up) suggests CHF, ascites, pregnancy, obstructive lung disease, or respiratory muscle weakness.
- **Platypnea** (worsening dyspnea in upright position) suggests AV malformations at lung bases, interatrial shunts, and cirrhosis.

- Dyspnea on exertion suggests a cardiac source, pulmonary HTN, or exercise-induced asthma.
- Dyspnea independent of activity suggests mechanical (aspiration), allergic, or pyschological problems.
- **Trepopnea** (dyspnea in one lateral position but not the other) signifies unilateral disease such as pleural effusion or obstruction of the proximal tracheobronchial tree.
- **Associated symptoms** include wheezing, coughing, sputum production, pleuritic chest pain, anginal chest pain, fevers, peripheral edema, abdominal swelling, snoring, excessive daytime sleepiness, peripheral or proximal muscle weakness, and severe stress.
- **Exposures** include workplace, home, or specific areas therein; tobacco; inhalants; pets or animals; toxins; and seasons.
- **Medications** include beta blockers, methotrexate, bleomycin, nitrofurantoin, and amiodarone.

On **physical exam,** careful attention should be paid to the pulmonary and cardiovascular systems.

- Respiratory rate
- Body habitus: cachexia or obesity
- Posture: leaning forward on elbows with COPD, supine in bed, head upright
- Use of accessory muscles
- Pursed lips
- Extent and symmetry of chest expansion
- Crackles, rhonchi, and wheezes (localized or diffuse)
- Decreased breath sounds: pneumothorax or pleural effusion
- Pulmonary HTN: RV heave, increased P_2 sound
- RV failure: elevated jugular vein pressure (JVP), hepatojugular reflux, pedal edema
- Lower extremity edema: bilateral suggests CHF if other history and physical exam features corroborate; unilateral suggests thromboembolism
- LV failure: diffuse, laterally displaced point of maximal impulse, S_3 gallop, crackles, elevated JVP
- Clubbing: may be seen with malignancy
- Cyanosis: insensitive sign of severe hypoxemia

MANAGEMENT

Approach to the Patient with Acute Dyspnea

Acute dyspnea evolving over minutes to days requires urgent evaluation. It is almost always caused by an acute cardiac or pulmonary process. Always use the ABCs and be prepared to initiate basic cardiac life support and advanced cardiac life support.

Differential Diagnosis
The differential diagnosis includes the following common causes:

1. Cardiac
   a. Pulmonary edema (or even simply elevated left-sided filling pressures) from myocardial dysfunction, including **ischemia,** and valvular dysfunction
   b. Pulmonary embolism
   c. Pericardial disease
2. Pulmonary
   a. Infection: bacterial, fungal, viral, TB
   b. Pulmonary embolism
   c. Obstructive lung disease: COPD, asthma
   d. Chest wall trauma
   e. Pneumothorax
   f. Pleural effusions
   g. Noncardiogenic pulmonary edema, ARDS

h. Upper airway obstruction
i. Pulmonary hemorrhage
j. Rapid progressive inflammation (e.g., aspiration, bronchiolitis obliterans–organizing pneumonia, eosinophilic pneumonia, inhaled toxicants)
k. Respiratory muscle weakness

Evaluation

The evaluation of acute dyspnea includes

1. ABCs: establish airway and ensure oxygenation
2. Directed history and physical exam to establish probable cause [remember that wheezing can reflect COPD or CHF ("cardiac asthma"); use other cues in the history and physical exam to help discriminate]
3. All patients should receive
   a. Chest x-ray to look for hyperinflation, parenchymal infiltrate, pleural effusion, pneumothorax, enlarged cardiac silhouette and pulmonary edema, diffuse interstitial infiltrates, or foreign body.
   b. ABG measurements to obtain an objective measurement of oxygenation, pH, and PCO_2. Pulse oximetry is often not sufficient for two reasons: First, the patient may not be dyspneic because he or she is hypoxemic. **Remember that a patient with normal oxygenation and a metabolic or respiratory acidosis can be dyspneic, because of the need to exhale CO_2 to raise the pH.** Second, in cases of methemoglobinemia, the apparent O_2 saturation is high, but the actual PO_2 is low.
   c. ECG to assess for acute changes of ischemia, infarction, or pericardial disease.
   d. Consider further testing based on clinical scenario, including $\dot{V}/\dot{Q}$ scan, echocardiogram, and peak-flow measurement.

Approach to the Patient with Chronic Dyspnea

Differential Diagnosis

The differential diagnosis of chronic dyspnea is broad, and an extensive history and physical exam must be conducted to help guide the workup. The differential includes but is not limited to

1. Impaired lung or bellows function
   a. Diffuse airway obstruction: asthma, COPD
   b. Focal airway obstruction: vocal cord paralysis or destruction, tracheal stenosis, endobronchial tumor
   c. Restriction of lung mechanics
   d. Interstitial lung disease: pulmonary fibrosis, pneumoconiosis, lymphangitic carcinomatosis, pulmonary vasculitis
   e. Extrapulmonary restriction: kyphoscoliosis, pleural effusion, fibrothorax
   f. Neuromuscular weakness: amyotrophic lateral sclerosis, phrenic nerve dysfunction, myopathy, myasthenia gravis, neuropathy
   g. Gas exchange problems with normal lung mechanics: right-to-left shunt [atrial septal defect/ventricular septal defect, hereditary hemorrhagic telangiectasias (or Osler-Weber-Rendu), hepatopulmonary syndrome]
2. Impaired cardiovascular function
   a. Myocardial dysfunction: cardiomyopathies (systolic and/or diastolic dysfunction); congenital anomalies with systemic and/or pulmonary ventricular dysfunction, intracardiac right-to-left shunt; arrhythmias
   b. Valvular disease
   c. Pericardial disease: constrictive pericarditis
3. Pulmonary vascular disease: pulmonary embolism, pulmonary HTN, central venous obstruction
4. Altered central ventilatory drive (central sleep apnea, obesity hypoventilation syndrome, idiopathic hyperventilation)

5. Metabolic disorders
   a. Increased metabolic needs: hyperthyroidism, obesity
   b. Anemia
   c. Metabolic acidosis: renal failure
6. Physiologic considerations: deconditioning, high altitude, vigorous exercise, pregnancy

Evaluation

The evaluation for chronic dyspnea includes

- A careful and comprehensive history and physical exam to limit the broad differential diagnosis
- Diagnostic tests to confirm clinical impression, investigate uncertain causes, or quantify degree of impairment

Initially, all patients should receive

- Pulmonary function tests (lung volumes, diffusing capacity, and ambulatory ABG), which may help distinguish obstructive lung disease, restrictive lung disease, and interstitial lung disease
- Chest x-ray
- ECG
- Blood chemistries and CBC (may reveal renal failure, acidosis, anemia, or polycythemia)

Other tests that should be considered for selected patients based on clinical suspicion include

- Bronchoprovocation studies
- $\dot{V}/\dot{Q}$ scan
- Chest CT
- Esophageal pH monitoring
- Thyroid function testing
- Echocardiogram (LV function, pulmonary artery pressure calculation)
- Bronchoscopy
- Lung biopsy
- Laryngoscopy

Treatment

Treatment of chronic dyspnea involves establishing the diagnosis and directing treatment specific to it. See chapters throughout Part II of this manual, which describe treatment for each of the major cardiovascular disease entities. In addition, see *The Washington Manual™ Pulmonary Medicine Subspecialty Consult* and *The Washington Manual™ General Internal Medicine Subspecialty Consult* for treatment of noncardiac causes of dyspnea.

KEY POINTS TO REMEMBER

- The etiologies for dyspnea are broad and need to be considered in every patient. History and physical exam are critically important. Cues from these sources will almost always lead you to the diagnosis.
- Acute dyspnea evolving over minutes to days requires urgent evaluation.

REFERENCES AND SUGGESTED READINGS

Altose MD. Assessment and management of breathlessness. *Chest* 1985;88[Suppl 2]:77S.
Manning HL, Schwartzstein RM. Pathophysiology of dyspnea. *N Engl J Med* 1995;333:1547–1553.
Sietsema K. Approach to the patient with dyspnea. In: Kelley WN, ed. *Textbook of internal medicine*. Philadelphia: Lippincott–Raven, 1997:1908–1912.
Tobin MJ. Dyspnea. Pathophysiologic basis, clinical presentation and management. *Arch Intern Med* 1990;150:1604–1613.

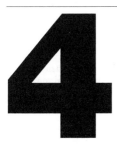

Diagnosis and Management of Syncope

Alan Zajarias

INTRODUCTION

Syncope is defined as a transient loss of consciousness (LOC) associated with inability to maintain postural tone secondary to decrease in cerebral perfusion.

Epidemiology

Syncope is responsible for 1% of hospital admissions and 3–6% of ER visits, and it is experienced by 3% of the general population. Prognosis depends on its etiology. Syncope of unknown etiology carries a 6% 1-yr mortality rate and a 4% incidence of sudden cardiac death. Cardiac syncope has an 18–33% 1-yr mortality rate and a 24% incidence of sudden cardiac death. Vasovagal, cardiac, and orthostatic hypotension are the most common causes.

CAUSES

It is important to define the underlying cause of syncope for two reasons: to assess the risk of sudden cardiac death and to improve quality of life by eliminating or limiting the episodes. The most common etiologies are neurocardiogenic (20%) and cardiovascular (20%), followed by orthostatic (10%), neurologic (10%), and psychiatric (10%).

Neurocardiogenic Syncope

Classification
VASOVAGAL SYNCOPE. Vasovagal syncope is the most common cause of neurocardiogenic syncope. It is postulated to be due to an exaggeration of the Bezold-Jarisch reflex. Excessive venous pooling in the lower extremities (LEs) decreases the ventricular volume and enhances ventricular contractility. Receptors in the inferoposterior wall of the LV sense the change in inotropism and transmit via nonmyelinated C fibers to the nucleus of the tractus solitarius, which stimulates vagal efferent fibers, triggering a vasodepressor, cardioinhibitory, or mixed response. Peripheral vasodilatation and bradycardia cause transient hypotension, a decrease in cerebral blood flow, and a transient LOC. Patients with cardiac transplants (denervated hearts) may still experience vasovagal syncope; thus, other mechanisms may involve excessive secretion of nitric oxide or beta-endorphins and serotoninergic pathways. Vasovagal syncope is often precipitated by emotional situations, pain, blood loss, dehydration, or standing motionless for a prolonged period, and it is associated with rising from a warm bed in the morning after alcohol ingestion. Patients usually refer to the following sequence of events: weakness, apprehension followed by nausea, diaphoresis, pallor, a change in visual fields followed by lightheadedness, and finally LOC. LOC is abrupt, lasting seconds. Consciousness is regained after recumbence, without memory loss or sensory clouding.
SITUATIONAL SYNCOPE. Situational syncope (5%) is associated with a specific activity, such as exercise, micturition, defecation, or cough (tussive) that activates neural receptors in the walls of the bladder, GI tract, and tracheobronchial tree, with completion of the neural pathway described above.

CAROTID SINUS SYNCOPE. **Carotid sinus syncope** is responsible for <1% of syncope cases. **Cardioinhibitory** (bradycardic, 70% of carotid sinus syncope), **vasodepressor** (hypotensive, 10% of carotid sinus syncope), or mixed response can be elicited after carotid sinus massage. A 3-sec asystolic pause and drop in BP of 50 mm Hg or 30 mm Hg with symptoms define a positive carotid sinus stimulation. Occasionally, a head and neck malignancy may compress the carotid sinus. An individual also may have a hypersensitive carotid sinus. These often warrant a pacemaker if the response is cardioinhibitory.

Diagnosis
The goal with a neurocardiogenic event is to document the correlation between symptoms and the event. A **Holter monitor** is provided for 24–48 hrs for continuous monitoring of heart rhythm and rate. Its advantage is that a patient is not required to activate it for a recording to occur. Disadvantages of a Holter monitor include limited monitoring time and variability among patients in their ability to document events appropriately. A **continuous-loop event monitor** is usually provided for 30 days and is often worn intermittently. This monitor continuously records data but saves rhythm and rate information only if the save button is pressed, which usually preserves the prior 2 mins and following 1 min. The patient (or a bystander) activates the device with symptoms of palpitations, near syncope, or syncope. The information can be transmitted transtelephonically.

The **head-upright, tilt-table test** is occasionally used if history and physical exam, ECG, and monitoring are not yielding adequate information. It is sometimes used to assess recurrent syncope in the setting of a structurally normal heart or in the presence of an abnormal heart after more malignant causes of syncope have been eliminated. The rationale behind this test is that vasovagal syncope may be induced in susceptible patients by elicitation of Bezold-Jarisch reflex. Protocols vary but generally last 35–45 mins and use an angle of 60–80 degrees. The addition of isoproterenol, nitrates, or adenosine increases the diagnostic yield. **Patients with structural heart disease or other causes of syncope, however, need to be excluded with appropriate testing.** The test has a specificity of 90% and sensitivity of 32–85%. Low sensitivity renders the test of limited usefulness, especially given the fact that the results often do not impact the management of suspected neurocardiogenic syncope. For example, if an event is vagal by history but ECG monitoring is negative, the event is likely vasodepressor in nature and should be treated accordingly. However, indeterminate monitoring may warrant a tilt-table test.

Finally, patients are occasionally offered an implantable recorder intended for long-term evaluation of rare events commonly missed by event monitors. The REVEAL (Medtronic) is an example of such a monitor; it is placed subcutaneously and maintains ECG data only.

Treatment
Neurocardiogenic syncope generally has a favorable long-term prognosis. The treatment of neurocardiogenic syncope involves a variety of approaches. First, patient education is important in avoiding precipitating activities or situations, as is sitting or lying when prodromes occur to prevent recurrences. Patients should avoid blood pooling in the LE by continuously contracting the muscles in the LE or using support stockings (e.g., thromboembolic disease hose) to the knees or thighs. Pharmacotherapy commonly starts with **beta blockers,** which act by decreasing cardiac inotropy that in turn abrogates the initiation of the Bezold-Jarisch reflex. Often, agents with intrinsic sympathomimetic activity, such as pindolol (Visken) (5–10 mg PO/day) or acebutolol (Sectral) (400–800 mg PO/day), are used to prevent bradycardia. Metoprolol (Lopressor, Toprol-XL), 50 mg PO/day, or atenolol (Tenormin), 25 mg PO/day, may also be given. Evidence proven by randomized, placebo-controlled trials is lacking or not convincing. **Anticholinergic agents,** such as propantheline bromide (Pro-Banthine, Propanthel) or scopolamine (Transderm Scop), have been used in small, uncontrolled trials with small benefits. Disopyramide (Norpace, Norpace CR) showed no benefit in a placebo-controlled trial and thus cannot be recommended. **Alpha-adrener-**

gic agonists, such as midodrine (ProAmatine), are used in orthostatic hypotension. Midodrine, which is a strong venoconstrictor, is well tolerated at doses of 2.5 mg PO bid–40 mg PO qd. Side effects include supine HTN, urinary frequency, piloerection, and worsening angina. **Selective serotonin reuptake inhibitors** may also be used: Paroxetine (Paxil, Paxil CR) had a 35.3% reduction in the incidence of repetitive vasovagal syncope episodes after 25 mos of follow-up compared with placebo. **Fludrocortisone (Florinef)** is a synthetic mineralocorticoid that increases blood volume by augmenting sodium reabsorption and has been proved to be as beneficial as atenolol; it should be dosed at 50 μg PO/day and titrated to 500 μg PO/day. **Theophylline and enalapril** have been shown to prevent recurrence of vasovagal syncope in small uncontrolled trials.

Permanent pacemaker implantation has been shown to decrease incidence of syncope in patients with predominantly cardioinhibitory response. In the VASIS trial, 42 patients with vasovagal syncope were randomized to receive pacemakers or conventional therapy. After 3.7 yrs of follow-up, the pacemaker group had less syncopal recurrence (5% vs 61%). The VPS study randomized 54 patients with recurrent syncope to receive pacemakers or placebo. The pacemaker group had a lower rate of recurrent syncope (22% vs 70%). **It is important to note that patients with vasodepressor syncope do not benefit from pacemaker implantation.** The American College of Cardiology (ACC)/American Heart Association (AHA) have established extensive guidelines for permanent pacemaker implantation in the setting of bradycardia and, in particular, in the setting of neurocardiogenic syncope and a hypersensitive carotid sinus. See Chap. 14, Bradycardia and Permanent Pacemakers (Table 14-2).

Orthostatic Syncope

The normal response to standing is characterized by carotid sinus and aortic-arch receptor stimulation enhancing adrenergic stimulation and renin-angiotensin-aldosterone system activation, which promote arteriolar vasoconstriction. Reflex venous constriction and abdominal and LE muscle contraction increase blood return. Finally, an increase in heart rate maintains adequate cardiac output. Failure of any of these mechanisms leads to orthostatic syncope, which is seen in 24% of elderly patients with syncope.

The **etiology** includes **hypovolemia,** in which LOC is preceded by nausea, pallor, diaphoresis, and tachycardia. **Autonomic dysfunction** usually lacks these symptoms and is associated with Shy-Drager syndrome; amyloidosis; endocrine causes, such as diabetes mellitus, adrenal insufficiency, or pheochromocytoma; or central or peripheral neurologic disease, such as Parkinson's, Wernicke-Korsakoff encephalopathy, tabes dorsalis, cerebrovascular accident, Guillain-Barré syndrome, or inflammatory myelopathy. **Miscellaneous causes** include anemia, electrolyte abnormalities, and **medications** (calcium channel blockers, arterial vasodilators, diuretics, ganglionic blockers, tricyclic antidepressants, and phenothiazines).

Diagnosis is made by assessment of orthostatic vital signs. A decrease in systolic BP of 30 mm Hg or 15 mm Hg in diastolic BP after 3 mins of standing raises suspicion of the diagnosis.

Treatment is directed toward the precipitating cause. Compression stockings in patients with autonomic dysfunction may be used. Avoiding dehydration and maintaining adequate antihypertensive medicine titration is fundamental. Finally, the use of midodrine, fludrocortisone, or high salt and volume intake to promote volume expansion may be helpful in refractory cases.

Cardiovascular Syncope

The **etiology** of cardiovascular syncope is a decrease in cardiac output. It may be due to a decrease in diastolic filling, as is seen in tachyarrhythmias, constrictive pericarditis, pericardial tamponade, and restrictive cardiomyopathy. Alternatively, obstruction of blood flow may be causative. **Valvular disease** (mitral, aortic, or pulmonary stenosis or atresia), **HCM,** or **mass effect** (atrial myxoma or ball thrombus) is common causes. **Ischemia** causes systolic dysfunction or bradycardia due to right coronary artery lesions or vagal response to angina, high-grade AV block, and VT. 7% of patients >65 yrs with MI present with syncope. The **pulmonary vasculature** is also attributable to syncope, as in primary pulmonary HTN, pulmonary embolus, or Eisenmenger syndrome.

Arrhythmias often precipitate syncope and are responsible for 15% of syncopal events. **Tachyarrhythmias** >180 bpm effectively decrease cardiac output (less if accompanied by loss of atrial contraction). Supraventricular tachycardias and AF occasionally cause syncope. More commonly, **VT** or **VF** causes a syncopal event. An acute MI can produce VT, which will produce syncope or even sudden death. Syncope in patients with ischemic or nonischemic cardiomyopathy, Wolff-Parkinson-White syndrome, long QT syndrome, Brugada syndrome, arrhythmogenic RV dysplasia, HCM, or a history of re-entrant ventricular arrhythmias **should be strongly suspected as due to ventricular arrhythmias. Torsades de pointes** is triggered by hypocalcemia, hypokalemia, hypomagnesemia, types IA or III antiarrhythmics, tricyclic antidepressants, fluoroquinolones, phenothiazines, and many other drug classes. "Quinidine syncope" was a common occurrence in the past, when this IA antiarrhythmic was used for the management of AF, and is due to torsades de pointes that spontaneously converts to sinus rhythm. Familial long QT syndromes also predispose to torsades de pointes (see Chap. 15, Tachyarrhythmias, Sudden Cardiac Death, and Implantable Cardioverter-Defibrillators).

Bradyarrhythmias, such as sick sinus syndrome, can be associated with sinus node arrest, sinoatrial exit block, or prolonged sinus recovery time after paroxysmal supraventricular tachycardia. **Stokes-Adams attacks** are syncopal events due to high-grade heart block. **Pacemaker malfunction** may also cause bradyarrhythmias or tachyarrhythmias (pacemaker-mediated tachycardia) that yield syncope.

Shunting (intracardiac or atrioventricular malformation) decreases the effective forward cardiac output. If right-to-left, the shunt may decrease the O_2 saturation of blood, causing cerebral hypoxia.

Workup of Cardiovascular Syncope

HISTORY. Patients with cardiac syncope generally have a known history of cardiac disease, previous MI, congestive heart failure (CHF), and cardiomyopathy. Postexertional syncope is common with conditions that cause a gradient across the aortic valve, such as HCM or aortic stenosis (AS), as well as some arrhythmias. Syncope occurring after lying down may be due to myxoma or ball thrombus. Palpitations may occur if syncope is associated with arrhythmias. Arrhythmia-mediated episodes are sudden and self-limited, without aura, and often occur at rest; on termination, patients are oriented but tired. Pallor or cyanosis is absent. If cerebral hypoxia is prolonged, syncope may be accompanied by seizure activity. Tachyarrhythmias (especially VT/VF) usually lack prodrome (*unlike* neurocardiogenic syncope). **Family history** should be carefully examined for sudden cardiac death, long QT syndromes, Brugada syndrome, HCM, premature CAD, or arrhythmogenic RV dysplasia. A history of **medications** should be carefully taken as well.

PHYSICAL EXAM. Vital signs, including orthostatic BP and heart rate, are of utmost importance. In addition, place special emphasis on cardiac auscultation by searching for evidence of murmurs or other abnormalities. Low cardiac output may decrease intensity of murmurs.

DIAGNOSIS. The **ECG** is suggestive in 5% of cases. Because it is risk free and inexpensive, it should be obtained in all patients. Abnormalities in electrical conduction, previous MI, LVH, a long QT interval, or evidence of VT may lead to the appropriate diagnostic tests or therapeutic interventions. **Echocardiogram** with Doppler interrogation is useful to determine ventricular function, valvular abnormalities (especially aortic stenosis), HCM or atrial myxoma, or intracavitary thrombus. Unsuspected findings are obtained in 5–10% of patients. Exercise testing may be used for patients with structurally normal hearts to evaluate for myocardial ischemia or exercise-induced arrhythmia or to reproduce exercise-induced syncope. It is recommended that an echocardiogram be obtained before the stress test in patients with exertional syncope to rule out HCM. A **Holter monitor** (24–48-hr continuous monitor) or **loop monitor** (when activated, records the heart rhythm before and after the symptoms) diagnose up to 45% of arrhythmic syncope. Equally important, symptoms occur in up to 17% without arrhythmia, ruling out arrhythmic syncope. The presence of sinus pauses >2 secs, high-grade AV block, and runs of nonsustained VT should be investigated. It is important to note that a nonarrhythmic episode of syncope does not rule out the possibility that a given patient may also be predisposed to arrhythmic syncope. This is particularly important to recognize in patients with structurally abnormal hearts or in those with an ECG that reveals an obvious predisposing cause of syncope (such as long QT or Brugada syndrome). The implantable monitor (e.g., REVEAL) is useful for rare events in people with no indication of malignant arrhythmias.

Signal-averaged ECG predicts inducibility by electrophysiologic studies (EPS). It obtains a series of QRS complexes and averages them, searching for late potentials in the terminal portion of the QRS. It is 90% sensitive and 95–100% specific in predicting inducibility of ventricular arrhythmias in EPSs. In the absence of late potentials, it has a 95% negative predictive value. A positive signal-averaged ECG suggests the need for EPSs. Signal-averaged ECG is rarely used in clinical practice.

EPSs are most useful in patients suspected of having cardiac syncope with known CAD, decreased ventricular function, and episodes of nonsustained VT, because these patients are at increased risk of sudden death. Syncopal patients with CAD, prior MI, and decreased LV function are referred for EPS if the history is unclear, even in the absence of nonsustained VT. The EPS is positive if there is inducible monomorphic VT. It is important to mention that the negative predictive value of EPS in patients with structurally normal hearts, or in those with nonischemic cardiomyopathy, is usually very poor, unless a rhythm is suspected that can be treated with radiofrequency ablation.

EPSs are occasionally used to detect conduction system disease in syncopal patients. Unfortunately, the yield is poor, because conduction defects do not necessarily correspond to the cause of the syncopal event. Nevertheless, an EPS is positive when there is a prolonged corrected sinus recovery time (>1000 msecs), the HV interval (*H*is to *ven*-tricle, the time required for an impulse to conduct from the AV node to the Purkinje system) is >90 msecs, and there is spontaneous or induced infrahisian block.

TREATMENT. The treatment of syncope secondary to cardiac disease naturally depends on the cause. Aortic stenosis may require surgical replacement, and other cardiac structural abnormalities may require repair. Syncope in patients with HCM requires a careful assessment to determine whether the event was hemodynamic (perhaps associated with exercise) or arrhythmic, because the treatment of these causes differs markedly (see Chap. 12, Assessment and Management of the Dilated, Restrictive, and Hypertrophic Cardiomyopathies).

Arrhythmic cardiac syncope addresses the role of implantable devices. The indications for pacemakers (see Chap. 14, Bradycardia and Permanent Pacemakers) and implantable cardioverter-defibrillators (ICDs) (see Chap. 15, Tachyarrhythmias, Sudden Cardiac Death, and Implantable Cardioverter-Defibrillators) have been outlined by the ACC/AHA guidelines.

Neurologically Mediated Syncope

Neurologic syncope is generally accompanied by focal neurologic deficits and associated with TIAs, space-occupying lesions, normal-pressure hydrocephalus, or strokes. **It is important to recall that the state of consciousness requires only one cerebral hemisphere and the brainstem to be perfused and functioning.** Vascular insufficiency, when associated with defects in anterior cerebral circulation, is manifested by focal neurologic deficit and seizures (but not syncope); when it involves the posterior circulation (vertebrobasilar system), it is accompanied by dizziness, vertigo, or drop attacks (syncope). Subclavian stenosis, when manifested by a BP differential drop in the left arm, may signify **subclavian steal**, which causes left arm activity-dependent reduction in blood flow to the brainstem via the collateralizing vertebral artery. **Syncope must be differentiated from seizures,** which are generally preceded by an aura, consist of unconsciousness that lasts >5 mins (syncope usually lasts no more than 1 min) and is accompanied by postictal confusion, sleepiness and/or paralysis, incontinence, and tongue biting. Evaluation with EEG or head CT is indicated if there is a strong suspicion of neurologic involvement by exam or history (e.g., seizure and/or focal signs). Carotid U/S with Doppler flow assessment is appropriate only if a transient ischemic attack or stroke is causative in the presentation; direction of vertebral blood flow (antegrade or retrograde) can also be evaluated for a crude assessment of the posterior circulation. As with any cerebrovascular-based process, urgent or emergent evaluation by a neurologist is essential.

Psychiatric Disease Manifested as Syncope

Major depression, conversion disorders, and anxiety disorders may be manifested by syncope. Patients with psychiatric disorders and syncope generally present with many symptoms and repetitive episodes of syncope, and they are younger than patients with other types of syncope. Syncopal episodes are generally preceded or accompanied by perioral or finger paresthesias. In one analysis, psychiatric illness was seen in 24% of patients presenting with vertigo, dizziness, and syncope, compared to 5% of patients presenting with syncope alone. Symptoms may be reproduced in the tilt-table test without change in BP or heart rate. Hyperventilation for 3 mins resulting in presyncope or syncope has a 59% positive predictive value in young patients suspected of psychiatric disorders. Referral to a psychiatrist is appropriate if the condition consists of repetitive syncopal events that lack cardiovascular or neurologic basis, but the workup should definitively establish this to be the case.

DECISION TO HOSPITALIZE THE SYNCOPAL PATIENT

Patients should be hospitalized for evaluation in the presence of a history of CAD, valvular disease, CHF, or ventricular arrhythmia. In addition, ECG findings of ischemia, serious brady- or tachycardia, long QT, or bundle-branch block; frequent spells with high suspicion of CAD or arrhythmia; age >70 yrs; the presence of orthostatic hypotension; and suspected intoxication of antiarrhythmic medication all warrant admission for workup. Patients should not drive if arrhythmic etiology is suspected until after their evaluations. If a ventricular arrhythmia is suspected, patients may not drive for at least 6 mos after ICD implantation.

KEY POINTS TO REMEMBER

- The most important management principles are to make use of a thorough history and physical exam and to rule out organic heart disease. Syncope in the presence of organic heart disease carries a very poor prognosis, whereas the patient with a normal heart who passes out usually has a favorable outcome.
- History and physical exam identify a potential cause of syncope in 45% of patients. The ECG adds an additional 5%.
- Guided questions should be used to elicit postural symptoms, exertional symptoms, palpitations, postictal or situational symptoms, frequency of attacks, medications used, and family history of syncope or sudden death. Exertional events may indicate aortic stenosis, pulmonary HTN, mitral stenosis, CAD, or HCM. Sudden events are usually due to cardiac arrhythmias. Premonitory nausea and malaise often predict vagal events.
- Aura, confusion, postictal paralysis or fatigue, urinary or stool incontinence, and tongue biting are suggestive of seizure activity. Ventricular arrhythmias can yield seizure activity due to hypoxia, but these events do not carry the prodromal, classic, primary neurologic seizure symptoms. They often are associated with postictal symptoms.
- Collateral history from family members or bystanders may prove to be important in aiding the diagnosis.
- On physical exam, it is crucial to obtain BP in both arms while the patient is supine and after 3 mins of standing. Change >20 mm Hg in systolic BP may indicate orthostatic syncope. Variance of 20 mm Hg between arms is suggestive of subclavian stenosis and may suggest subclavian steal.

- Syncope in elderly patients can be multifactorial. Always place medication-induced syncope, orthostatic syncope (volume depletion), or carotid hypersensitivity high in the differential diagnosis. AV block, sick sinus syndrome, and ventricular arrhythmias in patients with CAD and LV dysfunction are also common in the elderly.
- A neurologic workup, including head CT and carotid Dopplers, is usually not indicated unless there are focal neurologic signs and/or seizure activity. A unilateral hemispheric cerebrovascular accident causes profound neurologic symptoms but not syncope.
- The cause of syncope is undiagnosed in 40% of presentations.

REFERENCES AND SUGGESTED READINGS

Assessment Project of the American College of Physicians. Diagnosing syncope. Part 1: value of history, physical examination, and electrocardiography. *Ann Intern Med* 1997;126:989–996.

Assessment Project of the American College of Physicians. Diagnosing syncope. Part 2: unexplained syncope. *Ann Intern Med* 1997;127:76–86.

Benditt DG, Ferguson DW, Grubb BP, et al. Tilt table testing for assessing syncope. *J Am Coll Cardiol* 1996;28(1):263–275.

Benditt D, Lurie K, Fabian W. Clinical approach to diagnosis of syncope. An overview. *Cardiol Clin* 1997;15:165–175.

Conolly SJ, Sheldon R, Roberts R, et al. The North American Vasovagal pacemaker study (VPS): a randomized trial of permanent cardiac pacing for the prevention of vasovagal syncope. *J Am Coll Cardiol* 1999;33:16–20.

Di Girolamo E, Di Iorio C, Sabatini P, et al. Effect of paroxetine hydrochloride, a selective serotonin reuptake inhibitor, on refractory vasovagal syncope: a randomized double-blind placebo-controlled study. *J Am Coll Cardiol* 1999;99:1452–1457.

DiCarlo L, Morady F. Evaluation of the patient with syncope. *Cardiol Clin* 1985;3:499–514.

Fenton A, Hammill S, Rea R, et al. Vasovagal syncope. *Ann Intern Med* 2000;133:714–725.

Hammill S, Thomas J. Syncopal disorders. In: Giuliani E, ed. *Mayo Clinic practice of cardiology*. St. Louis: Mosby, 1996.

Kapoor W. Syncope. *N Engl J Med* 2000;343:1856–1862.

Mosqueda-Garcia R, Furlan R, Tank J, et al. The elusive pathophysiology of neurally mediated syncope. *Circulation* 2000;102:2898–2906.

Parry SW, Kenny RA. The management of vasovagal syncope. *QJM* 1999;92:697–705.

Sutton R, Brignole M, Menozzi C, et al. Dual-chamber pacing in the treatment of neurally mediated tilt-positive cardioinhibitory syncope: pacemaker versus no therapy. A multicenter randomized study. The Vasovagal Syncope International Study (VASIS) Investigators. *Circulation* 2000;102:294–299.

Cardiovascular Emergencies

Ryan G. Aleong

INTRODUCTION

This chapter describes the initial assessment and management of several cardiac emergencies. For further discussion of each of these conditions, see the respective chapters in Part II.

BRADYCARDIA

Bradycardia is due to sinus node dysfunction or AV block. For a full discussion of sinus node dysfunction and its etiologies, see Chap. 14, Bradycardia and Permanent Pacemakers, and Chap. 24, Procedures in Cardiovascular Critical Care (Intraaortic Balloon Pump, Swan-Ganz Catheterization, and Temporary Transvenous Pacemaker).

Clinical Presentation

Symptoms include syncope, presyncope, fatigue, angina, and shortness of breath. Patients may be asymptomatic. Tachycardia-bradycardia (AF with a rapid ventricular response in the setting of sick sinus syndrome, which results in long pauses and bradycardia after spontaneous conversion; see Chap. 14, Bradycardia and Permanent Pacemakers) may present with palpitations. BP, O_2 saturation, and other vital signs should be assessed. The patient should be examined for signs of **decreased cardiac output,** including pulmonary edema and altered mental status.

An **ECG and rhythm strip** should be examined. An ECG finding of inappropriate sinus bradycardia is a sinus rate <60 bpm that does not increase with activity. In sinus arrest, pauses of >3 secs are seen. Tachycardia-bradycardia syndrome is characterized by episodes of sinus or junctional bradycardia alternating with episodes of atrial tachycardia or AF.

Initial Management of Severe Bradycardia (Heart Rate <40 bpm)

- Assess airway, breathing, and circulation.
- Place a monitor/defibrillator on the patient.
- Ensure adequate IV access and oxygenation.
- If the patient has symptoms of bradycardia and is hemodynamically compromised,
  - Give atropine, 0.5–1.0 mg IV. Doses can be repeated q3–5mins up to a total dose of 0.04 mg/kg. The **exception** to using atropine is **bona fide** type II second-degree AV block, which may be worsened by atropine.
  - If BP is still unimproved, start dopamine (Intropin), 2–20 mg/kg/min, to keep systolic BP >90 mm Hg.
  - If BP is still unimproved, start transcutaneous pacing. Zoll pads are placed on the anterior and posterior chest walls. The patient should be adequately sedated. High outputs are usually required (100–200 mA).
  - If BP still unimproved, start epinephrine, 2–10 μg/min, to keep systolic BP >90 mm Hg.
  - Prepare patient for transvenous pacing.

- Plan to have the patient monitored in an ICU.
- Stop all medicines that may be causing bradycardia or hypotension. Check electrolytes and, if applicable, also digoxin level, TSH, and other clinically indicated tests.
- The Fab fragments of digoxin antibodies (Digibind) may be required in life-threatening digoxin toxicity. It should be noted that this therapy can trigger heart failure (HF) or hypokalemia (and associated arrhythmias) and is very expensive, so its use should be limited to cases in which definitive therapy (i.e., transvenous pacer) is not available or other effects of digoxin toxicity (delirium, hallucinations, vomiting) are problematic.
- See Chap. 24, Procedures in Cardiovascular Critical Care (Intraaortic Balloon Pump, Swan-Ganz Catheterization, and Temporary Transvenous Pacemaker), for the technique of temporary pacer placement.
- For indications on placing a permanent pacemaker, see Chap. 14, Bradycardia and Permanent Pacemakers.

ACUTE CORONARY SYNDROMES AND ACUTE MYOCARDIAL INFARCTION

ST-segment–elevation MI (STEMI) along with the acute coronary syndromes (ACS), non–ST-segment MI (NSTEMI) and unstable angina form a continuum. Initial management consists of symptom recognition, evaluation of the ECG, and triaging to the appropriate reperfusion strategy. Differentiating STEMI from NSTEMI/unstable angina is important, as it determines the type of therapy required.

Clinical Presentation

Initial assessment consists of brief history and physical exam to elicit symptoms of cardiac ischemia/infarction and an evaluation of the patient's stability from a cardiac and pulmonary standpoint.

- The classic symptoms of an MI include an intense, left-sided, substernal chest discomfort radiating to the left arm and an impending sense of doom. Chest pain is often prolonged, lasting >20 mins, and is not relieved with rest or NTG. The pain may radiate to the jaw, right arm, both arms, or back. Associated symptoms include dyspnea, diaphoresis, nausea, and vomiting. The symptoms of a NSTEMI/unstable angina may wax and wane more compared with STEMIs. The symptoms of ACS may resemble stable angina, but they are more severe and prolonged. Differentiating STEMI, NSTEMI, and unstable angina requires ECG and cardiac enzymes.
- Identifying risk factors associated with coronary disease will help with the diagnosis. These include diabetes, smoking, high cholesterol, HTN, and a family history of CAD.
- The differential diagnosis of chest pain is broad and includes aortic dissection, pericarditis, esophagitis, myocarditis, pneumonia, cholecystitis, pancreatitis, and pulmonary embolism. If aortic dissection is strongly considered as a possible diagnosis, it should be aggressively pursued, because giving thrombolytic therapy to patients with an aortic dissection could prove disastrous.
- The physical exam in ACS patients should assess the hemodynamic stability of the patient and exclude other possible diagnoses. The BP, pulse, and O_2 saturation should be immediately obtained. Signs of HF, including an S_3, and pulmonary edema should be sought. Documenting a baseline physical exam will also help identify future potential complications of an MI (acute mitral regurgitation, acute VSD).
- The ECG triages patients in three groups: ST-segment elevation, ST-segment depression, and nondiagnostic or normal ECG. ST-segment deviation of at least 1 mm in two contiguous leads is considered significant. A new left bundle-branch block should also raise concern of an acute MI. ST-segment depression of ≥ 1 mm and T wave inversions in ≥ two contiguous leads suggests an unstable angina/NSTEMI syndrome. **Comparing the ECG to a baseline ECG** and one after relief of symptoms aids in the diagnosis.
- Check cardiac markers (troponin I, CK-MB, myoglobin).
- Electrolytes, coagulation markers, and a chest x-ray should also be reviewed.

Initial Management for All Ischemic Syndromes

Initial management for all ischemic syndromes includes O_2 and ASA for all patients. As long as the patient is not hypotensive, exhibiting evidence of an RV infarction, has a history of severe aortic stenosis or hypertrophic-obstructive cardiomyopathy, or has recently taken sildenafil (Viagra), nitrates should be rapidly delivered for control of chest discomfort. If the heart rate is >65 bpm and the systolic BP is >110 mm Hg, beta blockers should be used as well. Morphine may be given for analgesia as well as relief from pulmonary congestion.

Triage of the patient is critical. The initial triage decision is based on the initial ECG and groups patients into one of three pathways: ST elevation/new left bundle-branch block, ST depression/dynamic T wave changes, and nondiagnostic ECGs. Patients with STEMI or new left bundle-branch block benefit from early reperfusion with fibrinolytics or angioplasty. Patients who present with STEMI should be monitored in a cardiac ICU. ACS patients can go to a high-risk floor with telemetry, as long as they are free from angina, have stable vital signs, and are not in severe HF.

See Chap. 7, Acute Coronary Syndromes (Unstable Angina/Non–ST-Segment Elevation Myocardial Infarction), and Chap. 8, Acute ST-Segment Elevation Myocardial Infarction, for a complete discussion of the management ACS and acute MI.

WIDE-COMPLEX TACHYCARDIAS AND VENTRICULAR TACHYCARDIA

VTs are responsible for the majority of cases of sudden cardiac death and are divided into sustained and nonsustained VT. Sustained VT lasts for ≥ 30 secs and usually causes hemodynamic compromise. Further discussion of nonsustained VT and the different morphologies of VT appears in Chap. 15, Tachyarrhythmias, Sudden Cardiac Death, and Implantable Cardioverter-Defibrillators. The differential diagnosis of wide-complex tachycardia is

- Sinus tachycardia with aberrant conduction (e.g., underlying bundle-branch block)
- Supraventricular tachycardia (SVT) with aberrant conduction, including atrial flutter with a regular ventricular response and antidromic atrioventricular tachycardia
- VT
- AF with preexcitation (in the setting of Wolff-Parkinson-White syndrome)
- Hyperkalemia
- Pacemaker-mediated tachycardia (see Chap. 14, Bradycardia and Permanent Pacemakers)

Initial assessment and management should focus on recognition of any hemodynamic compromise and application of advance cardiac life support (ACLS) if necessary. Thereafter, attempt to differentiate VT from other causes of wide-complex tachycardia and treat promptly.

Clinical Findings

The clinical presentation of VT depends on the ventricular rate, the duration of the tachycardia, the underlying cardiac function, and the presence of other medical conditions. **In patients with known structural heart disease, especially coronary disease, VT is a more likely cause of wide-complex tachycardia.** Slow VT (rate, 100–150) may be well tolerated with minimal or no symptoms. Patients with underlying heart disease may initially tolerate slow VT; if it persists for hours or longer, however, they develop HF and, potentially, cardiogenic shock. At rates <200, symptoms of decreased cardiac output are generally present, including dyspnea, light-headedness, syncope, or cardiac arrest. **Always assess early for the possibility of renal disease and, thus, associated hyperkalemia.**

Physical exam should assess the hemodynamic stability via **rapid** assessment of the peripheral pulse, BP, and other signs of reduced cardiac output, such as poor mental status and LV failure. **The extent of hemodynamic instability does not distinguish the type of tachycardia (SVT vs VT).** Evidence of AV dissociation, which implicates VT as the cause of the wide-complex tachycardia, may be seen on physical exam, with resulting **intermittent cannon *a* waves** on exam of the jugular neck veins and variability in the intensity of S_1. Repetitive cannon *a* waves with each beat may signify AV nodal reentrant tachycardia, as the atria contract against a closed mitral valve.

The **ECG and the rhythm strip** allow for proper diagnosis of the cause of a wide-complex tachycardia and appropriate treatment. Comparison to the ECG during sinus rhythm is helpful, as a **significant change in the QRS morphology and/or a shift in axis are more suggestive of VT.** Findings suggestive of VT include (a) AV dissociation, (b) fusion/capture beats, (c) left bundle-branch block with right-axis deviation, and (d) positive or negative concordance of QRS in ECG leads V_1–V_6. Should these features not be present, VT is still not ruled out, and the Brugada criteria should be used (see Chap. 15, Tachyarrhythmias, Sudden Cardiac Death, and Implantable Cardioverter-Defibrillators).

Treatment

Pulseless VT or VF requires immediate electrical defibrillation with a Zoll defibrillator or automated external defibrillator. ACLS protocols call for the initial use of 200 J, but in the setting of pulselessness (i.e., death), you will not be faulted for starting at 360 J. In addition, CPR should be started immediately, rapid assessment of the airway should occur, the patient should be intubated, and IV access should be obtained. The cardiac rhythm is briefly assessed between shocks. Administer epinephrine, 1 mg IV q3–5 mins, or vasopressin (Pitressin), 40 U IV once. Lidocaine (1.0–1.5 mg/kg IV, repeat in 3–5mins to maximum dose, 3 mg/kg) or amiodarone (Cordarone, Pacerone) (300 mg IV, repeat at 150 mg) should be given for continued pulseless VT. Procainamide (Procan SR, Procanbid, Pronestyl, Pronestyl-SR), 20–30 mg/min, can also be considered. If hyperkalemia is even suspected, calcium and bicarbonate should be administered immediately.

Stable VT (defined as no HF, angina, or hypotension) is divided into monomorphic and polymorphic VT. Polymorphic VT with a prolonged QT interval should raise concern of torsades de pointes, in which the rhythm has an up and down, thick and thin pattern. Immediate treatment should include administering 4 g $MgSO_4$, overdrive pacing, isoproterenol (Isuprel), and lidocaine. Persistent **torsades de pointes is usually unstable and may require defibrillation.** Polymorphic VT with normal baseline QT interval and monomorphic VT with a poor ejection fraction are both treated with amiodarone, 150 mg IV over 10 mins, or lidocaine, 0.5–0.75 mg/kg IV push, as well as correcting electrolyte disorders and/or ischemia.

For patients with monomorphic VT and a normal ejection fraction, the first-line agents are procainamide and sotalol (Betapace, Betapace AF), with amiodarone and lidocaine considered acceptable alternatives. Amiodarone should be administered to patients with a depressed ejection fraction. Note that regardless of the type of stable VT, synchronized cardioversion should be considered.

If cardioversion is successful in restoring normal sinus rhythm, but the arrhythmia recurs, antiarrhythmics will be required to maintain sinus rhythm. On the other hand, if the arrhythmia does not respond to cardioversion, higher energy or repositioning of the pads/paddles is required.

PERICARDIAL TAMPONADE

Cardiac tamponade occurs with an increase in intrapericardial pressure due to accumulation of fluid in the pericardial space, which is characterized by (a) elevation of intrapericardial pressure, (b) limitation of RV diastolic filling, and (c) reduction of stroke volume and cardiac output.

Clinical Findings

The **presentation** often depends on the rate of accumulation of pericardial fluid. Acute pericardial fluid accumulation occurs in the setting of aortic dissection, intrapericardial rupture of aortic or cardiac aneurysm and trauma from penetrating wounds, invasive diagnostic procedures, or cardiac surgery. Small amounts of fluid in the pericardial space in an acute setting cause a substantial rise in the intrapericardial pressure. **Beck's triad** may be seen in this setting; it consists of (a) a decline in systemic arterial pressure, (b) elevation of systemic venous pressure, and (c) a small, quiet heart. Symptoms indicative of a low cardiac output may be seen, such as altered mental status; agitation; cool, clammy extremities; and anuria.

Patients in whom pericardial tamponade develops slowly *appear acutely ill but are not in extremis.* Symptoms include rapidly progressive dyspnea with fullness or tightness of the chest and occasionally dysphagia. Pericardial pain is usually absent. These patients may develop increased abdominal girth and lower extremity edema. A large number of processes cause slow accumulation of pericardial fluid (see Chap. 16, Disease of the Pericardium).

Physical Findings

The physical exam will be affected by how rapidly cardiac tamponade develops, as previously mentioned. A common physical finding is **jugular venous distension (JVD).** Careful scrutiny of the jugular venous pressure (JVP) will reveal the loss of the y descent, while the x descent is maintained. Other common physical findings include tachycardia, tachypnea, pulsus paradoxus, pericardial friction rub (rarely), and diminished heart sounds. Systemic arterial hypotension may not be seen initially and depends on the degree of compensatory adrenergic drive. **Pulsus paradoxus** is an important clinical finding in cardiac tamponade and is defined by a decrease in systolic BP by >10 mm Hg during inspiration. Physiologically, the inspiratory increase in systemic venous return increases the volume of the right side of the heart, causing bulging of the interventricular septum and a decrease in the LV volume. Pulsus paradoxus may be seen in other settings, including asthma, COPD, and pulmonary embolism, and may be absent in settings that do not allow for reciprocal inspiratory changes in ventricular filling, namely atrial septal defects, aortic regurgitation, and pulmonary HTN.

The differential diagnosis of patients with elevated JVP and hypotension includes cardiac tamponade, RV failure, and constrictive pericarditis. Kussmaul's sign, which is an increase of the JVP during inspiration, is associated with constrictive pericarditis and RV infarction/failure.

Diagnostic and Imaging Studies

ECG may show electrical alternans, which consists of regular alternation with every beat of the configuration or magnitude of the P, QRS, and/or T waves. Most commonly, alteration of the QRS complex is seen. This phenomenon occurs with a large pericardial effusion with the heart swinging in pendular motion. Electrical alternans is an insensitive sign of cardiac tamponade and occurs in approximately 20% of cases.

Echocardiography should be performed unless the patient is too unstable. Findings indicative of cardiac tamponade include

- Pericardial effusion; postsurgical effusions may be loculated behind the left atrium and may require TEE for visualization.
- RV diastolic collapse.
- Right atrial collapse in late diastole is a very sensitive marker but not very specific.
- An increase in tricuspid valve flow by >40% and a decrease in mitral valve flow by >25% during inspiration.
- Inferior vena cava plethora.

Right-heart catheterization can be used to confirm the diagnosis. There is equalization of the right atrial, pulmonary capillary wedge, pulmonary artery diastolic, and RV mid-diastolic pressures, which are raised to 10–30 mm Hg. The right atrial and wedge pressure tracing reveals an attenuated or absent y descent. Cardiac output is reduced, and systemic vascular resistance is elevated.

Initial Management

Medical treatment consists of **volume expansion** to increase preload with IV fluids. Maintain BP with norepinephrine (Levophed) and dobutamine (Dobutrex) as needed. Avoid NTG, nitroprusside (Nipride), and other vasodilators.

Drainage of the pericardial fluid must be considered immediately. The acuity of the patient's condition, availability of trained personnel, and etiology of the effusion should dictate whether needle pericardiocentesis or surgical drainage is performed.

Percutaneous **pericardiocentesis** should be done by trained personnel with hemodynamic monitoring and echocardiographic guidance. Considerations for this procedure include

- Materials, including (a) preprocedure: povidone-iodine solution, sterile gloves/gown, 1% lidocaine without epinephrine, and code cart; (b) procedure: pericardiocentesis kit or an 18-gauge, 8-cm thin-walled needle with blunt tip, no. 11 blade, multiple syringes, hemostat, and specimen collection tubes; and (c) postprocedure: sterile gauze, dressings, and sutures.
- Check coagulation profile (PT, PTT, platelets) as time permits.
- Patient is supine in bed with head of bed elevated $\geq$ 45 degrees.
- The pericardial space may be entered via several sites. Echocardiography should help to determine which approach is best. The subxiphoid approach (the intersection of the xiphoid process and left costal margin) is preferred in emergent situations, as it avoids coronary and internal mammary vessels.
- Clean and prep the area in a sterile fashion. Give local anesthetic with 1% lidocaine, first with a 25-gauge and then a 21-gauge needle.
- An 18-gauge Cook needle is attached via a three-way stopcock to a handheld syringe containing 1% lidocaine. For ECG guidance, the metal hub of the needle can be attached to the V lead of the ECG machine with a sterile connector. If echocardiographic guidance is performed, ECG guidance may add little.
- In the subxiphoid approach, the tip of the needle is directed posteriorly toward the patient's left shoulder. The needle is advanced at the intersection of the xiphoid process and the left costal margin at a 30-degree angle to the body. Gently aspirate while the needle is advanced. Periodically inject small amounts of lidocaine to ensure patency of the needle and to anesthetize the pericardium.
- Needle position in the pericardial space can be confirmed with injection of contrast dye under fluoroscopic observation, injection of agitated saline with echocardiographic observation, a pericardial catheter to compare pericardial pressures to ventricular pressures, and by observing whether the aspirated fluid clots (pericardial fluid should not clot).
- Once in the pericardial space, a guidewire is advanced through the pericardiocentesis needle, and its position is confirmed with echocardiography or fluoroscopy.
- After withdrawing the needle, a small nick is made in the skin with a no. 11 blade, and a no. 5- or 6-French (Fr) dilator is advanced over the guidewire to dilate the entrance site; then it is gently removed.
- A tapered, large-bore, 6- or 7-Fr catheter or a pigtail catheter is advanced over the wire. Once the catheter is in proper position, the guidewire is removed. Attach a 50-mL syringe.
- Removal of 50–100 mL of pericardial fluid should cause a hemodynamic improvement, whereas removing this amount of fluid from an intracardiac chamber will cause further deterioration. If there is no improvement, also consider a loculated effusion.
- Diagnostic studies to perform on pericardial fluid include (a) WBC count with differential and Hct; (b) glucose, total protein, lactate dehydrogenase; (c) gram stain and culture for bacteria, fungi, and AFB; (d) cytology; and (e) other studies dictated by clinical scenario.
- Drainage of the remainder of fluid may be done with manual suction or by connecting IV tubing and a vacuum bottle.
- When no further fluid can be aspirated, gently remove the catheter and apply pressure to the entrance site until hemostasis is achieved. If reaccumulation of fluid is

anticipated, the catheter is left in place until <30 mL/24 hrs is drained or for a maximum of 48–72 hrs.

- Postprocedure, a chest x-ray should be done to detect a pneumothorax, and a transthoracic echo should be ordered to detect any remaining pericardial fluid.

Complications of pericardiocentesis include cardiac puncture ± hemopericardium or MI, pneumothorax, VT, cardiac arrest, coronary artery laceration, bradycardia, trauma to abdominal organs, infection, fistula formation, and pulmonary edema. Complications are more likely with small, loculated, or posterior effusions. See Chap. 16, Disease of the Pericardium, for detailed discussion on etiology, pathophysiology, and management of pericardial effusion.

HYPERTENSIVE CRISIS

Classification

Hypertensive crises should be differentiated into hypertensive emergencies, urgencies, and pseudoemergencies. The distinction is important because it dictates how rapid BP should be lowered, whether the patient will need ICU monitoring, and whether parenteral or PO medications can be used.

Hypertensive Emergency
Hypertensive emergency occurs when uncontrolled HTN leads to acute end-organ damage, necessitating immediate BP reduction. Hypertensive emergencies may present as several different syndromes. Two special categories include accelerated or malignant HTN and hypertensive encephalopathy. Accelerated or malignant HTN is characterized by severe elevation of BP with retinopathy, renal failure, and other target organ damage. Retinal exudates, hemorrhages, arteriolar narrowing, and spasm are seen in accelerated HTN, whereas papilledema is seen in malignant HTN. Hypertensive encephalopathy is a condition in which markedly elevated BP causes cerebral edema, resulting in headache, papilledema, vision complaints, seizures, altered mental status, and other neurologic symptoms.

Hypertensive Urgencies
Hypertensive urgencies present with markedly elevated BP without evidence of acute end-organ damage. (See also Management of Hypertensive Urgency).

Pseudoemergencies
Pseudoemergencies are characterized by a massive sympathetic outflow related to pain, hypoxia, hypercarbia, hypoglycemia, anxiety, or a postictal state. Treatment of the underlying disorder should treat the elevated BP.

Pathophysiology

Any situation that causes HTN can result in a hypertensive emergency. Patients with chronic HTN may develop hypertensive emergency at higher pressures due to chronic end-organ changes. **Underlying renal artery stenosis and acute withdrawal of clonidine or beta-receptor antagonists are common causes of severe HTN.** During moderate increases in BP, the endothelium adjusts by releasing vasodilator molecules, such as nitric oxide. With more severe increases in BP, the endothelium becomes overwhelmed, resulting in local inflammation, increased endothelium permeability, inhibition of fibrinolytic activity, and activation of the coagulation cascade. The brain, heart, and kidney all have autoregulatory mechanisms to maintain a near-constant blood flow; these mechanisms are overwhelmed during dramatic increases in BP. The brain is particularly vulnerable, because it is enclosed in a fixed space and extracts maximal O_2 at baseline. Normally, as mean arterial pressure increases, cerebral vasoconstriction occurs to keep cerebral blood flow near constant. With hypertensive emergency, the autoregulation system fails, resulting in cerebral vasodilation and cerebral edema.

Clinical Presentation

The **history** should elicit symptoms suggestive of end-organ damage, specifically chest pain (myocardial ischemia or MI, aortic dissection), dyspnea (pulmonary edema), and neurologic symptoms, such as altered mental status or seizures. The history should address essential HTN and previous chronic end-organ damage. Obtain details about antihypertensive medication; degree of BP control; use of over-the-counter medicines, such as sympathomimetics; illicit drugs, such as cocaine; and tobacco use.

Physical exam should look for evidence of end-organ damage. Elevated BP should be confirmed in two readings separated by 15–30 mins. In addition, BP should be taken in both arms to look for potential evidence of aortic dissection as well as with orthostatics to assess volume status. A funduscopic exam is particularly useful to look for new exudates or hemorrhages indicative of hypertensive urgency or papilledema, which indicate a hypertensive emergency. The cardiac exam should look for evidence of HF (raised JVD, S_3, S_4, pulmonary edema). The neurologic exam should assess mental status, meningeal irritation, visual fields, or other focal neurologic signs.

Lab and other diagnostic tests should not delay treatment of hypertensive emergency. Blood counts should look for evidence of hemolysis, whereas chemistries should look for acute renal failure and hyper- or hypoglycemia. ECG may show evidence of myocardial ischemia or MI. Chest x-ray should be obtained to evaluate for pulmonary edema or wide mediastinum, and a UA should be obtained to look for hematuria or severe proteinuria. A head CT may be needed if a cerebrovascular accident is suspected.

Management of Hypertensive Emergencies

The patient should be admitted to an ICU setting. Placing an arterial line should be strongly considered. *In general, it is recommended to reduce the mean arterial pressure by no more than 20–25% or to reduce the diastolic pressure to 100–110 mm Hg within minutes to several hours.* More rapid reduction may worsen end-organ damage, particularly in the brain. Exceptions include aortic dissection, LV failure, and pulmonary edema, in which BP should be reduced quickly. The specific antihypertensive medication should be adjusted for the situation; however, some specific IV medications that can be used include those listed below.

Sodium Nitroprusside

Sodium nitroprusside (Nipride) (SNP) is a rapid arterial and venous dilator and is recommended for most hypertensive emergencies. SNP should be given IV starting at doses of 0.25 μg/kg/min and titrated q5mins to 10 μg/kg/min. Thiocyanate toxicity is an uncommon side effect and occurs with prolonged infusions (days) in patients with hepatic or renal insufficiency. Symptoms of thiocyanate toxicity include nausea, anorexia, headaches, and mental status changes. Monitoring for clinical signs of thiocyanate toxicity is recommended, as opposed to routinely monitoring levels, but traditionally, levels are monitored starting 24 hrs after initiation of the infusion. Treatment of toxicity involves discontinuing SNP and dialysis. SNP has been reported to potentially increase ICP, which must be kept in mind as a side effect when treating patients with hypertensive encephalopathy.

Labetalol

Labetalol (Normodyne, Trandate) is an alpha- and nonselective beta-antagonist with partial beta-2 agonist quality. Labetalol can be given as bolus doses of 20–40 mg IV q10–15mins or with an infusion of 0.5–2 mg/min. Labetalol does not increase ICP and may be considered in patients with hypertensive encephalopathy. Beta-antagonists should be used before nitroprusside in aortic dissection. Contraindications to labetalol include HF, bradycardia, AV conduction block, and COPD.

Esmolol

Esmolol (Brevibloc) is a rapidly acting, beta-1–selective agent with a short half-life that is also very effective in these settings. See tables on p. 121 or 237 for dosing.

Nitroglycerin

NTG is a weak systemic arterial dilator but should be considered when managing HTN associated with CAD. The usual initial dose is 5–15 μg/min. NTG has a rapid onset and offset of action.

Hydralazine

Hydralazine (Apresoline) is a direct arterial vasodilator. A starting dose of 10–20 mg IV may be given. The onset of action is 10–30 mins. Hydralazine causes a reflex tachycardia and is contraindicated in myocardial ischemia and aortic dissection.

Management of Specific Hypertensive Emergencies

Hypertensive Encephalopathy

The goal of treatment should be to lower mean arterial pressure by approximately 20% of diastolic pressure to 100 mm Hg (whichever is greater) in the first hour. The agents of choice are SNP and labetalol. CNS depressants, such as clonidine (Catapres), should be avoided. In patients having seizures, the use of antiepileptics may help to lower BP.

Neurologic Complications

Neurologic complications, including cerebrovascular accident, embolic stroke, intraparenchymal hemorrhage, and subarachnoid hemorrhage, require an increased mean arterial pressure to maintain cerebral perfusion pressure. Surgically correctable lesions, such as intracranial hemorrhage and neoplasms, should be identified. Guidelines from the American Heart Institute on BP management in acute stroke and intracranial hemorrhage state

- If systolic pressure is >230 mm Hg or diastolic pressure is >140 mm Hg on two separate readings 5 mins apart, start nitroprusside.
- If systolic pressure is 180–230 mm Hg, diastolic pressure is 105–140 mm Hg, or mean arterial pressure is ≥ 130 mm Hg, start IV labetalol, esmolol, or other easily titratable IV antihypertensive.
- If systolic pressure is <180 mm Hg and diastolic pressure is <105 mm Hg, defer antihypertensive treatment.
- If ICP monitoring is available, cerebral perfusion pressure should be kept >70 mm Hg (cerebral perfusion pressure = mean arterial pressure – ICP).

Aortic Dissection

Patients with type A dissections should be referred for emergent surgical correction and aggressively treated with antihypertensives. Type B dissections should be treated with antihypertensives. The goal of therapy is to reduce the stress on the aortic wall by lowering heart rate and BP and, consequently, dP/dT (the derivative of pressure over time, which correlates with contractility). Labetalol or esmolol should be started initially to lower heart rate, **followed** by SNP. See Chap. 20, Diseases of the Aorta, for a detailed approach to aortic dissection.

Left Ventricular Failure with Pulmonary Edema

LV failure with pulmonary edema requires rapid reduction in BP with SNP or NTG. Small doses of loop diuretics may be added.

Myocardial Ischemia

IV NTG will improve coronary blood flow, decrease LV preload, and moderately decrease systemic arterial pressure. Beta blockers may be added to decrease heart rate and BP. SNP should only be added for additional BP control after beta blockers to avoid reflex tachycardia.

Preeclampsia and Eclampsia

IV hydralazine and labetalol are the most common antihypertensives used. ACE inhibitors are contraindicated in pregnancy.

Pheochromocytoma Crisis

Pheochromocytoma crisis may present with a markedly elevated BP, accompanied by profound sweating, marked tachycardia, pallor, and numbness/coldness/tingling in hands and feet. Phentolamine (Regitine), 5–10 mg IV, should be given and repeated as needed. SNP may be added. A beta blocker may only be added after phentolamine to avoid unopposed alpha-adrenergic activity. Of note, labetalol (alpha- and nonselective beta blocker) and clonidine interfere with catecholamine assays used in the diagnosis of pheochromocytoma, so they should be held before the collection of samples.

Cocaine-Induced Hypertensive Emergency

Moderate HTN can be treated with benzodiazepines. Severe HTN should be treated with nondihydropyridine calcium channel blockers, such as IV diltiazem, NTG, nitr0prusside, or phentolamine. *Beta blockers should be avoided, given the risk of unopposed alpha-adrenergic activity,* although labetol, which has alpha antagonist activity, may be used.

Management of Hypertensive Urgency

The majority of patients with hypertensive urgency have a history of HTN and usually do not progress to hypertensive emergency. Mean arterial pressure should not be decreased by more than 15–20%. Lowering mean arterial pressure excessively will cause a hypotensive crisis or potentially worsen cerebral vascular disease or myocardial ischemia. Oral antihypertensives may be used to control BP in 3–4 hrs. Patients may be discharged to home with close follow-up. Medications to consider include

- Captopril (Capoten) at doses of 6.25–25 mg has an onset in 15–30 mins and lasts 4–6 hrs. Hypotension may be precipitated in patients who are hypovolemic or who have renal artery stenosis.
- Clonidine at doses of 0.1 mg may be given every hour until the appropriate response is achieved. Sedation and rebound HTN are primary concerns with clonidine administration.
- Labetalol may be given orally starting at a dose of 100 mg twice/day and titrated to achieve desired BP. Onset of action is 30 mins–2 hrs.
- Short-acting nifedipine (Procardia) has been shown to cause sudden severe hypotension, myocardial ischemia/MI, and decreased cerebral perfusion. Short-acting nifedipine should be avoided in treating hypertensive crises.

CARDIOGENIC SHOCK

The definition of *shock* is **inadequate perfusion of target organs to maintain normal function.** Patients have evidence of end-organ damage, including decreased urine output; cold, diaphoretic extremities; or altered mental status. Other causes of hypotension, such as hypovolemia and sepsis, should be excluded. Patients with shock, irrespective of the cause, should always be managed in an ICU.

Cardiogenic shock is estimated to occur in approximately 7.2% of patients who present with an MI and has a mortality rate ranging from 50–80%. There are multiple etiologies of cardiogenic shock; however, the most common cause is an extensive MI, which severely compromises LV function. Less common causes include RV infarction and mechanical complications, such as papillary muscle dysfunction or rupture, ventricular septal rupture, or free-wall rupture. Underlying cardiomyopathy is a common cause.

Cardiogenic shock usually develops after the patient has been hospitalized. In the SHOCK trial, 75% of patients developed cardiogenic shock after admission at a median of 7 hrs after infarction. Risk factors for developing shock include older age, diabetes, anterior infarct, and history of previous MI, peripheral vascular disease, decreased LV ejection fraction, and larger infarct.

Initial Evaluation

Diagnosis should be made by documenting decreased cardiac function and excluding other causes of hypotension, including hypovolemia, hemorrhage, sepsis, pulmonary embolism, tamponade, aortic dissection, and preexisting valve disease. Physical exam of patients with shock reveals cool, mottled extremities and an altered mental status. Pulses are diminished and rapid. Cardiac exam may reveal distant heart sounds with an S_3 or S_4. Pay close attention for systolic murmurs indicative of a new VSD or papillary muscle rupture (see Acute Mitral Regurgitation). JVD and pulmonary rales may also be present.

Lab testing may show arterial hypoxia, elevated creatinine, and lactic acidosis. Chest x-ray may reveal evidence of pulmonary congestion. Bedside echocardiography gives rapid information regarding LV systolic function and mechanical complications, including acute VSD, severe mitral regurgitation (MR), free-wall rupture, and tamponade. Placement of a pulmonary artery catheter is appropriate in this setting and allows for differentiation of LV and RV infarction, mechanical complication, and volume depletion. In addition, a pulmonary artery catheter will guide treatment when starting inotropes and/or giving volume repletion.

Initial Management

Maintenance of adequate oxygenation is critical. Patients may require intubation and mechanical ventilation. Placement of a central venous line (and likely a pulmonary artery catheter) and an arterial line is necessary to properly guide hemodynamic management. Monitoring urine output with a bladder catheter is critical. Fluid administration should be considered unless pulmonary edema is present or the pulmonary capillary wedge pressure (PCWP) is >18 mm Hg.

In the case of LV pump failure, the infarct size determines the extent of cardiac failure. Patients who present with cardiogenic shock usually have necrosis or stunning of at least 40% of the LV myocardium. As previously discussed, tissue hypoperfusion may present as oliguria; cool, mottled extremities; and altered mental status. Patients have a systolic BP <90 mm Hg, cardiac index <2.2 L/min/m^2, and an elevated PCWP >18 mm Hg.

Management

Volume
In patients without significant pulmonary edema and a pulmonary artery wedge pressure <15 mm Hg, **gentle** volume expansion to raise the wedge pressure to 18–20 mm Hg should be started. Closely monitor patients for evidence of pulmonary edema. In patients with pulmonary edema, diuresis with furosemide (Lasix) improves oxygenation. Start furosemide at 20 mg IV and closely monitor BP, as worsening hypotension may occur.

Inotropes and Vasopressors
Vasopressors are very useful in cardiogenic shock; however, titration should be done with a pulmonary artery catheter. If systolic BP is <70 mm Hg, start norepinephrine at 2 μg/min and titrate to 20 μg/min to achieve a mean arterial pressure of 70 mm Hg. If systolic BP is 70–90 mm Hg, start dopamine. At 2–5 μg/kg/min, dopamine increases cardiac output and renal blood flow through beta- and dopamine-specific receptors, respectively. At 5–20 μg/kg/min, dopamine has alpha-adrenergic stimulation leading to vasoconstriction.

Dobutamine (Dobutrex) increases cardiac output by increasing inotropy and decreasing afterload. With systolic BP >90 mm Hg, dobutamine is the preferred agent. Dobutamine is started at 2.5 μg/kg/min and **slowly** titrated to 15 μg/kg/min (usual maximum dose is 10 μg/kg/min). Given its effect on afterload, BP should be monitored closely. The phosphodiesterase inhibitor milrinone (Primacor) acts as an inotrope and vasodilator and may be added if other agents prove ineffective.

Intraaortic Balloon Pumps
Intraaortic balloon pumps (IABPs) decrease systolic afterload and augment diastolic perfusion pressure to improve cardiac output and coronary perfusion. In several trials,

use of IABPs has shown a trend toward lower mortality rates when used as a bridge to revascularization [see Chap. 24, Procedures in Cardiovascular Critical Care (Intraaortic Balloon Pump, Swan-Ganz Catheterization, and Temporary Transvenous Pacemaker)].

Reperfusion
Reperfusion with percutaneous coronary intervention is advised for coronary ischemia with signs of severe LV dysfunction and shock. Several trials have examined the benefit of revascularization (percutaneously or surgically) vs medical treatment in patients with cardiogenic shock. The SHOCK trial prospectively examined patients who developed cardiogenic shock within 36 hrs of acute MI and compared revascularization to aggressive medical management, which included IABP and thrombolysis in many patients. Although there was not a mortality benefit at 30 days, there were significant mortality benefits at 6 mos and 1 yr. Younger patients (<75 yrs) showed greater benefit with revascularization, whereas older patients had better outcomes with medical management. The SHOCK trial and several other trials may support an early revascularization approach in selected patients.

RIGHT VENTRICLE INFARCTION

RV infarction occurs in up to 30% of patients with an inferior MI and is hemodynamically significant in 10% of patients. RV infarctions occur with right coronary artery lesions proximal to the acute marginal branches or, less commonly, with occlusion of the left circumflex artery in patients with a left-dominant system. The incidence of RV infarction in association with LV infarction varies from 13–84% in different series. The hypotension associated with RV infarctions is multifactorial. Decreased RV systolic pressure decreases LV filling and cardiac output. With concomitant LV infarction, decreased interventricular septal contraction further decreases RV systolic function.

Clinical Presentation

The combination of hypotension, clear lung fields, and JVD is highly specific for RV infarction. Patients have symptoms of low cardiac output, which include cool, clammy extremities and altered mental status. Other physical exam findings include AV dissociation and an RV S_3. **Kussmaul's sign,** which is an inspiratory increase in jugular venous pressure, is associated with severe RV infarctions but is also a feature of constrictive pericarditis.

Diagnosis

ECG typically shows inferior ST elevations, which may also be seen in V_1 and occasionally V_2 and V_3. **ST depression** in leads V_1–V_2 signifies concomitant posterior LV injury and does not rule out RV involvement. Thus, with inferior ST elevations, **a right-sided ECG is mandatory.** ST elevation of ≥ 1 mm in V_4R has a sensitivity of 70% and a specificity of 100% in diagnosing ongoing RV infarction. AV block (first degree or Mobitz I second degree) is not uncommon and is due to the Bezold-Jarisch reflex.

Echocardiography shows RV dilation and dysfunction; right-to-left shunting (seen with saline contrast) occurs if a patent foramen ovale exists, due to elevated right-sided pressures. Pulmonary artery catheterization reveals elevated right atrial and RV end diastolic pressures with normal to low pulmonary artery wedge pressures and low cardiac output. (Noncompliance of the right atrial waveform with a y descent greater than the x descent may also be seen.) Complications of RV infarction include high-degree AV block or complete heart block, AF, ventricular septal rupture, RV thrombus with pulmonary embolism, and pericarditis.

Management

Revascularization is critical. Medical management consists of maintenance of RV preload IV fluid administration and avoidance of nitrates and diuretics. 1–2 L of normal saline may be necessary to correct hypotension. Closely monitor fluid administration, as extensive volume loading of the RV may cause the septum to shift toward the LV and decrease LV preload. Consider dobutamine inotropic support if fluid administration fails to correct hypotension. Maintain AV synchrony with AV pacing in the setting of AV conduction problems and prompt cardioversion for hemodynamically significant AF. IABPs may be useful in patients with elevated RV pressures and corresponding decreased right coronary artery perfusion pressures. Ultimately, reperfusion dramatically improves RV function and mortality.

ACUTE MITRAL REGURGITATION

Acute MR after an MI may be due to papillary muscle rupture or, more often, papillary muscle dysfunction. This complication usually occurs in the setting of an inferior MI or ischemia of the posteromedial papillary muscle, which has single blood supply from the posterior descending branch of a dominant right coronary artery. **Papillary muscle rupture usually occurs 2–7 days after an MI.** This complication occurs in approximately 1% of acute MIs. Papillary muscle dysfunction without rupture occurs in a larger percentage of patients after MI. If not related to myocardial ischemia, acute MR can also occur due to chordal rupture. Include endocarditis in the differential diagnosis. See Chap. 13, Valvular Heart Disease, for further details.

Clinical Presentation

Patients usually present with a new apical mid- or holosystolic murmur. However, a significant number of patients with severe acute MR do not have a murmur of MR on exam. A thrill is rarely present. Papillary muscle rupture presents with acute, severe pulmonary edema and hypotension as compared to papillary dysfunction, which causes less hemodynamic compromise. **A clue to diagnosis is acute CHF in the setting of a seemingly small inferior MI.**

Diagnostic Testing

ECG usually shows evidence of recent inferior MI. With papillary muscle rupture, chest x-ray shows pulmonary edema, which may be localized to the right upper lobe due to a regurgitant flow directed toward the right pulmonary veins. Doppler echocardiography generally establishes the diagnosis. In papillary muscle rupture, a flail mitral valve leaflet may be seen. The Doppler study shows severe MR in both papillary muscle dysfunction and rupture. Pulmonary artery catheterization shows elevated PCWPs with tall V (regurgitant) waves characteristic of acute MR.

Treatment

Papillary muscle rupture has 50% mortality without surgical intervention in the first 24 hrs; thus, consider immediate surgical intervention. Coronary angiography should be performed before surgery. Medical management consists of afterload reduction with nitroprusside in patients with adequate arterial pressure. **Nitroprusside** is started at 0.25 μg/kg/min and titrated to a mean arterial pressure of 70–80 mm Hg. In hypotensive patients, consider **insertion of an IABP** to reduce afterload and improve forward cardiac output. The severity of the MR guides treatment for patients with papillary muscle dysfunction without rupture. Treat patients with severe MR similarly to those with papillary muscle rupture. Patients with moderate regurgitation should have afterload reduction with an ACE inhibitor.

ACUTE AORTIC INSUFFICIENCY

The differential for acute severe AI includes, most notably, infective endocarditis and aortic dissection. Because of its acuity, the patient often rapidly decompensates hemodynamically, because the LV has not had time to accommodate to the large increase in end diastolic volume. Consequently, the PCWP increases, and pulmonary edema ensues. The patient may also be hypotensive due to the ventricle's inability to compensate for the sudden increase in volume. See Chap. 13, Valvular Heart Disease, and Chap. 17, Infective Endocarditis and Acute Rheumatic Fever, for further details.

Presentation

A patient who presents with fever, tachycardia, pulmonary edema, and a prominent murmur (systolic and/or diastolic) over the LV outflow tract should raise suspicion for acute AI due to perivalvular extension of AV endocarditis. **AV block** may also be present due to perivalvular abscess formation and consequent impairment of AV nodal function. It is important to note that not all patients with acute severe AI have a diastolic murmur, because the diastolic flow gradient between the aorta and the LV is very low in the acute case. In this situation, the patient's pulse pressure is very high, because the aortic diastolic pressure converges very closely to the LV end diastolic pressure.

Similarly, aortic dissection needs to be excluded in a patient presenting with tachycardia, pulmonary edema, and a prominent murmur (systolic and/or diastolic) over the LV outflow tract in the setting of severe, tearing chest pain radiating to the back.

Diagnosis

In addition to standard assessment with history, physical exam, and ACLS if appropriate, echocardiography should be performed very early in the presentation to assess the **severity** and **etiology** of AI. The latter often requires TEE for full assessment. Additional imaging of the aorta with contrast chest CT or MRI is usually required. As with severe acute MR, the murmur of AI may not be present with acute AI.

Treatment

Provide supportive care initially. **IABP is absolutely contraindicated.** If the BP tolerates, the patient likely requires diuresis. If the patient is bradycardic, pacing may be required to keep the heart rate elevated (and diastolic filling time short). Generally, acute severe AI urgently requires surgical replacement of the valve.

VENTRICULAR SEPTAL RUPTURE

Ventricular septal rupture is a complication that occurs in 1–3% of acute MIs and accounts for approximately 5% of infarct-related deaths. Ventricular septal rupture occurs with slightly higher frequency in anterior than inferior MIs. VSDs occur in the setting of large, single-vessel MIs with poorly developed collateral vessels (patients without prior infarcts). Acute VSDs tend to occur as a complication of the first MI and usually occur within 1 wk. Approximately 20–30% of acute VSDs develop in the first 24 hrs after an acute MI, with most occurring in the following days. The VSD may be a single, large defect or may be more irregular and serpiginous. Anterior infarctions tend to cause VSDs in the apical septum, whereas inferior infarctions cause perforation of the basal septum. Inferior MI–related VSDs have a worse prognosis than those derived from anterior MIs. Pathogenesis results from left-to-right shunting and the consequent increase in volume return to an LV that already may be compromised.

Presentation

Patients present with recurrent chest pain and a sudden deterioration with hypotension and pulmonary congestion. Ventricular septal rupture usually presents with a new, harsh holosystolic murmur, which is best heard at the lower left sternal border and is occasionally associated with a thrill.

Diagnosis

Use **Doppler echocardiography** to determine the site and size of the defect as well as the extent of left-to-right shunting. **Pulmonary artery catheterization** with oximetry demonstrates an increase in O_2 saturation between the right atrium and RV (usually >8%), due to shunting across the incompetent interventricular septum.

Treatment

Many patients (especially those who become hemodynamically unstable) will die from multiorgan failure without prompt surgical repair. Surgical mortality is higher among patients with cardiogenic shock and basal septal rupture associated with inferior infarctions. Temporary medical management consists of reducing systemic vascular resistance with IABP and, as BP allows, nitroprusside and diuresis. A notable research effort is being made toward percutaneous closure of these defects using catheter-delivered closure devices.

CARDIAC RUPTURE

Rupture of the heart has an incidence of approximately 3% in post-MI patients. This complication tends to occur with transmural MIs, with the most common site being the LV free wall. Rupture usually occurs within the first 2 wks after an MI. Risk factors include advanced age, female sex, and HTN. Systemic steroid use may predispose patients to cardiac rupture. Rupture may occur in a subacute fashion with temporary pericardial sealing and subacute tamponade.

Presentation

Patients with acute rupture generally present with electromechanical dissociation (EMD) or asystole followed by sudden death. Chest pain may precede the event. Patients with subacute rupture generally present with transient hypotension, EMD, nausea, and chest pain. Pulsus paradoxus, diminished heart sounds, a pericardial rub, and a new to-and-fro murmur may be appreciated in subacute rupture.

Diagnosis

In cardiac rupture, ECG may show low voltages, evidence of recent MI, and transient bradycardia. In subacute rupture, ECG may show persistent or new ST elevations. Echocardiography reveals pericardial tamponade in subacute rupture, which consists of right atrial and RV diastolic collapse, respiratory variation in mitral/tricuspid valve flow patterns, and inferior vena cava dilation. Pulmonary artery catheterization in subacute rupture reveals equalization of diastolic pressures, consistent with tamponade.

Treatment

Treatment with early pericardiocentesis (see Pericardial Tamponade) once the problem is recognized and emergent thoracotomy with surgical repair are essential. Vasopressors may be necessary while transferring the patient to surgery.

PSEUDOANEURYSM

An incomplete rupture of the heart may occur if an organizing thrombus and the pericardium seal the site of rupture. The pseudoaneurysm does not consist of any elements of the myocardial wall. Pseudoaneurysms may become quite large and often drain off a portion of each ventricular stroke volume. Given that pseudoaneurysms consist of thrombus, systemic emboli may occur.

Presentation

Pseudoaneurysms may be clinically silent, with some patients only having symptoms of HF. Some patients may have a to-and-fro murmur. Spontaneous rupture occurs in approximately 30% of patients presenting in a fashion similar to cardiac rupture, as discussed above.

Diagnosis and Treatment

Echocardiography and cardiac MRI usually make the diagnosis. Surgical repair is recommended for all patients, regardless of symptoms, given the substantial risk of evolution to cardiac rupture.

KEY POINTS TO REMEMBER

- Cardiac emergencies carry common themes irrespective of the cause: establishing a heart rhythm that supports a BP; controlling the airway and oxygenation; triaging patients to a cardiac ICU; establishing an underlying diagnosis with history, physical, and echocardiography; determining the role of ongoing ischemia; and involving cardiac surgical service promptly when indicated.
- Medical management of hypertensive urgencies and emergencies depends on the nature of a patient's presentation.
- See the chapters in Part II of this handbook for more details on each emergent entity.

REFERENCES AND SUGGESTED READINGS

Acute Coronary Syndromes (Acute Myocardial Infarction). Guidelines 2000 for Cardiopulmonary Resuscitation and Emergency Cardiovascular Care. *Circulation* 2000;102(suppl I):I172–I203.

Alexander RW, Pratt CM, Ryan TJ, et al. Diagnosis and management of patients with acute myocardial infarction. In: Fuster V, Alexander RW, O'Rourke RA, eds. *Hurst's the heart*. New York: McGraw-Hill, 2001:1275–1360.

Algorithm Approach to ACLS Emergencies. Guidelines 2000 for Cardiopulmonary Resuscitation and Emergency Cardiovascular Care. *Circulation* 2000;102[Suppl I]:I136–I165.

Collins R, Peto R, Baigent C, et al. Aspirin, heparin and fibrinolytic therapy in suspected acute myocardial infarction. *N Engl J Med* 1997;336:847–860.

Gupta AK, Thakur RK. Wide QRS complex tachycardias. *Med Clin North Am* 2001;85(2):245–266.

Hagan PG, Nienaber CA, Isselbacher EM, et al. The International Registry of Acute Aortic Dissection (IRAD): new insights into an old disease. *JAMA* 2000;283:897–903.

Hasdai D, Topol EJ, Califf RM, et al. Cardiogenic shock complicating acute coronary syndromes. *Lancet* 2000;356:749–756.

Hennekens CH, Albert CM, Godfried SL, et al. Adjunctive drug therapy of acute myocardial infarction—evidence from clinical trials. *N Engl J Med* 1996;335:1660–1668.

Hoit BD. Diseases of the pericardium. In: Fuster V, Alexander RW, O'Rourke RA, eds. *Hurst's the heart*. New York: McGraw-Hill, 2001:2061–2086.

Hollenberg SM, Kavinsky CJ, Parillo JE. Cardiogenic shock. *Ann Intern Med* 1999;131:47–59.

Klein AL, Scalia GM. Diseases of the pericardium, restrictive cardiomyopathy, and diastolic dysfunction. In: Topol EJ, ed. *Cardiovascular medicine*. Philadelphia: Lippincott Williams & Wilkins, 1998.

Myerburg RJ, Kloosterman EM, Castellanos A. Recognition, clinical assessment, and management of arrhythmias and conduction disturbances. In: Fuster V, Alexander RW, O'Rourke RA, eds. *Hurst's the heart*. New York: McGraw-Hill, 2001:797–874.

Prieto A, Eisenberg J, Thakur RK. Nonarrhythmic complications of acute myocardial infarction. *Emerg Med Clin North Am* 2001;19(2):397–415.

Ram CV. Immediate management of severe hypertension. *Cardiol Clin* 1995;13(4):579–591.

TIMI III Registry ECG Ancillary Study Investigators. The electrocardiogram predicts one-year outcome of patients with unstable angina and non-Q wave myocardial infarction: results of the TIMI III Registry Ancillary Study. *J Am Coll Cardiol* 1997;30(1):133–140.

Topol EJ, Van der Werf T. Acute myocardial infarction early diagnosis and management. In: Topol EJ, ed. *Cardiovascular medicine*. Philadelphia: Lippincott Williams & Wilkins, 1998.

Urban BA, Bluemke DA, Johnson KM, et al. Imaging of thoracic aortic disease. *Cardiol Clin North Am* 1999;17(4):659–680.

Vaughn CJ, Delanty N. Hypertensive emergencies. *Lancet* 2000;356:411–417.

Williams SG, Wright DJ, Tan LB. Management of cardiogenic shock complicating acute myocardial infarction: towards evidence-based medical practice. *Heart* 2000;83:621–626.

Wolbrette DL, Naccarelli GV. Bradycardias: sinus node dysfunction and AV conduction disturbances. In: Topol EJ, ed. *Cardiovascular medicine*. Philadelphia: Lippincott Williams & Wilkins, 1998.

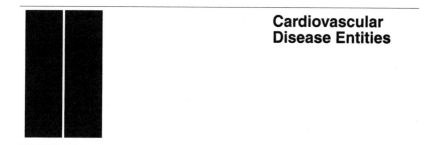

Cardiovascular Disease Entities

Stable Angina

Michael O. Barry and
Peter A. Crawford

INTRODUCTION

Typical angina is the symptom of chest discomfort (**usually not pain**) that usually lasts minutes and is precipitated by activity or stress and relieved by rest. The **Canadian Classification of Angina** is commonly employed to stratify patients into these groups:

I. Angina only with strenuous activity
II. Moderate activity, such as walking more than one flight of stairs, yields angina
III. Mild activity, such as less than one flight of stairs, yields angina
IV. Any activity, and even rest, yield angina

The symptomatic discomfort of angina pectoris is caused by inadequate oxygenation of the myocardium. In most situations, discomfort reflects underlying coronary atherosclerosis that involves at least a 50% luminal diameter, which corresponds to approximately 70% of the cross-sectional area. This stenosis reduces the maximal blood flow during exercise. The major determinant of total coronary flow is coronary vascular resistance. In response to exercise, adrenergic stimuli not only dilate peripheral arteries but also coronary arteries. The resulting decrease in coronary resistance permits the increased blood flow that is required to meet the myocardial demands of exercise and stress. It is important to realize that coronary atherosclerosis is a diffuse vascular disease associated with deficient endothelial-dependent relaxation. Moreover, it is clear that the reduction in coronary vascular reserve is not limited to angiographically abnormal vascular beds and may extend to apparently normal distant nonischemic coronary vascular regions.

Angina is a clinical diagnosis. It is considered to be **stable** when it remains reasonably constant and predictable in terms of severity, presentation, character, precipitants, and response to therapy. Frequently, the patient has multiple cardiovascular risk factors (hyperlipidemia, diabetes, HTN, smoking, obesity, and family history of premature CAD). **Remember that ischemic patients with diabetes often do not exhibit angina.**

Other Causes of Angina

A variety of other causes of coronary artery narrowing, other than atherosclerosis, exist (Table 6-1).

- **Congenital anomalies** of the coronary arteries can take many forms. Their prevalence is 1–2% of the general population. Anomalous origin of the left or right coronary artery from the contralateral sinus of Valsalva with passage between the aorta and pulmonary trunk may produce ischemia.
- **Bridging** of a coronary artery within the myocardium may produce symptoms of myocardial ischemia. The bridging occurs almost exclusively in the mid-portion of the left anterior descending vessel. There is systolic compression of the bridged segment with delayed diastolic relaxation, which causes the ischemic symptoms. Bridging is usually benign. Beta-adrenergic antagonists are helpful to increase diastolic filling, but nitrates can exacerbate the angina.

TABLE 6-1. ETIOLOGIES OF ISCHEMIA OTHER THAN ATHEROSCLEROSIS

Congenital coronary artery anomalies

Bridging coronary arteries

Coronary arteritis

Coronary artery ectasia

Radiation therapy

Syndrome X

Prinzmetal's variant angina

Cocaine

Aortic stenosis

HCM

From Topol E, ed. *Textbook of cardiovascular medicine.* Philadelphia: Lippincott Williams & Wilkins, 1998.

- **Coronary arteritis** is associated with collagen vascular diseases, such as SLE, polyarteritis nodosa, and scleroderma.
- **Coronary artery ectasia** is characterized by irregular, diffuse, fusiform dilatation of the coronary arteries. Thrombus and obstructive lesions are associated with these fusiform dilatations.
- **Radiation therapy** may produce coronary arterial fibrosis with intimal proliferation. This evolves at a variable time course and may lead to ischemia.
- **Cocaine** is associated with CAD due to the promotion of atherosclerosis as well as endothelial dysfunction.
- **Aortic stenosis** yields angina by subendocardial ischemia caused by wall stress.
- **HCM** also causes subendocardial ischemia by a similar mechanism to aortic stenosis, but also by microvascular disease that is an extension of the pathophysiology.
- **Prinzmetal's angina** and **syndrome X.**

Syndrome X

25% of patients with stable angina have coronary lesions on angiography that are inadequate to alter exercise-induced coronary flow. It was postulated that abnormalities in coronary vasomotor tone might mediate angina. Anginal pain in the presence of **normal coronary arteries** has been deemed syndrome X. It is believed that it is "microvascular angina," which is defective endothelial-derived dilatation of the coronary microcirculation. Evidence for myocardial ischemia in syndrome X patients is illustrated through the generation of reversible perfusion defects with thallium scintigraphy, MRI, or transient impairment of global or regional ventricular function by echocardiogram.

Another condition described as the metabolic syndrome X is characterized by the constellation of glucose intolerance, hyperinsulinemia, increased very-low-density lipoprotein, low HDL, HTN, and upper torso obesity.

Prinzmetal's Variant Angina

Prinzmetal's variant angina, or vasospastic angina, is a well-recognized but uncommon syndrome in which patients present with resting angina and ST-segment elevation. Variant angina is usually associated with an underlying noncritical stenosis; however, a substantial group has no evidence of underlying noncritical stenosis. There is postulated spasm of the artery, particularly around the area of noncritical stenosis, if present. Infusion of dopamine (Intropin), acetylcholine, or ergonovine (Ergotrate) is known to provoke coronary artery spasm angina. A mouse model of Prinzmetal's angina exists in which an inward rectifying potassium channel is disrupted, altering vascular tone.

TABLE 6-2. TYPES OF ANGINA

Type	Description
Stable angina	A predictable pattern regarding frequency and precipitating factors (sustained >3 mos)
New-onset angina	Recently developed angina within previous 3 mos
Emotional angina	Angina precipitated by certain psychological factors
Nocturnal angina	Angina that awakens
Anginal equivalents	Angina surrogates, including dyspnea, fatigue, abdominal pain, syncope, and diaphoresis
Crescendo angina	Change in the pattern of angina such that it comes on more easily, lasts longer, and/or is more frequent
Unstable angina	Sustained anginal pain (20–30 mins) that may or may not be associated with preceding crescendo angina
Postinfarct angina	Symptoms occurring within 24 hrs–30 days of an acute MI
Angina with normal coronary arteries	Syndrome X or microvascular angina
Variant angina	Prinzmetal's angina related to epicardial coronary spasm

Adapted from Topol EJ. Stable ischemic syndromes. In: Topol EJ, ed. *Textbook of cardiovascular medicine*. Philadelphia: Lippincott Williams & Wilkins, 1998:341.

Symptoms of Stable Angina

Several classes of angina can be organized into "types" (Table 6-2). The most important types to remember are **stable angina,** which occurs with a predictable amount of activity and is relieved by rest or NTG quickly, and **unstable angina,** which occurs with less activity than stable angina, angina at rest, or angina that lasts longer and is refractory to rest or NTG. **A patient who is having angina in bed is by definition experiencing unstable angina.**

Most describe angina as retrosternal chest discomfort or distress, not pain. Sometimes it is characterized as burning, tightness, heaviness, or choking or as a hot or cold sensation. **Location** of the symptoms also varies, ranging from exclusively in the chest to the epigastrium, neck, shoulders, back, or arms. **Duration** is usually 5–30 mins, not hours or seconds. Typically, the symptoms are produced by physical activity or emotional distress and are usually relieved by rest and/or NTG. The threshold at which they occur may be lowered by exposure to cold weather, ingestion of a meal, or smoking a cigarette. **Anginal equivalents** are dyspnea, weakness, extreme fatigue, or syncope. Atypical pain, which harbors some but not all of the above features, is more common in women and may be related to the higher prevalence of less common causes of ischemia, such as vasospasm and microvascular angina. **Nocturnal angina** is often precipitated by sleep apnea, but it can be an alarming sign of occlusive disease as well. **New-onset angina** has been associated with at least a doubling of the risk for nonfatal MI within the first year after onset. Noninvasive testing is usually helpful and feasible for risk stratification, but occasionally, direct interrogation of the coronary anatomy may be desirable. Most patients with angina have more than one cardiovascular-related illness, such as systemic HTN, hypercholesterolemia, prior MI, heart failure, or diabetes.

MANAGEMENT

Diagnosis

Electrocardiography (with and without Exercise)

ECGs usually show no acute ischemic change at rest among patients with stable angina. A variety of findings may be present if the patient had a previous MI (e.g., Q waves). Other possible changes include T wave inversion, ST-segment depressions, LVH, left bundle-branch block, or left anterior fascicular block.

In a patient with angina, **the likelihood of CAD with a normal ECG** depends on the following:

- The **description of the discomfort,** in which typical angina is more likely than atypical angina
- **Sex** of the patient, with men having greater likelihood than women
- **Age** of the patient, with older patients having greater likelihood than younger patients
- **Risk factors** exhibited (diabetes, lipids, HTN, smoking, family history)

Thus, a 35-yr-old female with no risk factors and an atypical story has approximately a 1% chance of having CAD, whereas a 65-yr-old male with a typical story and three risk factors has a 97% chance of having CAD.

The **exercise ECG** is helpful for detecting myocardial ischemia. Downsloping or horizontal ST-segment depressions (>1 mm) are indicative of ischemia (see Chap. 21, Noninvasive Cardiac Assessment for Coronary Artery Disease). However, ECG response is not the only criterion used in the test; other parameters used include symptomatic response, exercise capacity, and hemodynamic response (systolic BP and heart rate response). The exercise ECG has a sensitivity of approximately 70% and a specificity of approximately 70% to detect hemodynamically significant CAD.

Many patients are not good candidates for exercise ECG. These patients should have, in addition, cardiac imaging. Patients who should not receive exercise ECG include those with

- Complete left bundle-branch block
- Paced ventricular rhythm
- Preexcitation (Wolff-Parkinson-White syndrome)
- Resting ST-segment depressions >1 mm (including digoxin)
- LVH
- Mitral valve prolapse (MVP)
- Inability to exercise
- Angina who have undergone prior revascularization or in whom considerations of functional significance of lesions or myocardial viability are important

It is important to remember **Bayes' theorem,** which conveys that the posttest likelihood of a condition depends on both the pretest likelihood and the result of the test. This is a particular issue with tests that carry limited sensitivity and specificity. Therefore, in a patient who has a very low pretest likelihood of having CAD, the stress test does not confer useful additional information. Likewise, in a patient with a very high pretest likelihood of having CAD, the possibility of missing CAD is significant because of the limited sensitivity. Thus, stress testing is best used for those who have an intermediate likelihood of significant CAD. Of note, **the more severe the CAD, the more sensitive the stress test.**

Stress Echocardiography

Echocardiography is useful for detecting ischemia-induced regional wall motion abnormalities that occur at rest, with exercise, or with pharmacologic stress (commonly dobutamine) (Table 6-3). Exercise echocardiography has a sensitivity of approximately 75% and a specificity of 64–93%. Low-dose dobutamine can also be used to detect hibernating myocardium. Areas of hibernating myocardium exhibit poor or absent contraction at rest but normal contraction during dobutamine infusion, as opposed to infarcted tissue, which has no improvement with dobutamine. **Contractile reserve** can then be assessed by gradually increasing the dose of dobutamine. Limited contractile reserve suggests viability but also the possibility of ischemia; such territories benefit from revascularization [see Chap. 21, Noninvasive Cardiac Assessment for Coronary Artery Disease, and Chap. 22, Imaging and Diagnostic Testing Modalities (Nuclear Imaging, Echocardiography, and Cardiac Catheterization)].

Perfusion Scintigraphy

Myocardial perfusion scintigraphy with either the isotope thallium-201 or technetium-sestamibi (Cardiolite) is used to evaluate myocardial perfusion (see Table 6-3). Myocardial

TABLE 6-3. ADVANTAGES OF STRESS ECHOCARDIOGRAPHY AND STRESS PERFUSION IMAGING

Stress echocardiography	Stress perfusion imaging
Higher specificity	Higher technical success rate
Versatility: more extensive evaluation of cardiac anatomy and function	Higher sensitivity, especially with one-vessel coronary disease
Greater convenience, efficacy, and availability	Better accuracy in evaluating possible ischemia when multiple rest-LV wall motion abnormalities are present
Lower cost	More extensive published data available

From Gibbons RJ, Abrams J, Chatterjee K, et al. *ACC/AHA 2002 guideline update for the management of patients with chronic stable angina: a report of the American College of Cardiology/American Heart Association Task Force on Practice Guidelines* (Committee to Update the 1999 Guidelines for the Management of Patients with Chronic Stable Angina). 2002, with permission. Available at www.acc.org/clinical/guidelines/stable/stable.pdf

isotope uptake is proportional to the regional myocardial blood flow and depends on the presence of viable myocardium. During exercise or pharmacologic stress, the magnitude of the increase in blood flow to the nonischemic myocardial zones is greater than to the zones supplied by stenotic coronary arteries. Because of this heterogeneous blood flow distribution, the relative extraction of the isotope by nonischemic myocardium is greater than that by ischemic myocardium. During exercise, the isotope is administered IV. Stress images are obtained immediately; these images reveal a decreased uptake by the ischemic myocardium. In the case of thallium, redistribution images are obtained 4 hrs later, at which time the myocardium that was ischemic during stress is not ischemic and extracts the isotope. This reversible perfusion defect indicates the presence of viable myocardium. The most common stress agents used are adenosine or dipyridamole (Persantine), which are non–endothelium-dependent coronary vasodilators. These agents disproportionally increase blood flow to the nonischemic area, thus producing perfusion defects. The sensitivity approaches 90%, and the specificity is approximately 70% [see Chap. 21, Noninvasive Cardiac Assessment for Coronary Artery Disease, and Chap. 22, Imaging and Diagnostic Testing Modalities (Nuclear Imaging, Echocardiography, and Cardiac Catheterization)].

Contraindications to Stress Testing
ABSOLUTE

- MI in past 48 hrs
- Unstable angina, ongoing
- Poorly controlled CHF or arrhythmias
- Acute aortic dissection, pulmonary embolism, deep vein thrombosis
- Myocarditis, pericarditis
- Patient refusal

RELATIVE

- Significant valvular stenosis
- Systolic BP >200 mm Hg or diastolic BP >110 mm Hg
- Known left main CAD
- Significant arrhythmias
- HCM
- Mental impairment
- Electrolyte imbalances

Coronary Angiography
Coronary angiography remains the gold standard for evaluating obstructive coronary artery atherosclerosis. *The principal indication for angiography in patients with stable angina is consideration of coronary revascularization.* Patients with class III–IV angina

on maximal antianginal therapy, patients with high-risk criteria on noninvasive testing (see Chap. 21, Noninvasive Cardiac Assessment for Coronary Artery Disease), patients with angina and heart failure, and patients with angina who survived sudden cardiac death or serious ventricular arrhythmias carry class I indications for coronary angiography. In general, stenosis of $\geq 70\%$ of the luminal diameter, which corresponds to a reduction of $\geq 50\%$ of the cross-sectional area, is considered significant CAD. Remember that smaller lesions are often more likely to rupture, thrombose, and occlude than larger ones. **According to the American College of Cardiology (ACC)/American Heart Association (AHA) guidelines, coronary angiography is NOT indicated (class III indication) for stable angina responding to medical therapy** (see Treatment). You may see a different practice, depending on the attending cardiologist.

Risk Stratification

The average mortality rate associated with stable angina in patients with documented CAD ranges from 1–4%, but the prognosis varies widely depending on several factors, including (a) extent and severity of CAD, (b) LV systolic function, and (c) exercise capacity. Also important in the prognosis are cardiovascular risk factors, such as HTN, diabetes, hypercholesterolemia, smoking, peripheral vascular disease, and previous MI. Several prognostic indexes have been used to relate disease severity to risk of subsequent cardiac events. The simplest and most widely used is the classification of the disease into one-, two-, or three-vessel or left main CAD.

In the CASS registry of medically treated patients with chronic stable angina, the 12-yr survival rate of patients with normal coronary arteries was 91%, compared to 74% for those with one-vessel disease, 59% for those with two-vessel disease, and 40% with three-vessel disease.

The impact of **LV function is also important.** Data from the CASS registry revealed that as the LV function declines, so does the 12-yr survival rate. Additionally, as the number of coronary arteries involved and severity of LV dysfunction increase, the survival rate proportionally declines. Finally, maximum exercise capacity can be used to gauge prognosis. Exercise capacity is measured by maximal exercise duration, maximum metabolic equivalent level achieved, maximum heart rate, and double product. The **Duke Treadmill Score** combines this information and provides a way to calculate cardiovascular risk. The Duke Treadmill Score = (exercise time in mins) – (5 × the ST-segment deviation in mm) – (4 × the angina index). Angina score value of 0 is no angina, 1 if angina occurs, and 2 if angina is the reason for stopping the test. In general, a Duke score of ≥ 5 denotes low risk, $^-10$ to 4 denotes intermediate risk, and $<^-10$ denotes high risk for cardiovascular events (Table 6-4).

Treatment

The goals of therapy are to eliminate symptoms and reduce risk of development of unstable angina, MI, and death. In addition to pharmacologic and possible revascular-

TABLE 6-4. DUKE TREADMILL SCORE AND ASSOCIATED 4-YR SURVIVAL RATE AND ANNUAL MORTALITY PERCENTAGE

Duke Treadmill Score	4-yr survival	Annual mortality (%)
Low (≥ 5)	0.99	0.25
Moderate ($^-10$ to 4)	0.95	1.25
High ($<^-10$)	0.79	5.0

From Gibbons RJ, Abrams J, Chatterjee K, et al. *ACC/AHA 2002 guideline update for the management of patients with chronic stable angina: a report of the American College of Cardiology/American Heart Association Task Force on Practice Guidelines* (Committee to Update the 1999 Guidelines for the Management of Patients with Chronic Stable Angina). 2002, with permission. Available at www.acc.org/clinical/guidelines/stable/stable.pdf

ization therapy, coronary artery risk factor modification is essential. **ASA** and **beta blockers** are the preferred initial therapy. **Nitrates** should be added if there is an inadequate response to beta blockers. **Calcium channel blockers** are not the preferred initial therapy for stable angina, unless beta blockers are contraindicated.

Enteric-Coated ASA
Enteric-coated ASA is the cornerstone of treatment of chronic stable angina. ASA produces a sustained functional defect in the platelet activity through the irreversible inhibitor of cyclooxygenase, with resultant suppression of thromboxane A_2 production. The recommended dose ranges between 81–325 mg/day. Use of ASA in >3000 patients with stable angina was associated with a 33% reduction in the risk of an adverse cardiovascular events. When ASA cannot be used because of genuine allergy or GI complications, use ticlopidine (Ticlid), 250 mg PO bid, or clopidogrel (Plavix), 75 mg PO bid. The CAPRIE trial showed that clopidogrel had a favorable effect on vascular complications, similar to ASA. Of note, ticlopidine is a bid drug (clopidogrel is qd), and the side effects of neutropenia and thrombotic thrombocytopenic purpura are slightly more associated with ticlopidine than clopidogrel.

Beta-Adrenergic Blockers
Beta-blocking drugs decrease heart rate, BP, and contractility and, as a result, reduce myocardial O_2 consumption (Table 6-5). In patients with chronic, stable, exertional angina, beta blockers decrease the onset of angina, or the ischemic threshold is delayed or avoided. Beta blockers, in the absence of contraindications, should be considered initial therapy because of evidence demonstrating their ability to reduce cardiovascular mortality, especially among patients with a history of prior MI. Beta-blocking agents with beta$_1$ selectivity [such as metoprolol (Lopressor, Toprol-XL) and atenolol (Tenormin)] are preferable in patients with asthma, COPD, insulin-dependent diabetes, or peripheral vascular

TABLE 6-5. DOSING OF COMMONLY USED BETA BLOCKERS

Beta blocker	Dose and frequency
Atenolol	25–200 mg PO qd
Beta$_1$ selective	
Excreted by kidneys (hydrophilic)	
Metoprolol	50–400 mg PO bid
Beta$_1$ selective	qd formulation available
Excreted by liver (hydrophobic)	
CNS side effects	
Propranolol	40–640 mg PO qd–tid (depending on
Excreted by liver (hydrophobic)	formulation)
CNS side effects	
Labetalol	200–2400 mg PO bid
Alpha$_1$/beta$_1$/beta$_2$ antagonist	
Carvedilol	6.25–50 mg PO bid
Alpha$_1$/beta$_1$/beta$_2$ antagonist	
Nadolol	20–320 mg PO qd
Excreted by kidneys (hydrophilic)	

From Gibbons RJ, Abrams J, Chatterjee K, et al. *ACC/AHA 2002 guideline update for the management of patients with chronic stable angina: a report of the American College of Cardiology/American Heart Association Task Force on Practice Guidelines* (Committee to Update the 1999 Guidelines for the Management of Patients with Chronic Stable Angina). 2002, with permission. Available at www.acc.org/clinical/guidelines/stable/stable.pdf

TABLE 6-6. BETA BLOCKER SIDE EFFECTS

Fatigue and exercise intolerance

Depression

Insomnia and nightmares

Bronchospasm

Claudication

Conduction delays

Acute LV dysfunction

Decreased reaction to hypoglycemia

disease. Recall that with increasing dosage, some of the beta$_1$ selectivity is lost. The resting heart rate goal for patients on beta blockers is 45–60 bpm, and with moderate exercise (two flights of stairs), the heart rate should be <90 bpm. Upward titration of beta blockers should occur over 6–12 wks. Also, if side effects warrant discontinuation of beta blockers (Table 6-6), attempt to wean patients over 2–3 wks to prevent worsening angina or precipitation of an ischemic event.

Nitrates

Nitrates have multiple hemodynamic effects, including reducing preload and afterload, which reduce myocardial O_2 consumption. Nitrates also dilate epicardial coronary arteries through a smooth-muscle relaxant effect and, in turn, produce a favorable redistribution of transmural coronary flow. It is important to note that nitrates yield symptomatic improvement, but *no mortality benefit is conferred*.

A variety of nitrate preparations are available, ranging from the rapid-acting sublingual NTG to long-acting preparations (Table 6-7). For angina prophylaxis, long-acting nitrate preparations are usually preferable. The major drawback of long-term continued therapy is nitrate tolerance. To prevent nitrate tolerance, ensure a nitrate-free period of approximately 10 hrs, usually including sleeping hours. The most common side effects of nitrate therapy are throbbing headache, flushing, and light-headedness. These symptoms dissipate with continued nitrate use. Nitrates **should not be used** if a patient has a history of severe aortic stenosis or hypertrophic obstructive cardiomyopathy. Sildenafil (Viagra) should not be used in patients taking nitrates, due to high risk of severe hypotension.

Calcium Channel Blockers

The dihydropyridines [nifedipine (Procardia), amlodipine (Norvasc), felodipine (Plendil)] exert a much greater inhibitory effect on vascular smooth muscle than on the myocardium;

TABLE 6-7. NITRATES

Medication	Route	Dose	Duration of effect
NTG	Sublingual	0.3–0.6 mg	7 mins
	Spray	0.4 mg	7 mins
	Ointment	2% 6 × 6 in.	7 hrs
	IV	5–200 μg/min	Tolerance in 7–8 hrs
Isosorbide dinitrate (Isordil)	PO	5–80 mg, 2–3 times daily	Up to 8 hrs
Isosorbide mononitrate (Imdur or Monoket)	PO	60–240 mg, once daily	12–24 hrs

From Gibbons RJ, Abrams J, Chatterjee K, et al. *ACC/AHA 2002 guideline update for the management of patients with chronic stable angina: a report of the American College of Cardiology/American Heart Association Task Force on Practice Guidelines* (Committee to Update the 1999 Guidelines for the Management of Patients with Chronic Stable Angina). 2002, with permission. Available at www.acc.org/clinical/guidelines/stable/stable.pdf

TABLE 6-8. DOSING OF COMMONLY USED CALCIUM CHANNEL BLOCKERS

Calcium channel blocker	Dose and frequency
Diltiazem	120–540 mg PO qid (qd formulations available)
Nondihydropyridine	
Negative inotrope	
AV nodal blocker	
Verapamil	120–480 mg PO tid (qd formulations available)
Nondihydropyridine	
Negative inotrope	
AV nodal blocker	
Amlodipine (dihydropyridine)	2.5–10 mg PO qd
Felodipine (dihydropyridine)	2.5–20 mg PO qd
Nifedipine (dihydropyridine)	30–120 mg PO tid (qd formulation recommended)[a]
Nicardipine (dihydropyridine)	60–120 mg PO tid (qd formulations available)
Isradipine (dihydropyridine)	5–20 mg PO bid (qd formulations available)
Nisoldipine (dihydropyridine)	10–60 mg PO qd

[a]Short-acting form contraindicated in CAD.
From Gibbons RJ, Abrams J, Chatterjee K, et al. *ACC/AHA 2002 guideline update for the management of patients with chronic stable angina: a report of the American College of Cardiology/American Heart Association Task Force on Practice Guidelines* (Committee to Update the 1999 Guidelines for the Management of Patients with Chronic Stable Angina). 2002, with permission. Available at www.acc.org/clinical/guidelines/stable/stable.pdf

this effect is the direct opposite of that of the nondihydropyridine verapamil or diltiazem class of calcium channel blockers. Therefore, the dihydropyridines promote coronary and peripheral vasodilatation without causing significant negative inotrope activity. They are second line compared to beta blockers.

Peripheral vasodilatation may promote adrenergic tachycardia, especially with short-acting dihydropyridines, which are, therefore, contraindicated. In addition to negative inotropic properties, nondihydropyridines also have significant negative chronotropic effects (Table 6-8).

Risk Factor Modification
Cardinal risk factors for CAD include smoking, HTN, diabetes, hypercholesterolemia, obesity or a sedentary lifestyle, and strong family history (see Chap. 9, Primary and Secondary Risk Factor Stratification and Modification).

Of all the interventions to reduce coronary risk, none has more potential to improve life expectancy than smoking cessation. Use whatever means possible to promote smoking cessation, including nicotine replacement or bupropion (Wellbutrin) (see Chap. 9, Primary and Secondary Risk Factor Stratification and Modification, p. 96). Stress lipid, diabetes, and HTN control. Encourage moderate exercise, particularly isotonic exercise. Patients should avoid strenuous activity, which may produce angina symptoms; this is usually done by not exceeding 75% of maximal predicted heart rate.

Pharmacologic Therapy vs Revascularization
In patients with stable exertional angina, medical therapy is as effective as angioplasty. In the randomized RITA-II trial of medical therapy vs percutaneous transluminal coronary angioplasty (PTCA) for patients with class II or III angina, medical therapy was associated with a decreased risk of death or nonfatal MI. The AVERT and ACME trials showed similar results. Nevertheless, data show PTCA provides faster and better relief of anginal symptoms compared to medical therapy. Therefore, the typical indication for catheter-based revascularization is angina that **fails to respond ade-**

quately to medical management and in which the coronary lesion is amenable to intervention. The definition of inadequate response varies among patients. It could mean persistent exertional angina with triple therapy (beta blockers, nitrates, and calcium channel blockers) or a patient who cannot tolerate the medications.

Revascularization

Two proven forms of revascularization have been developed for the treatment of chronic stable angina: catheter-based techniques (PTCA) with stenting and rotational atherectomy and coronary bypass grafting.

Indications for revascularization include

- >50% left main occlusion
- Three-vessel CAD and ejection fraction <50%
- Two-vessel CAD involving left anterior descending coronary artery
- Proximal left anterior descending coronary artery involvement
- Moderate or large area of hibernating myocardium [see Stress Echocardiography, and Chap. 22, Imaging and Diagnostic Testing Modalities (Nuclear Imaging, Echocardiography, and Cardiac Catheterization)]
- Sustained VT or sudden cardiac death
- High-risk factors on stress testing [see Chap. 21, Noninvasive Cardiac Assesment for Coronary Artery Disease, and Chap. 22, Imaging and Diagnostic Testing Modalities (Nuclear Imaging Echocardiography, and Cardiac Catheterization)]
- Class III–IV angina despite maximal medical therapy

Catheter-Based Revascularization/Percutaneous Coronary Intervention

Catheter-based revascularization is ideal for candidates for percutaneous coronary intervention (PCI) who have angina, are <75, have single- or two-vessel CAD, and do not have diabetes. For most lesions in vessels with diameters >2.5 mm, **stents** are deployed after PTCA, because long-term patency rates and overall outcomes are improved. Three major **complications** of PCI exist. The first is abrupt closure of the vessel **(stent thrombosis)**, which usually presents with acute ischemic chest pain and an injury pattern on the ECG within the first week of stent deployment. The use of heparin-coated stent, IV glycoprotein IIb/IIIa receptor blockers, and PO clopidogrel reduces the risk of this complication. The second complication, **restenosis**, is a distinct and more common problem; it is defined as >50% loss in the diameter of the vessel. It is much more common without stents; with stenting, the incidence is <20% (more common in diabetics). The mechanism of restenosis with stents is *neointimal hyperplasia* caused by proliferation of smooth muscle and inflammatory cells. Restenosis occurs between 2–6 mos of the initial procedure; it responds to repeated angioplasty and stenting, as well as irradiation techniques (brachytherapy). Recently, the FDA approved the use of antineoplastic drug-eluting stents. An early trial from the RAVEL group has shown 0% restenosis rates at 6 mos with sirolimus (rapamycin)-eluting stents. The third complication is **coronary artery dissection,** which often can be repaired with multiple stents but can necessitate bypass surgery.

Two U.S. trials—the multicenter BARI and the single-center EAST—evaluated PTCA vs coronary artery bypass grafting (CABG) in patients with multivessel disease. The results of these trials at approximately 5 yrs showed that early and late survival rates are equivalent for PTCA and CABG groups. However, subgroup analysis showed a clear survival benefit with CABG for diabetics and patients with severe multivessel disease. Of note, the BARI and EAST trials studied PTCA without stenting; many believe the addition of stenting drastically changes the long-term results of angioplasty, particularly with drug-eluting stents.

Coronary Artery Bypass Grafting

Arterial grafts (e.g., left internal mammary artery) have been shown to have excellent long-term patency (90% at 10 yrs), whereas saphenous vein grafts have approximately 50% patency at 10 yrs. CABG has been shown to prolong life in patients with

- >50% left main stenosis.
- Critical stenosis (>70%) in all three major coronary arteries with or without LV dysfunction, or in two arteries, with one being the proximal left anterior descending. The survival benefit is greater for CABG in patients with LV ejection fraction <50%.

- Diabetes with diffuse coronary disease; such patients have shown significant survival benefit (25% at 5 yrs) from CABG (BARI trial).

KEY POINTS TO REMEMBER

- Angina is a substernal sensation that may signify CAD. It is **stable** when a similar amount of activity yields it, and it resolves with rest or NTG. It is **unstable** when it occurs at rest, with less activity than baseline, or does not resolve.
- The workup of angina includes history and physical exam, followed by ECG. Certain patients should undergo stress testing.
- It is imperative to manage modifiable risk factors (smoking, diabetes, HTN, lipids, weight). Smoking is the most important risk factor to modify.
- Patients should be referred for coronary angiography only in certain settings, such as class III–IV angina refractory to medications.
- ASA, beta blockers, and nitrates form the cornerstone of pharmacotherapy for stable angina. Calcium channel blockers are reserved for refractory angina and patients unable to take beta blockers.
- Revascularization is indicated in patients with high-grade stenoses, particularly of the left main and left anterior descending coronary arteries, especially if there is concomitant LV dysfunction or a known large territory of ischemia. The choice of method (percutaneous vs surgical) depends on the number and type of lesions, the presence of diabetes and/or LV dysfunction, and operator experience.

REFERENCES AND SUGGESTED READINGS

Cameron A, Davis KB, Green G, et al. Coronary artery bypass surgery with internal thoracic artery grafts: effects on survival over a 15-year period. *N Engl J Med* 1996; 334:216–219.

CAPRIE Steering Committee. A randomized, blinded trial of clopidogrel versus aspirin in patients at risk of ischemic events. *Lancet* 1996;348:1329–1339.

Gianrossi R, Detrano R, Mulvihill D, et al. Exercise-induced ST depression the in diagnosis of coronary artery disease: a meta-analysis. *Circulation* 1989;80:87–98.

Gibbons RJ, Abrams J, Chatterjee K, et al. *ACC/AHA 2002 guideline update for the management of patients with chronic stable angina—summary article: a report of the American College of Cardiology/American Heart Association Task Force on Practice Guidelines* (Committee on the Management of Patients With Chronic Stable Angina). *Circulation* 2003;107(1):149–158.

Gibbons RJ, Abrams J, Chatterjee K, et al. *ACC/AHA 2002 guideline update for the management of patients with chronic stable angina. A report of the American College of Cardiology/American Heart Association Task Force on Practice Guidelines* (Committee on the Management of Patients With Chronic Stable Angina), 2002. Available at http://www.acc.org/clinical/guidelines/stable/stable.pdf.

Goldman L, Braunwald E. *Primary cardiology*. Philadelphia: WB Saunders, 1998.

Miki T, Suzuki M, Shibasaki T, et al. Mouse model of Prinzmetal angina by disruption of the inward rectifier Kir6.1. *Nat Med* 2002;8:466–472.

Morice MC, Serruys PW, Sousa JE, et al. A randomized comparison of a sirolimus-eluting stent with a standard stent for coronary revascularization. *N Engl J Med* 2002;346:1773–1780.

RITA-2 Trial Participants. Coronary angioplasty versus medical therapy for angina: the second Randomized Intervention Treatment of Angina. *Lancet* 1997;350:461–468.

The Bypass Angioplasty Revascularization Investigators (BARI). Comparison of coronary bypass surgery with angioplasty in patients with multi-vessel disease. *N Engl J Med* 1996;335:217–225.

Topol E. *Textbook of cardiovascular medicine*. Philadelphia: Lippincott Williams & Wilkins, 1998.

Younis LT, Chaitman BR. Management of stable angina pectoris. *Cardiology* 1995;1:61–64.

Yusuf S, Zucker D, Peduzzi P, et al. Effect of coronary artery bypass graft surgery on survival: overview of 10-year results from randomized trials by the Coronary Artery Bypass Graft Surgery Trialists Collaboration. *Lancet* 1994;334:563–570.

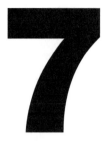

Acute Coronary Syndromes (Unstable Angina/ Non–ST-Segment Elevation Myocardial Infarction)

Christopher R. Leach

INTRODUCTION

Unstable angina (UA) is a clinical syndrome that shares a common pathophysiologic mechanism with other forms of acute myocardial ischemia called *acute coronary syndromes* (ACS) [1], namely non–ST-segment elevation MI (NSTEMI) and ST-segment elevation MI (STEMI). UA is often grouped with NSTEMI, the later being differentiated by the presence of chemical evidence of myocardial necrosis. As opposed to STEMI, which usually results from complete and prolonged occlusion of an epicardial blood vessel, UA/STEMI usually results from severe narrowing and/or transient occlusion of said vessel. If the stenosis is not severe enough or the occlusion does not persist long enough to cause myocardial necrosis, the syndrome is labeled UA.

Every year, UA results in >1,000,000 hospital admissions, compared with 300,000 for STEMI [2]. Up to 20% of patients who initially present with UA will later show evidence of myocardial necrosis; thus, this syndrome requires early diagnosis and aggressive treatment to minimize damage to the heart [3]. **It is important to note that although the short-term mortality of STEMI is greater than that of NSTEMI, the long-term mortality is the same.**

Definition

UA is a syndrome of myocardial ischemia that differs from chronic stable angina in that the latter tends to occur in vessels with significant stenoses that do not allow for blood flow to increase appropriately in the setting of increased O_2 demand. The result is dull chest or arm pain that occurs almost exclusively with exertion and is quickly relieved by rest. UA is instead caused by a sudden subtotal occlusion or a transient complete occlusion of a coronary vessel. It is differentiated from stable angina by meeting one of the following criteria: (a) new-onset exertional angina of <2 mos in duration; (b) angina that was previously stable but is now occurring with either increased severity of chest pain and/or frequency of episodes; (c) angina that occurs at rest; or (d) chest pain within 2 wks of previous MI. Short-term mortality is 2–4%, but long-term mortality is the same as that for STEMI.

Pathophysiology

Myocardial ischemia can be the result of either an increase in myocardial O_2 demand or a reduction in its supply. In the case of UA, the majority of cases are due to a sudden decrease in blood supply via partial occlusion of the affected vessel. The source of this blockage is most often a ruptured or eroded atherosclerotic plaque. Plaques are comprised of a lipid-rich core covered by a thin fibrin cap. They often do not appear to be severe when visualized with standard arteriography, with up to two-thirds of the plaques responsible for UA having a subcritical stenosis of <50% lumen diameter [4]. The plaque can rupture as a result of local factors, including inflammation or shear stress. Triggers for plaque rupture include increased heart rate, contractility, and BP.

After the plaque ruptures, *a series of events* begins that progresses toward vessel occlusion and risk of myocardial necrosis. By understanding this cascade, treatment can be initiated to attempt to reverse these events at each successive step. Once the fibrin cap becomes disrupted, the lipid-rich subendothelial components become exposed to the blood stream and act as a very potent substrate for thrombus formation. Tissue factor is exposed and initiates the intrinsic cascade, leading to increased thrombin levels and the deposition of fibrin. Concurrently, platelet adhesion commences, followed by release of dense granules containing multiple substances, including thromboxane A_2. The platelets express glycoprotein IIb/IIIa, which binds to fibrinogen and von Willebrand factor and results in platelet aggregation. In addition to the direct mechanical obstruction caused by the thrombus, the damaged endothelium decreases its production of natural vasodilators, such as nitric oxide. Platelets involved in the clot formation also release multiple vasoconstrictive factors, including thromboxane A_2 and serotonin. The result is local coronary vasoconstriction, which further reduces blood flow to the already at-risk, downstream myocardium. The occlusive matter, unlike in classic STEMI, is usu-ally a platelet-rich "white thrombus," which theoretically underlies the poor response of ACS to thrombolytics (see Thrombolytics below). The partial occlusion in ACS ushers an "ischemic cascade" within the supplied myocardium. The chronologic order is

Flow heterogeneity →
Diastolic dysfunction →
Wall motion abnormalities (may be very discrete) →
Detectable perfusion defect on nuclear imaging →
Increased primary capillary wedge pressure →
Ischemic ST changes →
Angina

Thus, angina is often the least specific measure of ischemia, as it is the last element of the cascade. Often, the partial occlusion of an epicardial coronary artery results in ischemia of the subendocardial myocardium, because this myocardium is the most downstream recipient of coronary flow and, therefore, the most vulnerable. Thus, infarctions in the absence of ST elevations were previously termed *subendocardial MIs*. This term has fallen out of favor, because it does not describe all infarctions that occur without ST elevation on the ECG.

A minority of patients present with UA from causes other than plaque rupture and thrombus formation (see Chap. 6, Stable Angina). Vasospastic angina is a rare variant that occurs in the absence of CAD. The mechanism is not well known but is thought to be related to dysfunctional endothelium resulting in local vasoconstriction severe enough to cause ischemia or even infarction. Most other patients have what is called **secondary angina.** Their chest pain arises from some other primary process that then results in an imbalance of O_2 supply and demand. An increase in O_2 demand, outpacing available supply, occurs in conditions such as fever, tachycardias, thyrotoxi-cosis, aortic stenosis, and severe HTN. Conditions in which a decrease in O_2 supply can also lead to secondary angina include anemia, hypotension, or hypoxemia.

PRESENTATION

Clinical Presentation

UA is a clinical diagnosis based predominantly on patient history and assisted by physical exam, ECG, and cardiac enzyme evaluation. As discussed earlier, patients with UA typically present with the chief complaint of chest pain or pressure. The pain is classically substernal or poorly localized, often with radiation to the left side of the chest, the neck or jaw, or the arms. Symptoms that may accompany UA include tran-sient nausea with or without vomiting, diaphoresis, and dyspnea. For the first episode of chest pain in any patient, the diagnosis of UA must be considered. If, however, the patient has a history of CAD or previous chest pain, the goal is to differentiate the character of this episode from his or her prior symptoms. Characteristics that can help differentiate UA from chronic stable angina include

- Chest pain that occurs at rest
- Pain that awakens the patient from sleep

- Episodes lasting >20 mins
- Pain that develops with less exertion than previously experienced

UA also may not be relieved by rest or may require greater doses of NTG to make a patient pain free.

The majority of patients with UA/NSTEMI (up to 80%) have known CAD. As a group, they tend to be older, have a higher percentage of women, and a higher incidence of diabetes and HTN than patients presenting with STEMI. Cocaine use has been known to cause ACS due to coronary vasospasm as well as increasing O_2 demand by increasing BP and heart rate. It is important to rule out cocaine use, especially among young patients (<40 yrs) without a history of coronary disease (see Cocaine and Unstable Angina).

The physical exam in patients with UA is rarely specific or sensitive. Often, there are no helpful physical findings. Abnormalities that can support the diagnosis include the finding of extra heart sounds (S_3/S_4), elevated jugular venous pressure, pulmonary rales, or a transient mitral regurgitation murmur. The exam can sometimes be helpful to exclude other diagnoses, such as costochondritis, pneumothorax, acute pericarditis, pneumonia, or aortic dissection; however, the history and physical exam are not adequate to rule out the diagnosis of ACS. In one study of patients who eventually proved to have UA or acute infarction, 22% described their pain as sharp or stabbing, and 13% described a pleuritic quality to their pain. In addition, 7% had chest pain that was reproducible with palpation [1]. Therefore, the diagnosis of UA must be rigorously ruled out with ECGs and cardiac enzymes in individuals who present with the complaint of chest pain.

MANAGEMENT

Electrocardiogram

Approximately 50% of patients with UA/NSTEMI present with significant ECG abnormalities [2], including transient ST-segment elevations and ST depressions, as well as T wave inversions. ST depressions of as little as >0.05 mV in two contiguous leads have been shown to be a sensitive indicator of myocardial ischemia. Symmetrical T wave inversions of >0.2 mV across the precordium are fairly specific for myocardial ischemia and are particularly worrisome for a critical lesion in the LAD. However, although less significant T wave abnormalities are a sensitive marker for ischemia, they are too nonspecific to help confirm the diagnosis on their own. ECG changes can also be helpful in determining prognosis in UA/NSTEMI. Based on data from the GUSTO IIb trial, the 30-day incidence of reinfarction or death in patients presenting with ECG changes and symptoms consistent with ACS was 9.4% in patients with ST elevation, 10.5% in those with ST depressions, and only 5.5% in those with T wave inversions alone [5]. Prolonged ST-segment elevation or the finding of a new left bundle-branch block should prompt concern for STEMI, and the patient should immediately be evaluated for possible revascularization via thrombolytics or percutaneous coronary intervention (PCI). Even among those UA patients with a completely normal resting ECG, up to 6% will eventually rule in for NSTEMI [1].

Cardiac Markers

Enzyme markers of myocardial necrosis are of critical importance in the diagnosis of ACS. By definition, NSTEMI occurs when, usually in the setting of UA symptoms, a patient has significant increases in cardiac enzyme assays, confirming myocardial damage. The most common enzyme markers are creatine kinase, creatine kinase isozymes, troponins (Tpn), and myoglobin.

- **Creatine kinase/CK-MB:** Creatine kinase is present in both skeletal and myocardial muscle cells; as such, it is no longer considered a sensitive or specific test for diagnosing ACS. However, the CK-MB isozyme, which is more specific for myocardial damage, continues to be an important tool in identifying patients with acute infarction.

The isozyme is readily detectable in the blood of normal subjects at low levels, but elevated levels rarely occur outside of ACS. An elevated level is usually present within 4–6 hrs after injury, with a peak level attained in approximately 10–18 hrs. Obtain serial measurements on presentation and repeat in 8–12 hrs. This assay is also very useful for postinfarct ischemia, because a fall and subsequent rise suggest reinfarction; in the acute setting, Tpn I does not fall rapidly enough for this assessment.

- **Tpn T and I:** Tpn components present in the peripheral blood are highly specific markers of myocardial necrosis. Two components of the Tpn complex are available as immunoassays: Tpn T and I. Both subunits have equal sensitivity and specificity. Tpn C, the third subunit, is also found in smooth muscle and is, therefore, unsuitable for this assay. Serum Tpn levels are usually undetectable; thus, any elevation is considered abnormal. Levels usually can be detected as early as 3 hrs after myocardial damage. Peak levels occur 10–12 hrs after the event, and Tpns can remain elevated for 10–14 days. The latter attribute makes measuring Tpn levels helpful in diagnosing myocardial damage even days after the initial ischemic event. Detectable Tpns that do not meet criteria for NSTEMI still have prognostic value: Tpn I levels as low as 0.4 ng/mL have been shown to carry an increased risk of mortality at 42 days [6]. Likewise, **the relationship between Tpn levels and 6-wk mortality is linear.** Similar to CK-MB, check Tpn levels in a serial fashion, with the initial level obtained on arrival and a repeat level obtained in 8–12 hrs.
- **Myoglobin:** A heme-binding protein that is found in both myocardium and skeletal muscle, myoglobin has the advantage of being released into the bloodstream earlier than CK-MB or Tpns. It can be detected in the serum as early as 2 hrs after the event. However, the low specificity makes myoglobin an inadequate test for the diagnosis of myocardial damage in ACS.

Diagnostic Testing

Noninvasive Testing

Many patients present with chest discomfort or dyspnea and a nondiagnostic ECG. Once the discomfort is controlled, the patient is admitted to the hospital for diagnosis and management. Some patients maintain refractory symptoms, despite a nondiagnostic ECG. For these patients, who usually have atypical angina but positive risk factors, or typical angina but no risk factors, nuclear perfusion imaging can be performed by injecting technetium-sestamibi IV while they are having discomfort (the **Pain-Mibi protocol**). They can then be imaged after the pain has resolved. Likewise, echocardiography can be used to assess for wall-motion abnormalities. If the patient is experiencing pain in the face of a negative Pain-Mibi or echocardiogram and a negative ECG, it is very unlikely that their pain is due to ischemic angina. **Do not forget etiologies such as aortic dissection or pulmonary embolism, however!**

To risk-stratify patients whose chest discomfort is controlled and in whom NSTEMI has been ruled out, stress testing is often performed. If a patient has two negative Tpn I measurements >12 hrs apart, stress testing generally can be safely performed if the patient is not having ongoing symptoms. If a patient has a positive Tpn I and a noninvasive management plan is undertaken (see below), a patient may have a submaximal or pharmacologic stress test 72 hrs after the peak Tpn I, assuming there are no ongoing symptoms. There are a variety of stress testing options, ranging from exercise ECG to the addition of echocardiography and nuclear scintigraphy imaging modalities, to evaluate patients who present with UA [see Chap. 6, Stable Angina; Chap. 21, Noninvasive Cardiac Assessment for Coronary Artery Disease; and Chap. 22, Imaging and Diagnostic Testing Modalities (Nuclear Imaging, Echocardiography, and Cardiac Catheterization)].

Exercise ECG stress testing has a sensitivity ranging from 75–90% but is generally accepted to be approximately 70%, with a corresponding specificity approaching 80% [7]. It is recommended as an adequate evaluation for ischemia in most patients. The addition of imaging increases the sensitivity and specificity of the exam to detect ischemia; it also helps localize sites of hypoperfusion and provides information on other clinically important variables, such as LV function. There are certain abnormalities in the resting ECG that require the addition of an imaging modality to the ECG study [see Chap. 6, Stable

Angina; Chap. 21, Noninvasive Cardiac Assessment for Coronary Artery Disease; and Chap. 22, Imaging and Diagnostic Testing Modalities (Nuclear Imaging, Echocardiography, and Cardiac Catheterization)]. **Patients who develop ischemic changes at <6.5 metabolic equivalents (approximately 6 mins) are considered high risk and should be referred for cardiac catheterization and possible revascularization.** If the patient is not able to exercise long enough to obtain the target heart rate due to comorbidities or physical incapacity, a pharmacologic stress test is appropriate. Common tests include dipyridamole or adenosine nuclear studies and dobutamine echocardiograms.

There are some instances in which a particular study may have advantages. Exercise or dobutamine echocardiograms may be preferred over nuclear studies in women, especially when breast attenuation increases the likelihood of a false-positive exam. Avoid adenosine in patients with a history of reactive airway disease, as it can trigger bronchospasm; dobutamine is a better option in such patients [8].

Diagnostic Left-Heart Catheterization
Coronary angiography is useful in providing detailed diagnostic information in patients with symptoms of UA. Indications for catheterization in UA/NSTEMI include

- Elevated troponins
- Recurrent symptoms despite medical therapy
- High-risk clinical findings, such as congestive heart failure (CHF), hypotension, arrhythmias
- Positive results on noninvasive testing, with high-risk findings
- Reduced ejection fraction (<35%)
- New ST-segment depression

Angiography should also be strongly considered in patients with a history of revascularization either by coronary artery bypass grafting (CABG) or percutaneous transluminal coronary angioplasty (PTCA). **Patients who have received stent implantation within the previous 6 mos and present with UA harbor in-stent restenosis until proven otherwise and usually warrant cardiac catheterization.** Early catheterization in **all** patients presenting with symptoms of ACS is a matter of controversy historically and is discussed later (see Early Invasive vs Conservative Treatment).

Angiographic findings in patients with the diagnosis of UA/NSTEMI show that up to 20% have no significant (>60% luminal stenoses) CAD, 40% have single-vessel disease, 30% have two-vessel disease, and 15% have three-vessel disease [9]. Typical findings of culprit lesions include

- Evidence of new thrombus formation in a location consistent with ECG or imaging studies
- Eccentric stenoses with uneven edges
- Haziness in the area of a subcritical stenosis, indicating possible plaque rupture

Women and nonwhites are more likely not to have significant epicardial disease. However, it has also been noted that up to one-third of these patients will have evidence of impaired coronary blood flow (i.e., slow washout of dye injection). This may be a result of microvascular disease and warrants continued aggressive medical treatment.

Risk Stratification
ACS is a broad continuum of cardiac events with a diverse range of outcomes. A tool to stratify patients based on risk of adverse outcomes may help identify patients who would benefit from additional treatment modalities. The **TIMI risk score** was developed as a method to differentiate patients based on simple criteria that are easily obtainable on arrival in the ER. Using the data from the ESSENCE and TIMI 11B trials, seven criteria were shown to be significant predictors of death, MI, or emergent revascularization [10]. Increasing risk score has been shown to correlate in a linear fashion with poor outcomes (Table 7-1). This score is an effective tool to gauge prognosis at presentation with UA/NSTEMI; studies have shown that it may be a useful way to discriminate which patients will benefit from an invasive strategy [10,11]. By calculating the TIMI risk score at the

TABLE 7-1. CALCULATING TIMI RISK SCORE[a]

Risk factors

Age >65 yrs

Known CAD (>50% stenosis)

Severe anginal symptoms (>two episodes of chest pain in last 24 hrs)

ST deviation on admission ECG

Elevated serum cardiac markers

Use of ASA in the 7 days before presentation

≥ 3 risk factors for CAD

  Family history

  Diabetes

  HTN

  Hypercholesterolemia

  Current smoker

[a]Each positive risk factor is worth one point; points are added together to determine TIMI risk score. Adapted from Antman EM, Cohen M, Bernick PJ, et al. The TIMI Risk Score for Unstable Angina/ Non-ST Elevation MI. *JAMA* 2000;284:835–842.

bedside, patients who are likely to benefit most from more aggressive therapy can be quickly identified and treated (see Early Invasive vs Conservative Treatment).

Treatment

Medical therapy for UA/NSTEMI is based on the two simultaneous goals of antithrombotic treatments to **limit clot formation** and antianginal therapy to make the patient **chest-pain free.** It is extremely important to initiate treatment immediately when ACS is suspected based on clinical presentation. Definitive diagnostic testing should not delay treatment.

Antithrombotic Therapy

Antithrombotic therapy includes several agents.

- **ASA:** Several trials have demonstrated ASA as having significant benefit in patients with UA/NSTEMI, and its administration in this setting is a class I indication. Incidence of death or subsequent MI is reduced by approximately 50% in these studies [1]. ASA blocks production of thromboxane A_2, thereby inhibiting platelet aggregation. Onset occurs within minutes of ingestion; it should be administered immediately by EMS or on arrival to the ER. Optimal doses of ASA have not been determined, but a 160-mg or 325-mg tablet should be given immediately, and the patient should be instructed to chew the tablet to speed absorption. The only contraindications to ASA therapy are a history of documented drug allergy and active bleeding. ASA should be given in 81- to 325-mg PO daily doses and should be continued indefinitely in all patients at risk for or with known CAD.
- **Adenosine 5'-diphosphate (ADP) antagonists (thienopyridines):** Clopidogrel (Plavix) and its predecessor, ticlopidine (Ticlid), act by inhibiting ADP-mediated platelet aggregation. Trials of these medications for secondary prevention of atherosclerotic vascular disease show that they are equal to ASA in reducing the rates of recurrent MI, stroke, or death. In the CAPRIE trial, treatment with clopidogrel, 75 mg PO/day, resulted in a relative reduction of approximately 9% vs ASA in preventing recurrent MI or death [12]. The full effect of the medication on platelets is not obtained until 2 days of therapy, however, and the effect on mortality does not become significant until at least 2 wks after treatment is initiated. Clopidogrel, 75 mg PO/day, is preferred to ticlopidine,

because the latter has a significant risk of neutropenia and a small risk of thrombotic thrombocytopenic purpura. A loading dose of clopidogrel (300 mg) to accelerate onset of effect was used for UA/NSTEMI in the CURE trial [13]. Long-term outcomes were improved with clopidogrel, compared to placebo, in the settings of conservative and invasive strategies; however, the likelihood of bleeding was higher (PCI-CURE trial) [14]. This issue is of particular concern for patients who may be candidates for CABG, based on their diagnostic and therapeutic courses. Because ADP antagonists can take days to reverse, their detrimental influence on surgery can be cumbersome. **Thus, for patients in whom a noninvasive management plan is intended or in whom CABG is unlikely (i.e., percutaneous revascularization is more likely), use of clopidogrel early in ACS is a class I indication. It should be withheld from patients in whom elective CABG is intended. Its use is also first line if there is an ASA allergy.**

- **Heparin:** Unfractionated heparin (UFH) acts by accelerating the action of anti-thrombin to inactivate thrombin, factor IXa, and factor Xa. No trials prove the benefit of heparin administered alone in UA/NSTEMI; however, several trials have shown a trend toward mortality benefit from the combination of UFH with ASA. Metaanalyses of these trials show the combination had a relative risk (RR) reduction of death or MI by 33%, compared to ASA alone [15,16]. Therapy should be initiated in all patients with intermediate- or high-risk factors, especially in the setting of continued chest pain on arrival. IV Heparin should be given with a loading bolus of 60 U/kg, then a continuous infusion of 16 U/kg, adjusted to maintain a PTT of 1.5–2 × normal (approximately 50–70 secs). Repeat PTTs should be drawn every 6 hrs during the initiation of therapy to maintain therapeutic levels, but after the PTT has stabilized, checks can made every 12 hrs. Most studies have continued treatment for 2–5 days, and there is no evidence that longer treatment is beneficial.

- **Low-molecular-weight heparins (LMWH):** LMWH are obtained by shortening the polysaccharide tail on the heparin molecule. The result is a relative loss of the ability to inactivate thrombin and an increased ability to inactivate factor Xa, which means these molecules act more proximally in the coagulation cascade. Because cascades amplify, this may provide a theoretical advantage over UFH. The advantages are better bioavailability, allowing SC dosing, and less protein binding for a more predictable anticoagulant activity that does not require laboratory monitoring. Disadvantages include a long half-life that can make emergent coronary angiography or intervention more complicated and inability to reverse its effects in the event of a bleeding problem. LMWH require dose adjustment in patients with renal insufficiency, and they should *be used with significant caution (and dose reduction by >50%) in patients with a serum creatinine >2mg/dL or creatinine clearance <30 cc/min.*

  LMWH have been studied in randomized controlled trials in patients presenting with ACS. In the FRISC trial, patients with UA were randomized to receive dalteparin (120 IU/kg/bid) or placebo. The LMWH group had a 63% RR reduction in combined end point of MI or death [absolute risk (AR) reduction, 1.8% vs 4.8%, respectively] [17]. In studies comparing LMWH to UFH, results with enoxaparin (Lovenox) show slight superiority over heparin. In both ESSENCE and TIMI 11B, enoxaparin compared to UFH showed significant RR reduction in death, MI, or urgent revascularization [18,19]. Trials with dalteparin and nadroparin have failed to reproduce these results.

  LMWH are an appropriate alternative to UFH in the treatment of UA/NSTEMI. Based on available data, enoxaparin should be given at a dose of 1 mg/kg every 12 hrs SC. Treatment should be continued for up to 5 days during initial hospitalization. Data from the FRISC II trial show potential benefit from treatment as long as 1 mo after hospitalization. LMWH have some caveats, however. First, because the level of anticoagulation cannot be easily monitored (LMWH do not raise the PTT or activated clotting time and can only be monitored with an anti-Xa assay), these medications are less desirable for some operators who perform coronary angiography and percutaneous interventions. Second, reproducibility among LMWH has been problematic. Third, a serum creatinine of >2 mg/dL renders safe use of LMWH more challenging. Fourth, few studies have demonstrated safety of concomitant use of LMWH and glycoprotein IIb/IIIa inhibitors (see below); however, this has been circumvented by two trials (NICE 3 and INTERACT) that show safety and efficacy of concomitant enoxaparin and glycoprotein IIb/IIIa inhibitor use [20]. Finally, the long half-life can create difficulty with removing the arterial introducer sheath at the end of the case. Despite these drawbacks, in the correct patient population, concomitant LMWH and glycoprotein IIb/IIIa inhibitor use may become the standard of care for high-risk ACS patients.

• **Glycoprotein IIb/IIIa antagonists:** Glycoprotein IIb/IIIa receptors are present on the platelet surface. They bind fibrinogen and other ligands and represent the final common pathway for platelet aggregation. Glycoprotein IIb/IIIa inhibitors work by blocking this receptor. Abciximab (ReoPro) is a murine antibody Fab fragment with nonspecific affinity for the GIIb/IIIa site. It has been studied predominantly in the setting of percutaneous interventions, where it has been shown to improve outcomes in patients with refractory UA undergoing coronary intervention. In the CAPTURE trial, abciximab administered for 24 hrs before PTCA showed a RR reduction of 29% vs placebo for death, MI, or revascularization (AR, 11.3 vs 15.9, respectively) [21]. Multiple trials have shown abciximab confers this benefit and is superior to other IIb/IIIa inhibitors in this setting [22]. *It is important to note, however, that it provides no benefit in patients not undergoing percutaneous intervention* (GUSTO IV-ACS) [23] *and is a class III indication in this setting.*

Eptifibatide (Integrilin) and tirofiban (Aggrastat) are the other glycoprotein IIb/IIIa inhibitors available for the treatment of UA/NSTEMI. Eptifibatide is a peptide sequence similar to one of the fibrinogen-binding sites for GIIb/IIIa. Tirofiban is a nonpeptide mimetic for a similar sequence. Each acts as a competitive inhibitor at the receptor site, and both have been shown to reduce the risk of death or MI in patients with ACS. In the PRISM-PLUS trial, patients with recent anginal symptoms and either ST/T wave changes or elevated cardiac enzymes were randomized to receive tirofiban, heparin, or both. The group treated with tirofiban and heparin showed a 32% risk reduction, compared to heparin alone (AR, 12.9 vs 17.9), for the combined end point of death, MI, or refractory ischemia [24]. The PURSUIT trial compared eptifibatide with placebo in similar patients already being treated with ASA and heparin. The eptifibatide group showed a small but statistically significant advantage over placebo (RR, 9%; AR, 14.2 vs 15.7) [25].

Consider glycoprotein IIb/IIIa inhibitors in the treatment of all high-risk patients with UA/NSTEMI, specifically those with significant ST/T changes or elevated CK-MB/Tpns. Administration of these agents is a class I indication in patients planned for coronary intervention, and a IIa indication in those not immediately planned for intervention (except in the case of abciximab, in which noninterventional use is a class III indication). They need to be administered with ASA and UFH, and the heparin must be continued throughout the treatment period before and during coronary intervention. In the PRISM-PLUS trial, the group treated with tirofiban alone actually had increased mortality compared to the heparin-only arm. A landmark trial, TACTICS-TIMI 18 (see below) demonstrated that in patients with high TIMI risk scores who were treated with tirofiban and UFH, an early (within 48 hrs) invasive approach was superior to a conservative approach. LMWH may be suitable substitutes for UFH (see above). Tirofiban can be administered with a loading bolus of 0.4 μg/kg/min over 30 mins, followed by a maintenance infusion of 0.1 μg/kg/min. Both doses should be decreased by 50% in patients with creatinine clearances <30 mL/min. Eptifibatide is given with a loading bolus of 180 μg/kg over 2 mins, followed by an infusion at 2 μg/kg/min. The duration of treatment in major studies has been 72–96 hrs or at least 12 hrs after any percutaneous intervention.

Contraindications to treatment with either medication include active bleeding, thrombocytopenia, uncontrolled HTN, and surgery or cerebrovascular accident in the preceding 30 days. Glycoprotein IIb/IIIa inhibitors have been shown to have an increased risk of major bleeding requiring transfusion, but this risk is relatively small. There is no increased risk of intracranial bleeds with these agents, except perhaps marginally in the elderly. Eptifibatide and tirofiban are to be used with caution in renal failure and are contraindicated in end-stage renal disease; abciximab may be used in these settings, as it is not cleared by the kidney.

• **Direct thrombin inhibitors:** Hirudin acts by directly binding to thrombin and inactivating it. It has been studied in multiple trials as an alternative to treatment with heparin in patients with UA/NSTEMI. Studies such as GUSTO-IIB have failed to show a significant benefit of hirudin over heparin in ACS without ST-segment elevations. In the OASIS-2 trial, 10,000 patients randomized to recombinant hirudin vs heparin showed no benefit for the original end point of death or MI. However, a metaanalysis of several studies showed a statistically significant benefit in patients with ACS treated with hirudin, with a RR reduction of 22% [26]. These trials have also shown an increased risk of bleeding events requiring transfusions in patients treated with hirudin. Presently, hirudin is not indicated as an alternative to heparin in UA/NSTEMI, except in patients with a known history of heparin-induced thrombocytopenia. In such patients, an initial bolus of 0.4 mg/kg IV, followed by continuous infusion at a rate of 0.15 mg/kg/hr, is the recommended dosage. Similar to heparin, regular monitoring is required with a goal PTT of 1.5–2.5 × normal. See Chap. 8, Acute ST-Segment Elevation Myocardial Infarction, for a further discussion of direct thrombin inhibitors.

- **Thrombolytics:** Thrombolytic therapy has been extensively studied in patients presenting with ACS. The only patients who show a proven benefit from thrombolysis are those who present with persistent ST elevation or a new left bundle-branch block. Patients with ST depressions or T wave inversions did not benefit from this treatment. A metaanalysis of patients with UA undergoing thrombolytics treatment showed an increase in the rate of MI compared to medical therapy without these agents [9]. **Therefore, thrombolytic therapy is contraindicated in patients with UA/NSTEMI.**

- **Statins:** The roles of hydroxymethylglutaryl coenzyme A (HMG-CoA) reductase inhibitors (statins) in lowering LDL cholesterol and raising HDL cholesterol—primary and secondary prevention of complications from CAD—are well known (see Chap. 9, Primary and Secondary Risk Factor Stratification and Modification). The MIRACL trial determined that **early** (within 4 days of presentation) treatment with atorvastatin, 80 mg/day, did not reduce major adverse cardiac events but **did reduce recurrent ischemia in the first 16 wks** [27]. Statins "stabilize plaques" by presumed mechanisms, thereby preventing rupture, improving endothelial function, decreasing platelet aggregability and thrombus deposition, and reducing vascular inflammation.

Antianginal Treatment

In addition to treatment aimed at preventing or reducing thrombosis, antiischemic therapy focuses on improving the balance of O_2 supply to O_2 demand. Antianginal medications mostly work by favorably adjusting this ratio to reduce ischemia and resolve chest pain.

- **Nitrates:** NTG acts as a vasodilator on both the systemic and coronary circulation. By working predominantly as a venodilator, it reduces preload and thereby reduces O_2 demand. At the same time, NTG has an effect on the coronary arteries, leading to increased blood supply through the affected vessel as well as increased collateral flow. Trials such as ISIS-4 and GISSI-3, which were not specifically for UA/NSTEMI, showed no mortality benefit from nitrates in patients with MI [1]. There are no randomized controlled trials studying the effect of nitrates on mortality in the setting of UA. However, a large quantity of observational data and an understanding of its desirable physiologic effects make NTG a mainstay of treatment for myocardial ischemia. Its use in ACS is a class I indication.

  NTG can be administered initially via sublingual tablets or spray. Up to three 400-µg tablets can be administered 5 mins apart, with the goal of treatment being to make the patient chest-pain free. If the treatment is successful, the patient can be placed on a standing dose of PO or topical nitrates for the remainder of the rule-out period to prevent recurrent pain. Dose these medications in such a way as to provide a NTG-free period every 24 hrs to prevent developing tolerance. If chest pain is refractory to the initial treatment, initiate IV NTG at a dose of 10 µg/min, which can be rapidly titrated by 10-µg/min increments q5mins until the patient is chest-pain free or hypotension prevents further increases in dose. There is no maximum dose, but a rate of 200 µg/min should be considered high enough to warrant a change in therapy. Side effects generally include headache and hypotension; the latter can be pronounced, and therapy should held for systolic BP <100. *Nitrates are contraindicated if a patient has a history of severe aortic stenosis or hypertrophic obstructive car-*

diomyopathy. Also, remember that patients who have recently taken *sildenafil* (Viagra) cannot take nitrates, and vice versa, because of the risk of hypotension. See Chap. 6, Stable Angina, for a list of nitrates used in angina.

- **Beta blockers:** Beta blockers act to reduce myocardial O_2 demand by inhibiting catecholamine-mediated effects on heart rate and contractility. They may also increase coronary blood flow by prolonging diastole. Trials of UA/NSTEMI have shown beta blockers to reduce the subsequent risk of progression to MI. They have a proven benefit on mortality for those patients who end up ruling in for infarction. For these reasons, beta blockers should be administered early in the treatment of UA/NSTEMI (class I indication), concurrently with nitrates. For patients with active chest pain, initial treatment should be with IV medication, such as metoprolol, 5 mg IV every 5 mins for three doses, or atenolol, 5–10 mg IV bolus. After the IV bolus or in patients without active chest pain, start PO metoprolol, 25–50 mg every 6 hrs, or atenolol, 50–100 mg qd, immediately. Side effects include hypotension, bradycardia, and AV block. Contraindications to treatment with beta blockers include symptomatic bradycardia, AV block, hypotension, and acute pulmonary edema. A history of COPD or reactive airways disease is **not** an absolute contraindication, and patients with a stable respiratory status can receive a trial of low-dose (i.e., metoprolol, 12.5 mg bid) beta blockers to see if they tolerate the medication. See Chap. 6, Stable Angina, for a list of beta blockers used in angina.

- **Morphine:** Morphine sulfate is recommended for the relief of chest pain in patients with ACS due to its analgesic and anxiolytic properties, which reduce sympathetic drive. It is also thought to improve myocardial O_2 demand by reducing preload. No clinical trials show any clinical benefit of morphine in the setting of ACS. Morphine's physiologic effects can be obtained with equal effect by other antianginals, such as NTG for preload reduction and beta blockers to reduce sympathetic drive. This can be accomplished with the effect of possibly masking ongoing ischemia with morphine's analgesic properties. Therefore, it may be considered prudent to withhold morphine therapy until maximal antianginal therapy has been reached with beta blockers and nitrates. Nevertheless, if these are unsuccessful, particularly if agitation and/or pulmonary congestion are present, its use is a class I indication. When needed, morphine can be dosed in 2–4–mg IV boluses with repeated doses as needed to relieve the pain. Morphine causes nausea and vomiting in 20% of patients and also can lead to hypotension and respiratory depression.

- **Calcium channel blockers:** Calcium channel blockers can be used as a third-line agent in patients continuing to have chest pain in the setting of adequate doses of beta blockers and nitrates. These medications have been shown to help with vasospastic angina. In that instance, verapamil (240–480 mg PO/day) is the agent of choice instead of beta blockers. Otherwise, no data show significant morbidity or mortality benefit with the use of calcium channel blockers. For short-acting dihydropyridines, such as nifedipine, these agents are associated with an increased risk of death when used in the setting of acute MI and are contraindicated. Avoid all calcium channel blockers in patients with CHF or conduction abnormalities. See Chap. 6, Stable Angina, for a list of calcium channel blockers used in angina.

- **ACE inhibitors:** ACE inhibitors have been studied in the setting of acute MI but not in UA. Trials to date have failed to show a short-term benefit from ACE inhibitors; however, multiple trials support a long-term benefit in mortality in patients with STEMI and a reduced ejection fraction <40%. The HOPE data showed patients with known CAD or diabetes and an additional cardiovascular risk factor gained significant benefit from treatment with daily ramipril [28]. This effect was in the setting of normal LV function. As a majority of the patients presenting with UA/NSTEMI fulfill these criteria, consider adding an ACE inhibitor to their medical regimens by discharge. They should be used even earlier in patients with LV dysfunction and/or diabetes presenting with ACS and persistent HTN despite nitrates and beta blockers (class I). See Chap. 10, Management of Acute and Chronic Heart Failure, for dosing information.

Early Invasive vs Conservative Treatment and Revascularization

Since the mid-1990s, debate has existed over the usefulness of more aggressive treatment of UA/NSTEMI through more liberal use of invasive techniques. An early invasive strategy was developed in which all patients presenting with UA/NSTEMI were evaluated with coronary angiography and possible revascularization within 48 hrs of initial presentation, in addition to receiving standard medical treatment. Early conservative therapy was based on medical treatment as reviewed above, with progression to angiography and revascularization only in patients who met specific criteria and were deemed to be failing medical treatment. These criteria varied between studies but usually included recurrent chest pain not resolved with adequate medical treatment; chest pain with new ECG changes; a positive stress test result based on ECG abnormalities, hemodynamic instability, or imaging showing two or more areas of reversible hypoperfusion; or recurrent chest pain after discharge requiring readmission to hospital.

The initial studies failed to show any benefit in early invasive treatment. In TIMI 11B, patients with UA/NSTEMI were randomized in two × two fashion to thrombolysis vs placebo and early invasive vs early conservative treatment, as described above. The outcomes at 6 wks showed no significant difference between the two groups in the combined end point of mortality, MI, or recurrent ischemia (16.2% vs 18.1%, respectively) [9]. The VANQWISH study involved 920 Veterans Affairs patients with NSTEMI by positive CK-MB who were assigned to either an early invasive or a conservative medical approach. Again, the combined end point of death or MI did not differ between the groups at the end of the study [29]. However, data for mortality at 30 days and 1 yr showed a significant hazard for the invasive group.

More recent studies have shown different results. In the FRISC II trial, results from nearly 2500 patients with UA and NSTEMI showed a significant benefit at 6 mos in the invasive group for the end point of death or MI (RR, 22%; AR, 9.4% vs 12.1%) [30]. The TACTICS-TIMI 18 study examined 2200 patients with UA/NSTEMI with either ECG changes or positive cardiac biomarkers, all of whom were treated with the glycoprotein IIb/IIIa inhibitor tirofiban in addition to ASA, heparin, and beta blockers. The investigators showed a 22% RR reduction in the group who underwent early invasive treatment as compared with conservative therapy (AR, 15.8% vs 19.4%) [11]. The TACTICS-TIMI 18 study also used the TIMI risk score to stratify patients based on their presenting data (see Risk Stratification). By re-examining the data based on risk score, the patients with high (5–7 points) and intermediate (3–4 points) scores benefited from early intervention, whereas the low-risk group (0–2 points) did not.

The reason for improved outcomes with an invasive approach in the more recent trials is not completely clear but most likely reflects improved interventional techniques (e.g., stents) as well as the introduction of new medical adjuncts that further improve intervention results (i.e., glycoprotein IIb/IIIa inhibitors, clopidogrel postintervention). Some controversy over the use of an early invasive approach still exists, but in light of the most recent data, intermediate- and high-risk patients may benefit from coronary angiography within the first 48 hrs of presentation, with revascularization as indicated. An early invasive strategy is a class I indication in the presence of recurrent angina despite maximal medical therapy, with elevated cardiac biomarkers in the serum, new ST depression, CHF symptoms in the setting of ACS, high-risk findings on stress testing, LV ejection fraction <40%, sustained ventricular arrhythmias, hemodynamic instability, prior percutaneous intervention within 6 mos, or prior bypass surgery.

The decision to perform CABG vs PCI in the ACS patient depends on the coronary anatomy, LV function, and the presence of diabetes. Chap. 6, Stable Angina, gives an outline of the guidelines; it also reviews complications of PTCA/stents and discusses drug-eluting stents.

Cocaine and Unstable Angina

An estimated 25 million Americans have used cocaine, and it is the most commonly used illicit drug among patients seeking ER care [31]. The pathogenesis of cocaine-induced angina is likely secondary to a combination of increased myocardial O_2 demand from increased BP, heart rate, and contractility; marked vasoconstriction of epicardial vessels; and increased platelet aggregation. The risk of MI in patients otherwise at low risk for cardiac events is increased by a factor of 24 immediately after cocaine use; such patients can account for up to 25% of those presenting to urban hospitals with nontraumatic chest pain. The majority have few risk factors for heart disease, and 50% have no evidence of coronary disease when subjected to coronary angiography. However, long-term users have been shown to have premature arteriosclerosis at autopsy.

Patients who are at risk of cocaine-induced chest pain **should undergo the same diagnostic considerations as other patients with symptoms of UA.** Urine drug screens for cocaine metabolites should be positive in the majority of patients. Treatment is somewhat different. All patients should still receive ASA as discussed earlier, due to increased risk of platelet aggregation. Nitrates should also be given in the usual fashion. Beta blockers are relatively contraindicated in these patients, as they could lead to unopposed alpha-mediated constriction and worsen myocardial ischemia. The exception would be a medication such as labetalol that has both beta- and alpha-blocking properties. Calcium channel blockers, such as verapamil, can also be used to reduce myocardial O_2 demand. **Benzodiazepines** can be used in this syndrome as an anxiolytic and to reduce ischemia. After the acute event, patient education and chemical dependency counseling are important to prevent recurrent events.

Discharge

After appropriate medical treatment, ACS patients with noninvasive stress testing or coronary angiography/revascularization will be ready for discharge home. The timeline for these events can be as little as 24 hrs to several days if CABG is indicated. At discharge, it is important to evaluate the patient for aggressive risk-factor modification to minimize the chance of recurrent events. Address diabetes education and glucose control, smoking cessation, improved BP control, education on diet and exercise, and lipid-lowering therapy if LDL is not below the National Cholesterol Education Program goal before discharge. Continue patients on medical regimens that have shown benefit in reducing mortality in patients with CAD, including ASA (81–325 mg/day), adequate doses of beta blockers, and ACE inhibitors. Add a statin in all patients with elevated LDL and perhaps even in those with a normal lipid profile and demonstrated CAD. In addition, discharge patients with medications to alleviate ischemic symptoms. All patients with CAD should be discharged with either sublingual or spray versions of NTG for symptom control. Education on the symptoms that should prompt the patient to immediately seek medical attention is also important to maximize his or her ability to be proactive in managing chronic disease and preventing slow response to MI symptoms. For further discussion, see Chap. 9, Primary and Secondary Risk Factor Stratificaion and Modification, for management of key risk factors as well as cardiac rehabilitation.

KEY POINTS TO REMEMBER

- UA and NSTEMI are treated similarly because they are driven by the same underlying pathophysiology. Together they are known as ACS.
- All patients should receive ASA and beta blockers, as well as nitrates for angina suppression, **early** in the presentation.
- Patients at higher risk, as assessed by TIMI risk score, benefit from an invasive strategy, including UFH or LMWH, an IV glycoprotein IIb/IIIa inhibitor, clopidogrel, and coronary angiography with revascularization. Carefully tailor therapy plans to individual patients.
- Low-risk patients can be risk stratified with stress testing before discharge.
- The role of LMWH over UFH in ACS is yet to be completely defined, although data are mounting in favor of the former.
- The role of preangiographic clopidogrel is targeted for patients unlikely to undergo CABG within 5 days of presentation (class I indication in nonsurgical patients). Although its early administration is associated with improved outcomes, the attendant bleeding risk, particularly if surgery is planned, makes it problematic in some settings. Clopidogrel is used as a class I indication for at least 4 wks after stent implantation.
- Do not forget the importance of secondary prevention. Urge patients to quit smoking, improve their diets, control their diabetes and HTN, enroll in cardiac rehabilitation,

and take a statin (see Chap. 9, Primary and Secondary Risk Factor Stratification and Modification).

SUGGESTED READING

Braunwald E, Antman EM, Beasley JW, et al. *ACC/AHA 2002 guideline update for the management of patients with unstable angina and non-ST-segment elevation myocardial infarction. A report of the American College of Cardiology/American Heart Association Task Force on Practice Guidelines* (Committee on the Management of Patients With Unstable Angina), 2002. Available at http://www.acc.org/clinical/guidelines/unstable/unstable.pdf.

REFERENCES

1. Braunwald E, Antman EM, Beasley JW, et al. ACC/AHA guideline update for the management of patients with unstable angina and non-ST-segment elevation myocardial infarction—2002: summary article: a report of the American College of Cardiology/American Heart Association Task Force on Practice Guidelines (Committee on the Management of Patients With Unstable Angina). *Circulation* 2002;106(14):1893–1900.
2. Cannon C, Braunwald E. Unstable angina. In: Braunwald E, ed. *Heart disease: a textbook of cardiovascular medicine*, 6th ed. Philadelphia: WB Saunders, 2001: 1232–1271.
3. Stone P, Thompson B, Anderson H, et al. Influence of race, sex and age on management of unstable angina and non-Q-wave myocardial infarction: the TIMI III Registry. *JAMA* 1996;336:1104–1112.
4. Yeghiazarans Y, Braunstein J, Askari A, et al. Unstable angina pectoris. *N Engl J Med* 2000;342(2):101–114.
5. Savonitto S, Ardissino D, Granger CB, et al. Prognostic value of the admission electrocardiogram in acute coronary syndromes. *JAMA* 1999;281(8):707–713.
6. Antman E, Tanasijevic M, Thompson B, et al. Cardiac-specific troponin I levels to predict the risk of mortality in patients with acute coronary syndromes. *N Engl J Med* 1996;335:1342–1349.
7. Ritchie J, Bateman TM, Bonow RO, et al. ACC/AHA guidelines for clinical use of cardiac radionuclide imaging: report of the American College of Cardiology/American Heart Association Task Force on Assessment of Diagnostic and Therapeutic Cardiovascular Procedures. *J Am Coll Cardiol* 1995;25:521–547.
8. Beller G, Zaret B. Contributions of nuclear cardiology to diagnosis and prognosis of patients with coronary artery disease. *Circulation* 2000;101:1465–1478.
9. TIMI IIIB Investigators. Effects of tissue plasminogen activator and a comparison of early invasive and conservative strategies in unstable angina and non-Q-wave myocardial infarction: results of the TIMI IIIB Trial. *Circulation* 1994;89: 1545–1556.
10. Antman E, Cohen M, Bernink PJ, et al. The TIMI Risk Score for unstable angina/non-ST elevation MI: a method for prognostication and therapeutic decision making. *JAMA* 2000;284(7):835–842.
11. Cannon C, Weintraub W, Demopoulos LA, et al. Comparison of early invasive and conservative strategies in patients with unstable coronary syndromes treated with the glycoprotein IIb/IIIa inhibitor tirofiban. *N Engl J Med* 2001;344:1879–1887.
12. CAPRIE Steering Committee. A randomized, blinded, trial of clopidogrel versus aspirin in patients at risk of ischaemic events (CAPRIE). *Lancet* 1996;348:1329–1339.
13. Yusuf S, Zhao F, Mehta SR, et al. Effects of clopidogrel in addition to aspirin in patients with acute coronary syndromes without ST-segment elevation. *N Engl J Med* 2001;345:494–502.
14. Mehta SR, Yusuf S, Peters RJ, et al. Effects of pretreatment with clopidogrel and aspirin followed by long-term therapy in patients undergoing percutaneous coronary intervention: the PCI-CURE study. *Lancet* 2001;358(9281):527–533.

15. Oler A, Whooley M, Oler J, et al. Adding heparin to aspirin reduces the incidence of myocardial infarction and death in patients with unstable angina: a meta-analysis. *JAMA* 1996;276:811–815.

16. Cohen M, Adams P, Parry G, et al. Combination antithrombotic therapy in unstable rest angina and non-Q-wave infarction in nonprior aspirin users: primary end points analysis from the ATACS trial. *Circulation* 1994;89:81–88.

17. FRISC Study Group. Low-molecular-weight heparin during instability in coronary artery disease. *Lancet* 1996;347:561–568.

18. ESSENCE Study Group. A comparison of low-molecular-weight heparin with unfractionated heparin for unstable coronary artery disease. *N Engl J Med* 1997; 337:447–452.

19. TIMI 11B Investigators. Enoxaparin prevents death and cardiac ischemic events in unstable angina/non-Q-wave myocardial infarction: results of the Thrombolysis In Myocardial Infarction 11B Trial. *Circulation* 1999;100:1593–1601.

20. Kereiakes DJ, Grines C, Fry EJ, et al. Enoxaparin and abciximab adjunctive pharmacotherapy during percutaneous coronary intervention. *Invasive Cardiol* 2001;13(4):272–278.

21. CAPTURE Investigators. Randomised placebo-controlled trial of abciximab before and during coronary intervention in refractory unstable angina: the CAPTURE study. *Lancet* 1997;349:1429–1435.

22. TARGET Investigators. Comparison of two platelet glycoprotein IIb/IIIa inhibitors, tirofiban and abciximab, for the prevention of ischemic events with percutaneous coronary revascularization. *N Engl J Med* 2001;344:1888–1894.

23. Simoons ML, GUSTO IV-ACS Investigators. Effect of glycoprotein IIb/IIIa receptor blocker abciximab on outcome in patients with acute coronary syndromes without early coronary revascularisation: the GUSTO IV-ACS randomised trial. *Lancet* 2001;357(9272):1915–1924.

24. PRISM-PLUS Study Investigators. Inhibition of the platelet glycoprotein IIb/IIIa receptor with tirofiban in unstable angina and non-Q-wave myocardial infarction. *N Engl J Med* 1998;338:1488–1497.

25. The PURSUIT Trial Investigators. Inhibition of platelet glycoprotein IIb/IIIa with eptifibatide in patients with acute coronary syndromes. *N Engl J Med* 1998; 339:436–443.

26. OASIS-2 Investigators. Effects of recombinant hirudin (lepirudin) compared with heparin on death, myocardial infarction, refractory angina, and revascularisation procedures in patients with acute myocardial ischaemia without ST elevation: a randomized trial. *Lancet* 1999;353:429–438.

27. Schwartz GG, Olsson AG, Ezekowitz MD, et al. Effects of atorvastatin on early recurrent ischemic events in acute coronary syndromes: the MIRACL study. A randomized controlled trial. *JAMA* 2001;285(13):1711–1718.

28. HOPE Investigators. Effects of an angiotensin-converting-enzyme inhibitor, ramipril, on cardiovascular events in high-risk patients. *N Engl J Med* 2000;342: 145–152.

29. VANQWISH Trial Investigators. Outcomes in patients with acute non-Q-wave myocardial infarction randomly assigned to an invasive as compared with a conservative management strategy. *N Engl J Med* 1998;338:1785–1792.

30. FRISC II Investigators. Invasive compared with non-invasive treatment in unstable coronary-artery disease: FRISC II Prospective Randomised Multicentre Study. *Lancet* 1999;354:708–715.

31. Lange R, Hillis LD. Cardiovascular complications of cocaine use. *N Engl J Med* 2001;345:351–358.

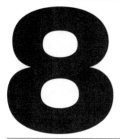

Acute ST-Segment Elevation Myocardial Infarction

Douglas R. Bree and
Peter A. Crawford

INTRODUCTION

CAD is the single largest killer of American men and women [1]. In the United States, approximately every 29 secs, a person suffers a coronary event, and approximately every minute, someone dies from one. An estimated 1.1 million Americans will suffer a new or recurrent coronary event this year, and >40% of these events will be fatal. Every year, roughly 220,000 people die of **acute MI (AMI)** without being hospitalized, usually due to cardiac arrest from VF. The effects of AMI are substantial, even if a patient survives the acute stage of the illness. Within 1 yr of an initial recognized MI, an estimated 25% of men and 38% of women will die. Within 6 yrs of the MI,

- 18% of men and 35% of women will have another heart attack
- 7% of men and 6% of women will experience sudden death
- 22% of men and 46% of women will be disabled with heart failure

Despite these grim statistics, the death rate from CAD has declined 26% since 1990.

CAUSES

Pathophysiology

An AMI is usually the result of formation of a coronary artery occlusion by thrombus formation from a previous atheromatous plaque. The setting for this event is believed to involve relatively mild to moderate immature plaques (i.e., those that at baseline do not significantly impede coronary flow) with thin fibrous caps and lipid-rich cores [2] that rupture in the acute setting of inflammation, shear forces, and local rheologic factors [3]. This initiates a sequence of platelet aggregation, fibrin deposition, and vasoconstriction that *completely occludes* the involved artery, predisposing to **transmural MI.** The pathologic entity in ST-segment elevation MI (STEMI) classically consists of the *fibrin-rich red thrombus,* which is believed to be part of the reason these presentations respond to thrombolytics (see Thrombolysis). The degree of infarction is determined by the area of myocardium supplied by the artery, the presence of collateral vessels to the area, and the amount of time the vessel remains occluded. The pathologic consequences of AMI are primarily determined by the *open artery hypothesis,* which maintains that the reestablishment of early, full, and sustained reperfusion will improve clinical outcomes [4]. The TIMI Study Group defined the coronary perfusion grading system that is most commonly used in the United States as follows [5]:

- **TIMI 3 flow:** full perfusion with normal flow
- **TIMI 2 flow:** perfusion of entire coronary bed but with delayed flow
- **TIMI 1 flow:** some penetration of contrast past obstruction but no perfusion of distal coronary bed
- **TIMI 0 flow:** complete coronary occlusion

Multiple studies have found that AMI has a consistent mortality gradient of improved survival with improved TIMI flow [6]. Achieving TIMI 3 flow over all lower flow scores yields particular benefit, with a recognized reduction in both short-term

[7] and long-term survival [8]. The open artery hypothesis, therefore, guides the management of AMI with the specific goal to achieve TIMI 3 flow in the infarct-related artery as rapidly and definitively as possible.

It is important to distinguish the pathophysiology of **acute STEMI** from **ACS** (unstable angina and NSTEMI) [see Chap. 7, Acute Coronary Syndromes (Unstable Angina / Non–ST-Segment Elevation Myocardial Infarction)]. Treatment for these processes is different, because the physiology is usually different. Occasionally, it can be difficult to discriminate between them (see Management), so the ability to assess these patients early is very important. **STEMI always should prompt you to think of rapid revascularization.**

History

The classic presentation of AMI is similar to angina; however, it is typically much more severe and prolonged. Patients complain of crushing, substernal- to left-sided chest discomfort that may radiate into the left arm, neck, shoulder, back, or jaw. It is common for patients to also experience associated symptoms of dyspnea, diaphoresis, nausea, vomiting, palpitations, and an impending sense of doom. The onset of discomfort may occur in the setting of exertion or rest but usually is differentiated from stable angina by failure to be relieved by rest and/or nitroglycerin (NTG), with pain symptoms lasting >20 mins. In patients with known cardiac disease and prior angina or MI, a reliable history can usually be obtained by inquiring if their current pain was similar to prior episodes. AMI may occur without classic chest discomfort, particularly in the elderly and diabetics.

Of great importance in the evaluation of possible AMI is the urgency with which the initial history should be obtained. A detailed and thorough history and physical exam are not advisable in the patient with ongoing pain and ECG changes; **focus on a targeted history and rapid ECG interpretation** (AHA guidelines recommend **within 10 mins of arrival**) [9]. If a patient's description of symptoms and ECG tracing are supportive of AMI, seek immediate assessment for revascularization [percutaneous transluminal coronary angioplasty (PTCA), thrombolytics].

Differential Diagnosis

Several other disease entities may mimic AMI and present with chest discomfort and ECG changes; patients need careful assessment with history, physical exam, and, in some cases, diagnostic tests.

Pericarditis
Chest pain associated with acute pericarditis is typically worse with recumbency and relieved by sitting upright and leaning forward. The ECG shows diffuse ST-segment elevation, also with possible PR segment depression and peaked T waves. Acute pericarditis may accompany AMI, and the initial approach must rule out AMI. A stat echocardiogram can be helpful in this regard, not for assessment of pericardial effusion but to assess focal wall motion abnormalities that would accompany AMI. See Chap. 16, Disease of the Pericardium, for an example of an acute pericarditis ECG and management of this condition.

Aortic Dissection
The pain of acute aortic dissection is typically a tearing, severe pain that radiates into the back. Suspect this condition in patients with this type of pain and a widened mediastinum on chest x-ray, and confirm the diagnosis with TEE, chest CT or MRI, or aortography. Dissections involving the ascending aorta may involve the coronary ostia [particularly the right coronary artery (RCA)], thereby producing associated compromised coronary blood flow and infarction. See Chap. 5, Cardiovascular Emergencies, and Chap. 20, Diseases of the Aorta, for workup and management discussions.

Pulmonary Embolism
Pulmonary embolism (PE) is very difficult to differentiate from AMI by history and physical exam alone. The onset of chest pain in PE usually involves shortness of breath.

TABLE 8-1. KILLIP CLASSIFICATION IN ACUTE MI

Class	Definition	Mortality (%)
I	No congestive heart failure signs	6
II	+ S_3 and/or basilar rales	17
III	Pulmonary edema	30–40
IV	Cardiogenic shock	60–80

From Killip T 3rd, Kimball JT. Treatment of myocardial infarction in a coronary care unit. A two-year experience with 250 patients. *Am J Cardiol* 1967;20:457.

A history of conditions that predispose to PE, such as recent surgery, immobilization, malignancy, and hypercoagulable states, helps suggest this diagnosis. The diagnostic evaluation may include $\dot{V}/\dot{Q}$ nuclear scanning, spiral CT, and pulmonary arteriogram. See Chap. 18, Pulmonary Hypertension, Right-Heart Failure, and Pulmonary Embolism, for the workup and management discussions.

PRESENTATION

Physical Exam

As with ACS, the initial physical exam is typically not helpful in determining the actual presence of AMI vs other causes of chest discomfort; however, it can be an important prognostic determinant of patient survival. The goals of the exam are determining patients' hemodynamic stability; assessing possible cardiogenic pulmonary edema; rapidly detecting mechanical complications of MI, such as **papillary muscle dysfunction, free-wall rupture,** and **ventricular septal defect (VSD);** and assessing possible other etiologies of acute chest discomfort. The **Killip classification** system and **TIMI risk score** [10] (Tables 8-1 and 8-2) are helpful in using physical exam findings to assess a patient's 30-day mortality.

TABLE 8-2. TIMI RISK SCORE FOR ST-ELEVATION MI

Risk factor (weight)	Risk score/30-day mortality (%)
Age 65–74 yrs (2 points)	0 (0.8)
Age ≥ 75 yrs (3 points)	1 (1.6)
Diabetes mellitus/HTN or angina (1 point)	2 (2.2)
Systolic BP <100 (3 points)	3 (4.4)
Heart rate >100 (2 points)	4 (7.3)
Killip classification II–IV (2 points)	5 (12.4)
Weight <67 kg (1 point)	6 (16.1)
Anterior STE or LBBB (1 point)	7 (23.4)
Time to Rx >4 hrs (1 point)	8 (26.8)
Risk score = total points (0–14)	>8 (35.9)

LBBB, left bundle-branch block; STE, ST-segment elevations.
From Morrow DA, Antman EM, Charlesworth A, et al. TIMI risk score for ST-elevation myocardial infarction: a convenient, bedside, clinical score for risk assessment at presentation. *Circulation* 2000;102:2031–2037, with permission.

MANAGEMENT

Diagnostic Workup

The diagnosis of AMI requires the presence of ≥ 2 of the following three criteria:

1. History of prolonged chest discomfort or anginal equivalent
2. ECG changes consistent with ischemia or infarction
3. Elevated cardiac enzymes

Electrocardiogram

- Suspicion of an AMI is raised by the following **injury patterns:**
- ≥ 1 mm (0.1 mV) of ST-segment elevation in ≥ two contiguous leads. The distribution of ST-segment elevation helps determine the occluded anatomy and prognosis, and it can alert the physician to potential complications of MI (Fig. 8-1). The leads that interrogate the reciprocal walls often show "reciprocal depression." Elevation in leads

   I, aVL suggest "high lateral wall" involvement, commonly caused by occlusion of a diagonal branch of the left anterior descending (LAD) or proximal left circumflex (LCx) coronary artery

   II, III, aVF suggest inferior involvement (RCA or LCx, if left dominant)

   V$_2$–V$_3$ suggest septal involvement (occlusion of LAD proximal to septal perforator branches)

   V$_2$–V$_4$: anterior wall involvement (LAD)

   V$_5$–V$_6$: lateral wall involvement (LCx)

- A **posterior MI** is suggested by **ST depression** in leads V$_1$–V$_3$, which interrogate the anteroseptum. The "reverse-mirror test" is useful to demonstrate this: The **ST depressions are actually ST elevations of the posterior wall,** and the increasing size of the R waves in these leads should be of concern, as they are actually posterior Q waves. ST-elevation in the inferior leads II, III, and aVF and/or the lateral leads V$_5$–V$_6$ often accompanies these changes in the setting of a posterior MI (inferoposterior and posterolateral MIs involving the RCA or obtuse marginal branch of the LCx) (Fig. 8-2). These changes help distinguish ST depressions in V$_1$–V$_3$ from the true ST depressions of anteroseptal ischemia, which is treated as an ACS (see Chap. 7, Acute Coronary Syndromes: Unstable Angina and Non–ST-Segment Elevation Myocardial Infarction).
- An **RV infarction** is suggested by ST elevation in leads V$_3$R and V$_4$R and occasionally V$_1$. ST elevations in the inferior leads should always prompt you to perform a right-sided ECG to assess for RV involvement with an inferior MI. Proximal RCA lesions may involve the RV, as the RV marginal branches from the RCA supply the RV. The RV is also perfused directly intracavitarily, because it is thin walled (Fig. 8-3). Although the principle of revascularization of the RV infarct is the same for other STEMIs, other aspects of treatment are unique (see Post–Acute Myocardial Infarction Complications).

With regard to ST elevation, it is critical to remember the difference between the acute injury pattern of MI and ST elevation in pericarditis. Chronologically, the ST segments normalize before T wave inversion in acute pericarditis, whereas the T waves invert before ST normalization in MI. Compare Figs. 8-1 (p. 74) and 16-1 (p. 202) for a clear demonstration.

Over 6–12 hrs, elevated ST segments resulting from occlusion of a coronary artery usually evolve to Q waves in the absence of spontaneous, medical, or mechanical reperfusion. Typically, this occurs in the presence of a transmural infarct, with loss of concomitant loss of R wave voltage, as the replacement of cardiac muscle with inflammatory and, ultimately, scar tissue ensues.

- Hyperacute T waves, either pointed tall or deeply inverted, are occasionally evident in the setting of severe acute ischemia and are usually transient. Other etiologies, such as electrolyte abnormalities and CNS disturbances, must be considered. See Fig. 1-1 (p. 5) for an example.

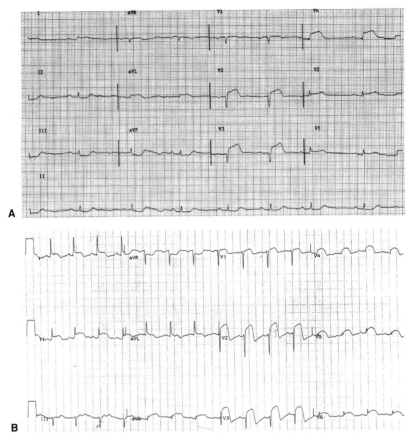

FIG. 8-1. A: Acute anterior injury pattern with reciprocal inferior depressions occurring in a patient with a totally occluded left anterior descending artery (LAD). **B:** Acute injury pattern with anterior, septal, lateral, and inferior wall involvement caused by left main or proximal LAD occlusion. Note the inferior ST elevations. In this patient, the LAD may be termed *wrap-around*, because it supplies a significant portion of the inferior wall after traversing the cardiac apex. Note that the T waves have begun to invert in the precordial leads, firmly distinguishing this pattern from that of acute pericarditis. Furthermore, Q waves are beginning to develop, indicating that this ECG was taken at least several hours into the clinical event.

- The finding of **new left bundle-branch block (LBBB)** in the setting of acute chest symptoms is managed similarly to ST elevation and is suggestive of occlusion of the proximal LAD.
- In the setting of an old LBBB or a paced rhythm, an acute injury pattern can be determined by the following specific criteria:
  - ST elevation >5 mm in right precordial leads (V_1–V_3) (ST elevation is discordant with QRS)
  - ST depression/T-wave inversion in V_1–V_3 (normally the ST is slightly elevated in these leads with an LBBB or paced rhythm)
  - ST elevation >1 mm that is concordant with QRS (leads V_4–V_6, where normally the ST is slightly depressed in leads with a large R wave with an LBBB or paced rhythm)

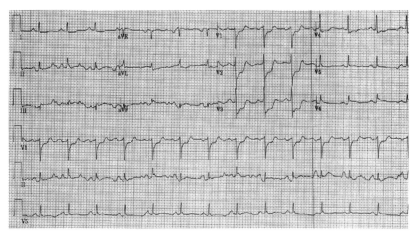

FIG. 8-2. Inferoposterolateral MI caused by occlusion of a large obtuse marginal branch in a left-dominant coronary system. Subtle ST elevation in the inferior leads is present, along with pronounced ST depression in leads V_1–V_4 and elevation in V_6.

Lab Data

- **Troponin:** The detection of elevated troponin I or T is a highly sensitive and specific marker for even minimal myocardial damage; however, it has limited efficacy in the early management of AMI due to significant lag time until abnormal levels are reached. Elevation of these enzymes requires 4–6 hrs to occur, peaks in 24–48 hrs, and slowly returns to normal in 7–10 days.
- **Creatine kinase:** As with troponins, detection of elevated CK-MB fraction is associated with a lag time of 4–6 hrs before elevation, thereby limiting its usefulness early on. CK-MB, however, differs from troponins by faster clearance, achieving normal levels approximately 72 hrs after an infarction. This can help determine the timing of a cardiac event and determine the severity. This assay is also very useful for postinfarct ischemia, because a fall and subsequent rise suggest reinfarction; in the acute setting, troponin I does not fall rapidly enough for this assessment.
- **Myoglobin:** Levels of myoglobin elevate more quickly than other enzymes—typically within 1–4 hrs. The specificity of this enzyme is less than that of troponins.

Other Diagnostic Options

Although not considered among the criteria for AMI diagnosis, echocardiography may be helpful when the diagnosis is in doubt. Segmental wall motion abnormalities suggest myocardial ischemia or MI (assuming there was no baseline wall motion abnormality) and can help localize the territory at risk. Another alternative diagnostic strategy in a patient with ongoing chest symptoms is nuclear imaging while a patient is experiencing symptoms [called a *Pain-Mibi study,* because sestamibi is injected as a tracer; see Chap. 22, Imaging and Diagnostic Testing Modalities (Nuclear Imaging, Echocardiography, and Cardiac Catheterization)]. An area of decreased perfusion on these images while the patient is resting and experiencing symptoms is supportive of cardiac ischemia or infarction.

Treatment

Primary goals in the management of AMI are rapid diagnosis, adequate pain relief, assessment and implementation of possible reperfusion strategies, administration of antithrombotic and antiplatelet therapy, use of proper adjunctive medications, and surveillance for complications of AMI. The ACC/AHA have outlined guidelines for the management of AMI that provide consensus recommendations according to the strength of evidence of various management practices (see the Preface) [9].

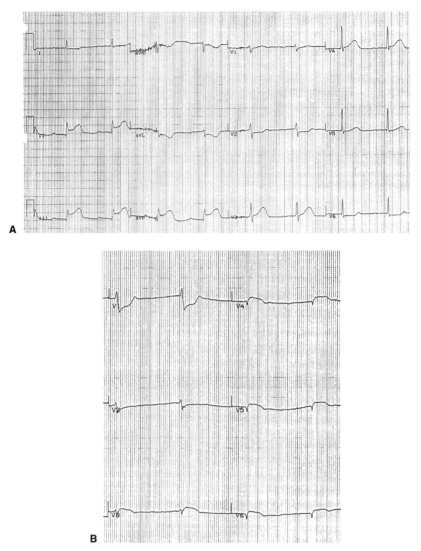

FIG. 8-3. Inferior MI with right ventricular infarction. **A:** Standard leads showing pronounced ST elevation inferiorly. **B:** Right-sided precordial leads show ST elevation in V_3R and V_4R corresponding to a right ventricular infarction.

Rapid Recognition
ERs should have a protocol that yields a targeted physical exam and 12-lead ECG within 10 mins of arrival, with a goal of door-to-needle time of <30 mins (class I).

Reperfusion
Patients <75 yrs who present with ST elevation in two contiguous leads (or LBBB not known to be old) within 12 hrs of the onset of the pain that prompted medical attention should be considered for reperfusion therapy (class I). The benefits of reperfusion are

most recognized in patients treated earliest and who are at greatest risk. Patients who present with MI symptoms >12 hrs and <24 hrs after pain onset should still be considered for reperfusion (class IIb), particularly in the setting of continued ST elevation, persistent symptoms, recurrent ischemia, LV dysfunction, widespread ECG changes, or prior MI, PTCA, or coronary artery bypass grafting (CABG). The optimal reperfusion strategy remains somewhat controversial, and management varies depending on various centers and resources. Thrombolytic therapy has advantages of faster administration and wider availability. The advantage of percutaneous coronary intervention (PCI) is increased early efficacy of opening occluded arteries and an improved survival. In a systematic review of ten randomized controlled trials [11], primary PTCA vs primary thrombolysis reduced mortality at 30 days after intervention, (4.4% in PTCA vs 6.5% in thrombolysis; absolute risk reduction, 2.1%; odds ratio; 0.66, 95% confidence interval, 0.46 to 0.94; number needed to treat, 48). The advantage of PTCA is somewhat clearer in regard to reducing risk of stroke, particularly for hemorrhagic strokes, with consistently lower rates in almost all trials. In a large trial, the collective rate of hemorrhagic stroke was 1.1% [12]. Given the likely benefit over thrombolytics and the established reduction in stroke, in larger centers with the capacity for PTCA and adequate experience, **PTCA with stenting is the reperfusion method of choice.** In centers without PTCA capabilities, data support transfer to PTCA facilities for patients with contraindications to thrombolytic therapy (class IIa). It is important to note that thrombolytic administration to patients presenting >24 hrs after symptom onset is a class III indication.

In patients in **cardiogenic shock,** the SHOCK trial demonstrated a significant reduction in 6-mo mortality in patients randomized to PTCA over thrombolytic therapy [13], and PTCA should be considered in patients in whom revascularization can be performed within 18 hrs of onset of shock (class I). Intraaortic balloon pump (IABP) insertion may be necessary as well.

Advances in mechanical and pharmacologic therapy for AMI have been rapid, and new interventions, such as intracoronary stenting, new fibrin-specific thrombolytics, and new antithrombotic and antiplatelet agents, have required new considerations in the optimal treatment of AMI. Many older trials used as a basis for therapy are now being rethought, and studies that include newer interventions are ongoing, continuing to help the management of AMI evolve.

The key consideration in the choice of reperfusion strategy in AMI is that the intervention should not be delayed by indecision on method. The approach to reperfusion therapy was recently framed as a pragmatic question by another author: Ask at the time of presentation, "At this time of day at this hospital, how can I most safely and quickly open this patient's artery with the best flow and keep the artery open?"[4].

Thrombolysis

The benefits of early (<12 hrs) thrombolytic therapy are well established in the medical literature, with pooled data from the FTT Collaborative Group displaying an 18% relative reduction in mortality [14]. The various thrombolytic agents have similar efficacy and vary predominantly by rate of administration. Large trials have failed to show any mortality benefit between different agents [15,16]. A practical note: Thrombolytics have not been shown to be successful in vein grafts; thus, **if a patient post-CABG presents with an AMI, the preferred mode of reperfusion is percutaneous coronary intervention (PCI).**

Agents
NON–FIBRIN SPECIFIC
Streptokinase (SK).   SK is administered as an IV infusion of 1.5 million U over 60 mins; patients previously exposed to SK should not receive further exposure due to development of antibodies. Allergic reactions are not uncommon. Benefits include low cost and lower incidence of intracranial hemorrhage; benefits were first shown in the initial GISSI-1 trial [17]. Currently, SK is rarely used.
FIBRIN SPECIFIC
Tissue Plasminogen Activator (tPA, alteplase).   The accelerated protocol is an IV bolus of 15 mg, followed by 0.75 mg/kg infusion over 30 mins, then 0.5 mg/kg over 60 mins. The GUSTO-1 trial [18] showed a 15% reduced 30-day mortality in

patients treated with tPA vs SK. However, tPA is considerably more expensive than SK and has a slightly higher risk of intracranial hemorrhage.

Reteplase (Retavase).   Reteplase is given as an IV bolus of 10 U over 2 mins, followed by a repeat bolus after 30 mins. The INJECT trial [19] showed comparable efficacy and safety as SK and as tPA in the GUSTO III trial [20], with easier bolus dosing due to longer half-life.

Tenecteplase (TNKase).   Tenecteplase is administered as a single IV bolus of 0.5 mg/kg. Advantages include improved fibrin specificity and high resistance to plasminogen activator inhibitor-1 (PAI-1). Initial reports from TIMI 10B show tenecteplase had similar rates to tPA of TIMI 3 flow and bleeding complications.

Contraindications
Absolute contraindications include previous hemorrhagic stroke, known intracranial neoplasm, active internal bleeding, and suspected aortic dissection. Multiple relative contraindications exist (Table 8-3).

Bleeding Risk
The overall risk of intracerebral hemorrhage is 0.7%, and overall, strokes occurred in 1.4%. Predictive factors for stroke and intracranial hemorrhage included age $\geq$ 65 yrs, weight <70 kg, HTN on admission, and use of tPA rather than other agents [21]. Major bleeding was increased by thrombolytic therapy.

After **successful** thrombolysis **(i.e., resolution of chest pain and ≥50% reduction in magnitude of ST elevations within 90 mins of administration),** there is no ACC/AHA guideline for cardiac catheterization to assess the anatomy of the affected artery or other arteries; routine coronary angiography in the absence of persistent ischemia or hemodynamic compromise is in fact a **class III indication.** In this setting, it is a class I indication to perform a submaximal (at 4–6 days) or symptom-limited (at 10–14 days) stress test after the event. Stress testing is contraindicated within 72 hrs of an AMI. The practice of attending cardiologists varies extremely on this issue. For patients with AMI who did not undergo primary angioplasty, class I indications for coronary angiogram include recurrent angina, congestive heart failure (CHF), arrhythmias, and a positive submaximal stress test.

TABLE 8-3. CONTRAINDICATIONS FOR USE OF THROMBOLYTIC AGENTS IN ACUTE MI

Absolute contraindications

　　Previous hemorrhagic stroke at any time; any other cerebrovascular events within 1 yr

　　Known intracranial neoplasm

　　Active internal bleeding (not including menses)

　　Suspected aortic dissection

Relative contraindications

　　Severe, uncontrolled HTN (BP >180/110 mm Hg)

　　History of cerebrovascular accident or known intracerebral pathologic condition not covered in contraindications

　　Current use of anticoagulants in therapeutic doses (INR >2); known bleeding diatheses

　　Recent trauma (within 2–4 wks), prolonged CPR (>10 mins), or major surgery (within 3 wks)

　　Noncompressible vascular punctures

　　Recent internal bleeding (within 2–4 wks)

　　Pregnancy

　　Active peptic ulcer disease

　　For streptokinase or anistreplase: prior exposure to either agent or prior allergic reaction

Direct Percutaneous Coronary Intervention

PCI is a suitable alternative to thrombolytic therapy (class I indication) if performed in a timely fashion by individuals skilled in the procedure (>75 PCIs/yr) and in high-volume centers (>200 PCIs/yr). Also consider PCI in patients who present with cardiogenic shock (class I) and in patients with thrombolytic contraindications (class IIa.) On identification of the culprit lesion, consider intervention if the lesion is amenable to angioplasty. If significant left-main disease or three-vessel disease is found, consider emergent CABG. The Stent-PAMI trial examined stenting (compared to PTCA alone) of culprit lesions in the setting of AMI [22] and found it reduces the combined end point of death, reinfarction, disabling stroke, and target-vessel revascularization significantly at 6 mos. The CADIL-LAC trial [23], among others, showed benefit in 6-mo major adverse cardiac events, comparing stenting over PTCA alone, primarily due to a reduced rate of need for target vessel revascularization. Percutaneous intervention on the non–infarct-related artery in the setting of an AMI is a class III indication. Complications of PTCA and stent implantation are discussed in Chap. 6, Stable Angina.

Rescue Percutaneous Transluminal Coronary Angioplasty

Thrombolytic therapy does not achieve coronary artery patency in 15–50% of patients [24]. Rescue percutaneous intervention is appropriate for patients who have received thrombolytic therapy but have ongoing symptoms and persistent ST elevation (>50% of original degree of elevation) 90 mins after administration. Patients with cardiogenic shock, CHF, refractory arrhythmias, and particularly patients with large anterior MIs also should potentially be assessed for mechanical reperfusion. Accelerated idioventricular rhythm (see Chap. 15, Tachyarrhythmias, Sudden Cardiac Death, and Implantable Cardioverter-Defibrillators, for an example) is considered a fairly specific indicator of reperfusion; however, most other arrhythmias are not considered reliable. CABG is indicated in the setting of failed PTCA in patients with ongoing signs and symptoms of ischemia or in similar patients whose coronary anatomy is not suitable for PCI.

Adjunctive Measures

During and after reperfusion, patients presenting with an AMI should be monitored in a cardiac ICU.

- **ASA (class I):** Administer a 325-mg dose of crushed ASA immediately to patients suspected of experiencing AMI. The only contraindication is hypersensitivity. ASA administration provided a decrease in vascular mortality by 23% and nonfatal infarct by 49% in the ISIS-2 study [25].
- **IV heparin:** The recommended dosing of heparin (class IIa) is a bolus of 60 U/kg (maximum 5000 U), followed by an infusion of 14 U/kg/hr (maximum, 1000 U/hr). Titrate the infusion rate to maintain an aPTT of 50–70 secs. Although early studies showed no mortality benefit to IV heparin, recent metaanalyses have suggested a mortality benefit. The use of heparin with SK has not been shown to provide any increased survival and had an increased rate of bleeding complications. Therefore, patients treated with SK are recommended not to receive heparin until 6 hrs post-SK infusion (class III indication to give heparin in this setting) and are not recommended to receive a bolused dose. With newer-generation thrombolytics, heparin is coadministered.
- **Glycoprotein IIb/IIIa inhibitors**
  - **In the setting of thrombolytic therapy:** Recent trials have been conducted that have evaluated the use of reduced-dose thrombolytic medications with abciximab in reduction of ischemic complications from AMI. The GUSTO V trial [26] compared full-dose reteplase with half-dose reteplase and abciximab. Researchers found similar mortality with a reduction in ischemic complications; however, an increased rate of nonintracranial bleeding was noted in the latter group. The ASSENT-3 trial [27] likewise showed half-dose tenecteplase with abciximab reduced ischemic complications, with a mild increase in bleeding episodes. Overall, the role of GPIIb/IIIa antagonists pre-PCI in the setting of thrombolytics is still evolving.
  - **In the setting of PTCA/stent:** The ADMIRAL trial [28] compared abciximab and stenting with placebo and stenting. The results showed a significant reduction in the composite end point of death, reinfarction, or urgent revascularization at 30 days

and 6 mos for the abciximab/stent group. Also notable was an improved patency rate before stenting and success rate of stenting in the abciximab/stent group.

- **Low-molecular-weight heparins (LMWH):** LMWH are an attractive antithrombotic alternative to heparin due to more predictable kinetics, easier administration, and no monitoring requirement. One arm of the ASSENT-3 trial [27] showed enoxaparin (Lovenox) with full-dose tenecteplase (TNKase) had significantly improved composite end point of mortality, in-hospital reinfarction, and in-hospital refractory ischemia with similar safety profile. In this study, patients received a 1-mg/kg SC dose of enoxaparin, followed by 30-mg IV bolus. The SC dose was then repeated q12h to hospital discharge (maximum, 7 days). LMWH is used by some operators poststent implantation. In general, the role of LMWH in acute STEMI is still developing.

- **Direct thrombin inhibitors:** Direct thrombin inhibitors include hirudin (Refludan), lepirudin (Refludan), argatroban, and bivalirudin (Angiomax). They act to directly inhibit the actions of thrombin and have several potential advantages over other antithrombotic regimens, including ability to inhibit both clot-bound and circulating thrombin, more predictable plasma levels, and absence of immune thrombocytopenia. Despite these advantages, early studies have failed to show significant mortality reduction. The HERO-2 trial is examining the efficacy of bivalirudin administered before SK, whereas prior studies examined thrombin inhibitors given after thrombolytics. At present, use of these agents is reserved primarily for patients who have previously suffered from heparin-induced thrombocytopenia and other operator- and patient-dependent settings.

- **Beta blockers (class I):** Beta blockers help reduce myocardial O_2 demand and potentially reduce infarct size; they afford a 15% relative reduction in major adverse cardiac events. Multiple studies have proved that beta blockade reduces mortality, recurrent ischemia, and arrhythmias. Contraindications include bradycardia (heart rate <55 bpm), hypotension (systolic BP <90 mm Hg), decompensated CHF, second- or third-degree AV block, and severe bronchospastic disease. Typical regimens include metoprolol, 5 mg IV q5min, three × as tolerated, titrated up to oral metoprolol (Lopressor), up to 50 mg q6h as BP and heart rate permit.

- **ACE inhibitors:** ACE inhibitors' benefits include a favorable impact on ventricular remodeling, improved hemodynamics, and prevention of heart failure. Debate over empiric ACE-inhibitor therapy for all AMI continues, but the evidence clearly shows that patients with ejection fraction <40% (class I), large anterior AMIs (class I), and prior MIs (class IIa) derive the most benefit from prompt ACE-inhibitor therapy. The SAVE, AIRE, and TRACE trials have demonstrated clear benefits in these groups. Contraindications include hypotension, acute renal failure, bilateral renal artery stenosis, and hyperkalemia. Multiple agents and regimens exist; captopril (Capoten), 6.25 mg PO tid/qid, titrated to maximal tolerated dose, has a short plasma half-life and, therefore, allows easier dose titration.

- **NTG:** Actions of NTG include venodilation and coronary artery dilation. Sublingual NTG is a first-line agent for relief of angina and should be given unless the patient has hypotension, marked sinus tachycardia, or sinus bradycardia or is suspected of having an RV infarct. Sublingual NTG may be given q5mins for three doses if BP permits. In patients who have responded to sublingual NTG, an infusion of IV NTG can be started at 10 μg/min and titrated to relieve symptoms with close monitoring of heart rate and BP. Nitrates are contraindicated in patients with history of severe AS or HCM. Patients who have taken sildenafil (Viagra) during the previous 24 hrs should not be given NTG due to the potential for severe hypotension. Effect of NTG on survival has not been confirmed by large, randomized trials; therefore, NTG is thought to be beneficial in patients with CHF, large anterior infarction, persistent ischemia, or HTN. Continued use >48 hrs after AMI is warranted for recurrent angina or persistent pulmonary congestion.

- **O_2:** O_2 administration provides increased O_2 supply to ischemic myocytes. The benefit of O_2 is greatest in patients with arterial O_2 desaturation, overt pulmonary congestion, and routinely during the first 2–3 hrs of AMI.

- **Morphine:** Morphine acts to provide analgesia for ischemic cardiac pain, produces a favorable hemodynamic effect, and reduces myocardial O_2 consumption. When pain is refractory to NTG and beta blockers, morphine can be given as 2–4 mg IV doses and repeated q10mins until pain is relieved or hypotension occurs.

- **Magnesium:** Studies have shown conflicting data regarding administration of empiric magnesium and mortality benefit. Use of magnesium presently is a class IIa indication when plasma magnesium level is documented to be low or with torsades de pointes (see Chap. 15, Tachyarrhythmias, Sudden Cardiac Death, and Implantable Cardioverter-Defibrillators, for an example).
- **Blood transfusion:** A retrospective cohort study of elderly patients with AMI showed a 30-day mortality benefit in patients with admission Hct of <33% if they were transfused [29].

Post–Acute Myocardial Infarction Complications
(See Chap. 5, Cardiovascular Emergencies, for additional details.)

- **Cardiogenic shock:** Cardiogenic shock typically occurs within the first 48 hrs. It can occur in 5–7% of AMIs, particularly large anterior MIs, and is usually due to myocardial ischemia; treatment consists of IABP, inotropes, pressors, Swan-Ganz catheter to optimize primary capillary wedge pressure (PCWP) between 18–20 mm Hg, and revascularization, if possible.
- **Free-wall rupture:** Free-wall rupture occurs 2–6 days after MI, more commonly in patients without prior angina or MI and with large infarcts by enzyme criteria. It may present as hypotension, cardiac tamponade, and pulseless electrical activity. Mortality is very high, and management consists of volume resuscitation, inotropes, pericardiocentesis, and surgical repair.
- **Pseudoaneurysm:** A contained rupture sealed by thrombus and pericardium can occur as a complication of an anteroapical MI. It is clinically silent but may be characterized by a to-and-from murmur. The thrombus present may yield systemic emboli. A hemodynamically significant pericardial effusion may result. Diagnosis is by echocardiography, and it is often found incidentally. Treatment is surgical in nearly all cases.
- **Ventricular septal defect:** VSD typically occurs 2–5 days after AMI and is more common in anterior MIs. It presents with new harsh holosystolic murmur with or without hemodynamic compromise, and diagnosis depends on echocardiography with Doppler and/or Swan-Ganz catheterization. Management involves IABP, inotropes, vasodilators, and surgical vs catheter-based closure.
- **Papillary muscle rupture:** Papillary muscle rupture usually occurs 2–7 days after MI and involves the posteromedial papillary muscle. It is most commonly due to inferior MI and presents with new holosystolic murmur (although this may not be present), cardiogenic shock, and pulmonary edema. Diagnosis can be made by echocardiography or Swan-Ganz catheter waveforms with prominent v waves; treatment involves afterload reduction with IABP or vasodilators, revascularization, and surgical repair.
- **Right ventricular infarct:** RV infarct occurs in the setting of inferior MI and is characterized by a triad of hypotension, elevated jugular venous pressure with Kussmaul's sign, and clear lung fields. It is diagnosed by right-sided ECG with ST elevation in V_3R and V_4R or by witnessed RV wall motion abnormality on echocardiography. Treatment includes volume loading to PCWP of 18–20 mm Hg, avoiding nitrates, and low-dose dobutamine if necessitated by hypotension.
- **Arrhythmias:** Arrhythmias occur very commonly after AMI; management of types of rhythm disturbance is addressed in other chapters. Accelerated idioventricular rhythm should not be treated unless it is causing hemodynamic disturbance. Prophylactic antiarrhythmic infusion after AMI to suppress VT/VF has not been shown to improve mortality and, therefore, is not given routinely.
  - **Bradycardias** may warrant a temporary transvenous pacer if associated with significant AV block [see Chap. 14, Bradycardia and Permanent Pacemakers, and Chap. 24, Procedures in Cardiovascular Critical Care (Aortic Balloon Pump, Swan-Ganz Catheterization, and Temporary Transvenous Pacemaker)].
  - AV block in association with an **inferior MI** usually portends a good prognosis, as the mechanism is ischemia of the AV node (the AV nodal branch derives from the RCA) and a compensatory Bezold-Jarisch reflex, which stimulates vagal tone.
  - AV block in association with an **anterior MI** usually portends a poor prognosis (permanent pacer likely required), as the mechanism is infarction of part of the distal

TABLE 8-4. FORRESTER CLASSIFICATION SYSTEM FOR ACUTE MI

Class	Cardiac index (L/min/m²)	PCWP (mm Hg)	Mortality (%)
I	>2.2	<18	3
II	>2.2	>18	9
III	<2.2	<18	23
IV	<2.2	>18	51

From Forrester JS, Diamond G, Chatterjee K, et al. Medical therapy of acute myocardial infarction by application of hemodynamic subsets (first of two parts). *N Engl J Med* 1976;295:1356.

conduction system. Close attention to electrolyte abnormalities and acid/base balance are essential.

- **Post–myocardial infarction pericarditis:** Post-MI pericarditis occurs 1–4 days after MI and may cause recurrent chest discomfort and widespread ST elevation. PR depression may occur on ECGs but is uncommon; pericardial rub may be found on exam. Treatment consists of high-dose ASA or NSAIDs. Steer clear of heparin to avoid hemorrhagic transformation.
- **Dressler syndrome:** Dressler syndrome presents 2–10 wks after MI with fever, malaise, and pleuritic chest discomfort. Often, patients have an elevated ESR, and echocardiography may demonstrate pericardial effusion. It is managed with high-dose ASA or NSAIDS.
- **Left ventricular thrombus:** LV thrombus may occur with large anteroapical MIs that produce akinetic or dyskinetic segments on echocardiogram or left ventriculogram. Treatment consists of anticoagulation with warfarin for 3–6 mos.
- **Ventricular aneurysm:** Ventricular aneurysm may occur acutely after an MI and cause significant hemodynamic compromise or develop more insidiously up to 6 wks after an MI. Persistent ST elevation after AMI is suggestive but not diagnostic of an aneurysm; echocardiography establishes the diagnosis and provides information regarding LV function and presence of thrombus. Treatment involves afterload reduction, preferably with ACE inhibitor to help reduce LV remodeling with warfarin; anticoagulation; and potentially surgical resection in selected cases.

Prognosis
Several systems are available to help determine prognosis after AMI:

- **Killip classification** relies on simple bedside physical exam findings of S_3, pulmonary congestion, and cardiogenic shock (see Table 8-1).
- **Forrester classification** relies on hemodynamic monitoring of cardiac index and PCWP (Table 8-4).
- **TIMI risk score** [10] is the most recent prognostic system devised and combines simple historical and exam findings assessed in patients with STEMI who were treated with thrombolytic therapy. Mean 30-day mortality was 6.7%. Note that this is a different risk score than that compiled for ACS [contrast Tables 8-2 (p. 72) and 7-1 (p. 61)].

Patients should be aggressively risk stratified secondarily to help prevent recurrent events. See Chap. 9, Primary and Secondary Risk Factor Stratification and Management, for management of key risk factors and cardiac rehabilitation.

ACKNOWLEDGMENT

The editor thanks Morton R. Rinder and Jane Chen for providing the ECGs for this chapter.

KEY POINTS TO REMEMBER

• Acute STEMI (AMI) most commonly occurs when a thin atheromatous plaque in a coronary artery ruptures, triggering platelet aggregation and thrombus formation. An occlusion can result, leading to ischemic injury of the supplied myocardium.
• After rapid recognition, optimal therapy depends on rapid revascularization, either via thrombolytics or PCI.
• Do not forget the importance of ASA and beta blockers, as well as nitrates for angina suppression **early** in the presentation.
• If it can be expeditiously delivered in an experienced setting, PCI with stent implantation yields a higher patency rate and improved long-term outcomes than thrombolysis. However, if this would impose too long a delay (>1 hr), administer a thrombolytic if there are no contraindications.
• Monitor patients who suffer an AMI in a cardiac ICU to observe for early complications, such as arrhythmias or cardiogenic shock. Other complications, including VSD, papillary muscle rupture, perforation, and pseudoaneurysm formation, are more likely to occur in subsequent days.
• RV infarct is managed similarly to other infarcts with regard to reperfusion, but management of hemodynamics is quite distinct. Avoidance of nitrates and fluid resuscitation are the mainstays of therapy. Be suspicious of an RV infarct in any patient with inferior ST elevations, particularly if he or she becomes hypotensive in response to NTG.
• Posterior MI is evidenced by ST **depression** in leads V_1–V_3. Suspect this, as opposed to anteroseptal ischemia, particularly if there are inferior ST elevations.

REFERENCES

1. American Heart Association. *2001 Heart and stroke statistical update*. http://www.americanheart.org
2. Antman EM, Braunwald E. Acute myocardial infarction. In: Braunwald E, ed. *Heart disease: a textbook of cardiovascular medicine*. Philadelphia: WB Saunders, 1997.
3. Ross R. Atherosclerosis: an inflammatory disease. *N Engl J Med* 1999;340(2):115–126.
4. Gibson CM. Primary angioplasty compared with thrombolysis: new issues in the era of glycoprotein IIb/IIIa inhibition and intracoronary stenting. *Ann Intern Med* 1999;130:841–847.
5. Cannon CP, Braunwald E, McCabe CH, et al. The Thrombolysis in Myocardial Infarction (TIMI) trials: the first decade. The TIMI Investigators. *J Interv Cardiol* 1995;8:117–135.
6. Lincoff AM, Topol EJ, Califf RM, et al. Significance of a coronary artery with thrombolysis in myocardial infarction grade 2 flow "patency" (outcome in the Thrombolysis and Angioplasty in Myocardial Infarction trials). *Am J Cardiol* 1995;75:871–876.
7. The GUSTO Angiographic Investigators. The comparative effects of tissue plasminogen activator, streptokinase, or both on coronary artery patency, ventricular function and survival after acute myocardial infarction. *N Engl J Med* 1993;329:1615–1622.
8. Lenderink T, Simoons ML, Van Es GA, et al. Benefits of thrombolytic therapy is sustained throughout five years and is related to TIMI perfusion grade 3 but not grade 2 flow at discharge. *Circulation* 1995;92:1110.
9. ACC/AHA Guidelines for the management of patients with acute myocardial infarction: executive summary and recommendations. *Circulation* 1999;100:1016–1030.
10. Morrow DA, Antman EM, Charlesworth A, et al. TIMI risk score for ST-elevation myocardial infarction: a convenient, bedside, clinical score for risk assessment at presentation. *Circulation* 2000;102:2031–2037.
11. Weaver WD, Simes RJ, Betriu A, et al. Comparison of primary coronary angioplasty and intravenous thrombolytic therapy for acute myocardial infarction: a quantitative review. *JAMA* 1997;278:2093–2098.

12. The GUSTO IIb Angioplasty Substudy Investigators. A clinical trial comparing primary coronary angioplasty with tissue plasminogen activator for acute myocardial infarction. *N Engl J Med* 1997;336:1621–1628.
13. Hochman JS, Sleeper LA, Webb JG, et al. Early revascularization in acute myocardial infarction complicated by cardiogenic shock. SHOCK Investigators. Should we emergently revascularize occluded coronaries for cardiogenic shock. *N Engl J Med* 1999;341:625–634.
14. Thrombolytic Therapy Trialists' (FTT) Collaborative Group. Indications for thrombolytic therapy in suspected acute myocardial infarction: collaborative overview of early mortality and major morbidity results from all randomised trials of more than 1000 patients. *Lancet* 1994;343:311–322.
15. The International Study Group. In-hospital mortality and clinical course of 20,891 patients with suspected acute myocardial infarction randomised between alteplase and streptokinase with or without heparin. *Lancet* 1990;2:71.
16. Third International Study of Infarct Survival (ISIS-3) Collaborative Group. ISIS-3: a randomized trial of streptokinase vs tissue plasminogen activator vs anistreplase and of aspirin plus heparin vs aspirin alone among 41,299 cases of suspected acute myocardial infarction. *Lancet* 1992;339:753.
17. Gruppo Italiano Per Lo Studio Della Streptochinasi Nell'Infarct Miocardico (GISSI). Effectiveness of intravenous thrombolytic treatment in acute myocardial infarction. *Lancet* 1987;2:871–874.
18. Global Utilization of Streptokinase and Tissue Plasminogen Activator for Occluded Coronary Arteries (GUSTO) Investigators. An international randomized trial comparing four thrombolytic strategies for acute myocardial infarction. *N Engl J Med* 1993;329:673–682.
19. International Joint Efficacy Comparison of Thrombolytics. Randomized, double-blind comparison of reteplase double-bolus administration with streptokinase in acute myocardial infarction (INJECT): trial to investigate equivalence. *Lancet* 1995;346:329.
20. The GUSTO III Investigators. A comparison of reteplase with alteplase for acute myocardial infarction. *N Engl J Med* 1997;337:1118–1123.
21. Simoons MI, Maggioni AP, Knatterud G, et al. Individual risk assessment for intracranial hemorrhage during thrombolytic therapy. *Lancet* 1993;342:523–528.
22. Grines CL, Cox DA, Stone GW, et al. Coronary angioplasty with or without stent implantation for acute myocardial infarction. *N Engl J Med* 1999;341:1949–1956.
23. Stone GW, Grines CL, Cox DA, et al. Comparison of angioplasty with stenting, with or without abciximab, in acute myocardial infarction. *N Engl J Med* 2002;346:957–966.
24. Goldman LE, Eisenberg MJ. Identification and management of patients with failed thrombolysis after acute myocardial infarction. *Ann Intern Med* 2000; 132:556–565.
25. ISIS Collaborative Group. Randomized trial of intravenous streptokinase, oral aspirin, both, or neither among 17,187 cases of suspected acute myocardial infarction. *Lancet* 1988;2:349–360.
26. The GUSTO V Investigators. Reperfusion therapy for acute myocardial infarction with thrombolytic therapy or combination reduced thrombolytic therapy and platelet glycoprotein IIb/IIIa inhibition: the GUSTO V randomised trial. *Lancet* 2001;357:1905–1914.
27. The Assessment of the Safety and Efficacy of a New Thrombolytic Regimen (ASSENT)-3 Investigators. Efficacy and safety of tenecteplase in combination with enoxaparin, abciximab, or unfractionated heparin: the ASSENT-3 randomised trial in acute myocardial infarction. *Lancet* 2001;358:605–613.
28. Montalescot G, Barragan P, Wittenberg O, et al. Platelet glycoprotein IIb/IIIa inhibition with coronary stenting for acute myocardial infarction. *N Engl J Med* 2001;344:1895–1903.
29. Wu WC, Rathore SS, Wang Y, et al. Blood transfusion in elderly patients with acute myocardial infarction. *N Engl J Med* 2001;345(17):1230–1236.

Primary and Secondary Risk Factor Stratification and Modification

Richard G. Garmany and Ryan G. Aleong

This chapter highlights the indices and predictors of cardiovascular risk and emphasizes mechanisms of modifying those risk factors, both primarily and secondarily, that portend a poor outcome.

HYPERLIPIDEMIA

Lipoprotein structure is a triglyceride core surrounded by a phospholipid layer containing apolipoproteins on the surface. Lipoproteins include chylomicrons, very-low-density lipoprotein (VLDL), intermediate-density lipoprotein (IDL), LDL, and HDL. The benefits of lowering cholesterol levels include decreased lipid deposition in plaques, which slows progression of atherosclerosis (according to angiographic studies). True regression is uncommon; however, lowering serum lipids slows progression significantly. This is unlikely to be the primary mechanism of the decrease in clinical events seen in patients who have undergone lipid-lowering therapy. Other mechanisms include

- Improved endothelial function is seen in studies of peripheral vessels in patients on statins.
- Decreased platelet thrombus formation is seen with reduction of hypercholesterolemia.
- Decreased vascular inflammation is supported by results of the CARE investigators showing decreased levels of CRP, a marker of inflammation in patients in the pravastatin (Pravachol) group over 5 yrs.

Guidelines for therapy from the Adult Treatment Panel III are based on a nine-step evaluation process:

- **Step 1:** Measure a fasting lipid profile, including total, LDL, and HDL cholesterol levels q5yrs for adults >20. Goals of therapy are listed in Table 9-1.
- **Step 2:** Determine the presence of CAD **equivalents,** conditions that confer the same degree of risk as a known history of heart disease, including
  - History of CAD
  - History of symptomatic carotid artery disease
  - History of peripheral vascular disease
  - History of abdominal aortic aneurysm
  - Diabetes mellitus (DM)

- **Step 3:** Determine the presence of other major **risk factors** that modify risk and may change LDL goals, including
  - Smoking
  - HTN (defined as BP >140/90 mm Hg or use of any antihypertensive medications)
  - HDL cholesterol <40 mg/dL (HDL >60 mg/dL removes one other risk factor from this list)
  - Family history of CAD in a first-degree male relative <55 yrs or a first-degree female relative <65 yrs
  - Age: males >45 yrs, females >55 yrs

- **Step 4:** If the patient has two or more risk factors from step 3 without a CAD risk equivalent from step 2 and does not have a history of CAD, use the Framingham

TABLE 9-1. CHOLESTEROL THERAPY GOALS

LDL cholesterol (mg/dL)	
<100	Optimal
100–129	Near optimal/above optimal
130–159	Borderline high
160–189	High
≥ 190	Very high
Total cholesterol (mg/dL)	
<200	Desirable
200–239	Borderline high
≥ 240	High
HDL cholesterol (mg/dL)	
<40	Low
≥ 60	High

From Expert Panel on Detection, Evaluation, and Treatment of High Blood Cholesterol in Adults. Executive summary of the third report of the National Cholesterol Education Program Expert Panel on Detection, Evaluation, and Treatment of High Blood Cholesterol in Adults (Adult Treatment Panel-III). *JAMA* 2001;285:2486–2497.

risk tables to determine 10-yr risk for CAD. There are separate tables for men and women. The three levels of 10-yr risk (>20%, 10–20%, or <10%) are used to guide lipid-lowering therapy decisions in step 5 (Table 9-2).
- **Step 5:** The risk category as determined in steps 2, 3, and 4 is used to establish the LDL goal, as well as guiding the LDL level for instituting therapeutic lifestyle changes (TLCs) and starting drug therapy (Table 9-3).
- **Step 6:** Initiate TLC if LDL is above goal. Features of TLCs include diet with recommended saturated fat <7% of calories and cholesterol <200 mg/day. Consider increased viscous (soluble) fiber (10–25 g/day) and plant stanols/sterols (2 g/day) as therapeutic options to enhance LDL lowering. Weight loss and increased physical activity are also components of TLC.
- **Step 7:** Consider adding drug therapy (Table 9-4) if LDL exceeds levels shown in Table 9-3. Consider administering drug therapy simultaneously with TLC for CAD and CAD equivalents. Consider adding drug to TLC after 3 mos for other risk categories.
- **Step 8:** Identify metabolic syndrome and treat, if present, after 3 mos of TLC. See Table 9-5 for clinical identification of metabolic syndrome.

  Treatment of metabolic syndrome involves treatment of the underlying causes by managing weight aggressively and increasing physical activity. Treat additional nonlipid risk factors if they persist despite lifestyle changes. This includes treating HTN, using ASA in patients with known CAD, and treating elevated triglyceride levels or low HDL levels as described in step 9.
- **Step 9:** Treat elevated triglycerides (Table 9-6, p. 91). Treatment of elevated triglycerides (≥ 150 mg/dL) is guided primarily by reaching LDL goal and includes weight management and increased physical activity. If triglycerides are ≥ 200 mg/ dL after LDL goal is reached, set secondary goal for non-HDL cholesterol (total – HDL) 30 mg/dL higher than LDL goal (Table 9-7, p. 92).

  If **triglyceride level is 200–499** mg/dL after LDL goal is reached, consider adding a drug if needed to reach the non-HDL goal. This may be accomplished by increasing the dose of LDL-lowering drug or adding nicotinic acid or fibrate to specifically target VLDL. **If triglycerides are ≥ 500** mg/dL, first lower triglycerides to prevent pancreatitis. This begins with a very-low-fat diet with <15% of calories from fat, in addition to intensive weight management and increased physical activity; fibrate or

TABLE 9-2. 10-YR RISK FOR DEVELOPING CAD, BASED ON FRAMINGHAM DATA

Men

Age (yrs)	Points	Age (yrs)	Points	Age (yrs)	Points
20–34	–9	50–54	6	65–69	11
35–39	–4	55–59	8	70–74	12
40–44	0	60–64	10	75–79	13
45–49	3				

Total cho-lesterol (mg/dL)	Points				
	Age 20–39 yrs	Age 40–49 yrs	Age 50–59 yrs	Age 60–69 yrs	Age 70–79 yrs
<160	0	0	0	0	0
160–199	4	3	2	1	0
200–239	7	5	3	1	0
240–279	9	6	4	2	1
280+	11	8	5	3	1

	Points				
	Age 20–39 yrs	Age 40–49 yrs	Age 50–59 yrs	Age 60–69 yrs	Age 70–79 yrs
Nonsmoker	0	0	0	0	0
Smoker	8	5	3	1	1

HDL in (mg/dL)	Points
≥ 60	–1
50–59	0
40–49	1
<40	2

Systolic BP (mm Hg)	If untreated	If treated
<120	0	0
120–129	0	1
130–139	1	2
140–159	1	2
160+	2	3

TABLE 9-2. CONTINUED

Point total	10-yr risk (%)
<0–11	<10
12–14	10–20
>15	≥ 20

Women

Age (yrs)	Points	Age (yrs)	Points	Age (yrs)	Points
20–34	–7	50–54	6	65–69	12
35–39	–3	55–59	8	70–74	14
40–44	0	60–64	10	75–79	16
45–49	3				

Total cholesterol (mg/dL)	Points				
	Age 20–39 yrs	Age 40–49 yrs	Age 50–59 yrs	Age 60–69 yrs	Age 70–79 yrs
<160	0	0	0	0	0
160–199	4	3	2	1	1
200–239	8	6	4	2	1
240–279	11	8	5	3	2
≥ 280	13	10	7	4	2

	Points				
	Age 20–39 yrs	Age 40–49 yrs	Age 50–59 yrs	Age 60–69 yrs	Age 70–79 yrs
Nonsmoker	0	0	0	0	0
Smoker	9	7	4	2	1

HDL in (mg/dL)	Points
≥ 60	–1
50–59	0
40–49	1
<40	2

Systolic BP (mm Hg)	If untreated	If treated
<120	0	0
120–129	1	3
130–139	2	4
140–159	3	5
≥ 160	4	6

TABLE 9-2. CONTINUED

Point total	10-yr risk (%)
<0–19	<10
20–22	10–20
>22	≥ 20

From Expert Panel on Detection, Evaluation, and Treatment of High Blood Cholesterol in Adults. Executive summary of the third report of the National Cholesterol Education Program Expert Panel on Detection, Evaluation, and Treatment of High Blood Cholesterol in Adults (Adult Treatment Panel-III). *JAMA* 2001;285:2486–2497.

nicotinic acid will be required in many of these patients. When the triglyceride level is <500 mg/dL, then address LDL-lowering therapy. Guidelines **for treatment of low HDL cholesterol** (<40 mg/dL) after reaching the LDL goal call for weight management and increased physical activity. If triglycerides are 200–499 mg/dL, achieve the non-HDL goal. If triglycerides are <200 mg/dL (isolated low HDL) in CAD or CAD equivalent, consider nicotinic acid or fibrate.

Several clinical trials have investigated lipid-lowering therapy. Those involving the use of statins in primary prevention of CAD (patients with no history of CAD) include **WOSCOPS,** which involved treatment of men with high cholesterol (mean LDL level, 192 mg/dL) with pravastatin and showed a 31% relative reduction in risk of nonfatal MI or death from CAD. The **AFCAPS/TexCAPS** study treated men and women with average LDL (130–190 mg/dL) with lovastatin and showed a 37% reduction in the risk for a first fatal or nonfatal MI. Studies of secondary prevention in patients with a history of CAD include **4S,** in which men and women with history of angina or MI and elevated cholesterol (mean LDL, 188 mg/dL) were treated with simvastatin, showing a 37% reduction of coronary death and nonfatal MI over placebo. It was also the first study to show a reduction of total mortality. The **CARE** study evaluated pravastatin in patients with average cholesterol levels and a history of MI 3–20 mos before randomization and showed a 24% risk

TABLE 9-3. LDL CHOLESTEROL GOALS

Risk category	LDL goal	LDL level at which to initiate therapeutic lifestyle changes	LDL level at which to consider drug therapy
CAD or CAD risk equivalents (see step 2) or 10-yr risk >20%	<100 mg/dL	≥ 100 mg/dL	≥ 130 mg/dL (100–129 mg/dL: drug optional)[a]
≥ 2 risk factors (see step 3) and 10-yr risk ≥ 20%	<130 mg/dL	≥ 130 mg/dL	10-yr risk 10–20%: ≥ 130 mg/dL 10-yr risk <10%: ≥ 160 mg/dL
0–1 risk factor[b]	<160 mg/dL	10-yr risk <10%: ≥ 160 mg/dL	190 mg/dL (160–189 mg/dL: LDL-lowering drug optional)

[a]Use clinical judgment to determine need for drug therapy in this group.
[b]Almost all people with 0–1 risk factor have a 10-yr risk <10%; thus, 10-yr risk assessment in people with 0–1 risk factor is not necessary.
From Expert Panel on Detection, Evaluation, and Treatment of High Blood Cholesterol in Adults. Executive summary of the third report of the National Cholesterol Education Program Expert Panel on Detection, Evaluation, and Treatment of High Blood Cholesterol in Adults (Adult Treatment Panel-III). *JAMA* 2001;285:2486–2497.

TABLE 9-4. DRUGS AFFECTING LIPID LEVELS

Drug class	Agents and daily doses	Lipid/lipoprotein effects	Side effects	Contraindications
HMG-CoA reductase inhibitors (statins)	Lovastatin (20–80 mg PO), pravastatin (20–40 mg PO), simvastatin (20–80 mg PO), fluvastatin (20–80 mg PO), atorvastatin (10–80 mg PO)	LDL ↓ 18–55% HDL ↑ 5–15% TG ↓ 7–30%	Myopathy Increased liver enzymes	Absolute: active or chronic liver disease Relative: concomitant use of certain drugs[a]
Bile acid sequestrants	Cholestyramine (4–16 g PO), colestipol (5–20 g PO), colesevelam (2.6–3.8 g PO)	LDL ↓ 15–30% HDL ↑ 3–5% TG unchanged or ↑	GI distress Constipation Decreased absorption of other drugs	Absolute: dysbetalipoproteinemia TG >400 mg/dL Relative: TG >200 mg/dL
Nicotinic acid	Immediate-release (crystalline) nicotinic acid (1.5–3 g PO), extended-release nicotinic acid (Niaspan) (1–2 g PO), sustained-release nicotinic acid (1–2 g PO)	LDL ↓ 5–25% HDL ↑ 15–35% TG ↓ 20–50%	Flushing Hyperglycemia Hyperuricemia (or gout) Upper GI distress Hepatotoxicity	Absolute: chronic liver disease, severe gout Relative: diabetes, hyperuricemia
Fibric acids	Gemfibrozil (600 mg PO bid), fenofibrate (200 mg PO), clofibrate (1000 mg PO bid)	LDL ↓ 5–20% (may be ↑ in patients with high TG) HDL ↑ 10–20% TG ↓ 20–50%	Dyspepsia Gallstones Myopathy	Absolute: severe renal disease, severe hepatic disease

HMG-CoA, 3-hydroxy-3-methylglutaryl-coenzyme; TG, total cholesterol goal; ↑, increased; ↓, decreased.

[a]Cyclosporine, macrolide antibiotics, various antifungal agents, and cytochrome P-450 inhibitors (fibrates and niacin should be used with appropriate caution).

From Expert Panel on Detection, Evaluation, and Treatment of High Blood Cholesterol in Adults. Executive summary of the third report of the National Cholesterol Education Program Expert Panel on Detection, Evaluation, and Treatment of High Blood Cholesterol in Adults (Adult Treatment Panel-III). *JAMA* 2001;285:2486–2497.

TABLE 9-5. CLINICAL IDENTIFICATION OF METABOLIC SYNDROME

Risk factor	Defining level
Abdominal obesity[a]	Waist circumference[b]
Men	>102 cm (>40 in.)
Women	>88 cm (>35 in.)
Triglycerides	≥ 150 mg/dL
HDL cholesterol	
Men	<40 mg/dL
Women	<50 mg/dL
BP	≥ 130/≥ 85 mm Hg
Fasting glucose	≥ 110 mg/dL

[a]Overweight and obesity are associated with insulin resistance and the metabolic syndrome. However, the presence of abdominal obesity is more highly correlated with the metabolic risk factors than is an elevated BMI. Therefore, the simple measure of waist circumference is recommended to identify the body-weight component of the metabolic syndrome.
[b]Some male patients can develop multiple metabolic risk factors when the waist circumference is only marginally increased, e.g., 94–102 cm (37–39 in.). Such patients may have a strong genetic contribution to insulin resistance and should benefit from changes in lifestyle habits, similar to men with categoric increases in waist circumference.
From Expert Panel on Detection, Evaluation, and Treatment of High Blood Cholesterol in Adults. Executive summary of the third report of the National Cholesterol Education Program Expert Panel on Detection, Evaluation, and Treatment of High Blood Cholesterol in Adults (Adult Treatment Panel-III). *JAMA* 2001;285:2486–2497.

reduction of fatal or nonfatal MI. In the **LIPID** study, patients with a history of ACS from 3–36 mos before randomization and a wide range of LDL values (130–170 mg/dL) were treated with pravastatin and found to have a 24% relative risk reduction of CAD mortality, including noncoronary mortality.

HYPERTENSION

- HTN detection begins with proper **BP measurements,** which should be obtained at each health care encounter. To measure BP, patients should be seated in a chair with their backs supported and their arms bared and supported at heart level. Patients should refrain from smoking or ingesting caffeine during the 30 mins preceding the measurement. Measurement should begin after at least 5 mins of rest. The appropriate cuff size must be used to ensure accurate measurement. The bladder within the cuff should encircle at least 80% of the arm. Many adults will require a large adult cuff.

TABLE 9-6. ADULT TREATMENT PANEL III CLASSIFICATION OF SERUM TRIGLYCERIDES

Serum triglyceride level (mg/dL)	Classification
<150	Normal
150–199	Borderline high
200–499	High
500	Very high

From Expert Panel on Detection, Evaluation, and Treatment of High Blood Cholesterol in Adults. Executive summary of the third report of the National Cholesterol Education Program Expert Panel on Detection, Evaluation, and Treatment of High Blood Cholesterol in Adults (Adult Treatment Panel-III). *JAMA* 2001;285:2486–2497.

TABLE 9-7. COMPARISON OF LDL CHOLESTEROL AND NON-HDL CHOLESTEROL GOALS FOR THREE RISK CATEGORIES

Risk category	LDL goal (mg/dL)	Non-HDL goal (mg/dL) (Total cholesterol − HDL)
CAD and CAD risk equivalent (10-yr risk for CAD >20%)	<100	<130
Multiple (2+) risk factors and 10-yr risk ≤ 20%	<130	<160
0–1 risk factor	<160	<190

From Expert Panel on Detection, Evaluation, and Treatment of High Blood Cholesterol in Adults. Executive summary of the third report of the National Cholesterol Education Program Expert Panel on Detection, Evaluation, and Treatment of High Blood Cholesterol in Adults (Adult Treatment Panel-III). *JAMA* 2001;285:2486–2497.

Record systolic BP and diastolic BP. The first appearance of sound (phase 1) is used to define systolic BP. The disappearance of sound (phase 5) is used to define diastolic BP. Two or more readings separated by 2 mins should be averaged. If the first two readings differ by more than 5 mm Hg, obtain additional readings and average them. Table 9-8 describes proper follow-up based on the BP values obtained.

- The Joint National Committee on Prevention, Detection, Evaluation, and Treatment of High Blood Pressure (JNC) 6 guidelines define optimal, normal, and high normal levels of BP, as well as three stages of HTN (Table 9-9). The MRFIT trial, an important, long-term, large-scale trial, related HTN to CAD and showed systolic BP was more closely related to CAD than diastolic BP.
- In addition to BP assessment, the **physical exam** should include funduscopic exam, vascular exam for bruits, cardiac exam for rhythm and extra heart sounds, lung exam for wheezes or crackles, abdomen exam for bruits or masses, peripheral pulse check, and neurologic exam.
- **Lab and diagnostic studies** to obtain in patients with newly diagnosed HTN include serum chemistries, UA, CBC, and ECG. Obtain additional studies as indicated on an individual basis.

TABLE 9-8. FOLLOW-UP FOR PATIENTS WITH HTN

Initial systolic BP (mm Hg)[a]	Initial diastolic BP (mm Hg)	Follow-up recommended[b]
<130	<85	Recheck in 2 yrs
130–139	85–89	Recheck in 1 yr
140–159	90–99	Confirm within 2 mos
160–179	100–109	Evaluate or refer to source of care within 1 mo
≥ 180	≥ 110	Evaluate or refer to source of care immediately or within 1 wk, depending on clinical situation

[a]If systolic and diastolic categories are different, follow recommendations for shorter follow-up (e.g., 160/86 mm Hg should be evaluated or referred to source of care within 1 mo).
[b]Modify scheduling of follow-up according to reliable information about post-BP measurement, other cardiovascular risk factors, or target organ disease.
From Sixth report of the Joint National Committee on Prevention, Detection, Evaluation, and Treatment of High Blood Pressure. *Ann Intern Med* 1997;157:2413–2446.

TABLE 9-9. CLASSIFICATION OF BP FOR ADULTS ≥18[a]

Category	Systolic BP (mm Hg)	Diastolic BP (mm Hg)
Optimal[b]	<120 and	<80
Normal	<130 and	<85
High normal	130–139 or	85–89
HTN[c]		
Stage 1	140–159 or	90–99
Stage 2	160–179 or	100–109
Stage 3	≥ 180 or	N ≥ 110

[a]Intended for patients who are not taking antihypertensive drugs and are not acutely ill. When systolic and diastolic BPs fall into different categories, the high category should be selected to classify the individual's BP status. In addition to classifying stages of HTN on the basis of average BP levels, clinicians should specify presence or absence of target organ disease and additional risk factors. This specificity is important for risk classification and treatment.
[b]Optimal BP with respect to cardiovascular risk is <120/80 mm Hg; however, unusually low readings should be evaluated for clinical significance.
[c]Based on the average of ≥ 2 readings taken at each of ≥ 2 visits after an initial screening.
From Sixth report of the Joint National Committee on Prevention, Detection, Evaluation, and Treatment of High Blood Pressure. *Ann Intern Med* 1997;157:2413–2446.

TABLE 9-10. COMPONENTS OF CARDIOVASCULAR RISK STRATIFICATION IN PATIENTS WITH HTN

Major risk factors

Smoking

Dyslipidemia

DM

Age >60 yrs

Sex (men and postmenopausal women)

Family history of cardiovascular disease: women <65 yrs or men <55 yrs

Target organ damage/clinical cardiovascular disease

Heart diseases

LVH

Angina or prior MI

Prior coronary revascularization

Heart failure

Stroke or TIA

Nephropathy

Peripheral arterial disease

Retinopathy

From Sixth report of the Joint National Committee on Prevention, Detection, Evaluation, and Treatment of High Blood Pressure. *Ann Intern Med* 1997;157:2413–2446.

TABLE 9-11. RISK STRATIFICATION AND TREATMENT[a]

BP stages (mm Hg)	Risk group A (no risk factors; no TOD/CCD)	Risk group B (at least one risk factor, not including diabetes; no TOD/CCD)	Risk group C (TOD/CCD and/or diabetes, with or without other risk factors)
High normal (130–139/85–89)	Lifestyle modification	Lifestyle modification	Drug therapy[b]
Stage 1 (140–159/90–99)	Lifestyle modification (up to 12 mos)	Lifestyle modification[c] (up to 6 mos)	Drug therapy
Stages 2 and 3 (≥ 160/≥ 100)	Drug therapy	Drug therapy	Drug therapy

CCD, clinical cardiovascular disease; TOD, target organ disease.
[a]For example, a patient with diabetes and a BP of 142/94 mm Hg plus LVH should be classified as having stage 1 HTN with TOD (LVH) and with another major risk factor (diabetes). This patient would be categorized as stage 1, risk group C, and recommended for immediate initiation of pharmacologic treatment. Lifestyle modification should be adjunctive therapy for all patients recommended for pharmacologic therapy.
[b]For patients with multiple risk factors, consider drugs as initial therapy plus lifestyle modifications.
[c]For those with heart failure, renal insufficiency, or diabetes.
From Sixth report of the Joint National Committee on Prevention, Detection, Evaluation, and Treatment of High Blood Pressure. *Ann Intern Med* 1997;157:2413–2446.

TABLE 9-12. CLINICAL SITUATIONS IN WHICH ANTIHYPERTENSIVE AGENTS MAY BE BENEFICIAL

Condition	Agent(s)
Heart failure	ACE inhibitors, beta blockers, angiotensin-receptor antagonists, diuretics
Acute coronary syndromes	Beta blockers, ACE inhibitors, calcium channel blockers, nitrates
Essential tremor	Nonselective beta blockers
Hyperthyroidism	Beta blockers
Diabetes	ACE inhibitors, angiotensin-receptor antagonists, low-dose diuretics
Sinus bradycardia, sick sinus syndrome, or AV blocks	ACE inhibitors, diuretics, alpha blockers
Atrial tachycardia	Beta blockers, calcium channel blockers
Osteoporosis	Thiazides
Hyperlipidemia	Alpha blockers, ACE inhibitors, angiotensin-receptor blockers
Migraine	Nonselective beta blockers, nondihydropyridine calcium channel blockers
Isolated systolic HTN	Diuretics, calcium channel blockers
HTN among blacks	Diuretics, calcium channel blockers, alpha blockers
Smokers	ACE inhibitors, calcium channel blockers, alpha-blockers

From Sixth report of the Joint National Committee on Prevention, Detection, Evaluation, and Treatment of High Blood Pressure. *Ann Intern Med* 1997;157:2413–2446.

**TABLE 9-13. CLINICAL SITUATIONS IN WHICH ANTIHYPERTENSIVE
AGENTS SHOULD BE USED WITH CAUTION**

Condition	Agent(s) to avoid
COPD, asthma	Beta blockers
Depression	Beta blockers, central alpha-agonists
Diabetes	Beta blockers, high-dose diuretics
Hyperlipidemia	Beta blockers without intrinsic sympathomimetic activity, high-dose diuretics
Gout	Diuretics
Second- or third-degree AV block	Beta blockers, nondihydropyridine, calcium channel blockers
Liver disease	Labetalol, methyldopa
Peripheral vascular disease	Nonselective beta blockers
Renal insufficiency	Use K^+-sparing diuretics, ACE inhibitors, and angiotensin-receptor antagonists judiciously (protective in this setting unless their effect on the efferent arteriole decreases glomerular filtration rate dramatically, a particular problem in the setting of renal artery stenosis and NSAID use); with atenolol, watch for bradycardia and hypotension carefully as it is renally cleared. Metoprolol (hepatically cleared) may be more appropriate.

From Sixth report of the Joint National Committee on Prevention, Detection, Evaluation, and Treatment of High Blood Pressure. *Ann Intern Med* 1997;157:2413–2446.

- JNC 6 **risk-group stratification** includes groups A, B, and C. This is based on the average of at least three readings on separate occasions, unless BP >160/115 mm Hg (Table 9-10). Based on this assessment and the level of BP, the patient's risk group can be determined, as shown in Table 9-11.
- **Lifestyle modification** should include low-salt diet, smoking cessation, weight loss, limiting alcohol intake, increasing physical activity, and adequate K^+ intake.
- **First-line agents for initial therapy: Thiazide diuretics** and **beta blockers** have been proved to reduce morbidity and mortality in patients with HTN and no target organ damage. Other possible choices include ACE inhibitors, angiotensin-receptor blockers, and calcium channel blockers. Based on the HOT trial data, consider daily **ASA** therapy in all patients with HTN. Table 9-12 lists clinical situations in which specific antihypertensive agents may be beneficial. Table 9-13 lists clinical situations in which specific antihypertensive agents should be used with caution.

DIABETES

Type I DM is an autoimmune-mediated destruction of insulin-producing cells typically occurring in children and young adults. Type II DM, usually occurring after age 30 yrs, is due to insulin resistance and strongly related to obesity.

The presence of diabetes leads to accelerated CAD. Diabetes also causes more severe CAD, including more diffuse disease and more coronary branches involved. In addition, patients with DM tend to have fewer coronary collaterals. Tight control of diabetes has been shown to prevent microvascular complications of types I and II DM and is recommended in patients at risk for CAD.

Additional risk-factor control is of added importance in diabetics. Give particular attention to controlling cholesterol, with the LDL goal in diabetics of <100 mg/dL. Address obesity, as this is well known to improve glycemic control. Recommendations for BP are

<130/80 mm Hg. If proteinuria exists, recommendations are <125/80 mm Hg. Most authorities recommend daily ASA for adults with diabetes.

OBESITY

Obesity is associated with hyperlipidemia, HTN, and DM. Waist-to-hip ratio has been found to be a better predictor of CAD than total weight or BMI. A combination of exercise and diet is recognized as the preferred treatment. Medical treatment includes orlistat (Xenical), which inhibits gastric and pancreatic lipases and blocks fat absorption.

NUTRITION

In the GISSI Prevenzione trial [1], fish oils (n-3 polyunsaturated fatty acids) exhibited a 2% reduction in cardiovascular deaths. The AHA Step I diet (primary prevention) mandates that <30% of total calories are derived from fat; <10% of calories are from saturated fat and <300 mg/cholesterol qd. The AHA Step II diet (secondary prevention) mandates <7% of calories from saturated fat and <200 mg/cholesterol qd.

SMOKING

Smoking is the largest cause of preventable death among older adults (secondhand smoke is the third-largest cause). Smoking leads to increases in BP and heart rate as well as platelet activation and coronary plaque destabilization. Risk of CAD increases in a **linear fashion** in relation to the number of cigarettes smoked daily. Smoking cessation leads to rapid decline in the risk of CAD, with significant reduction seen within 1 yr (25–50% risk reduction in cardiovascular events for primary and secondary prevention). 3 yrs after smoking cessation, the risk of CAD equals that of a nonsmoker.

Replacement therapy with the nicotine patch, nicotine gum, nicotine spray, and nicotine inhalers is available and has been shown to significantly increase the rate of cessation. Bupropion (Wellbutrin), used alone or in combination with replacement therapy, has also been shown to increase cessation rates. The standard regiment is 150 mg PO qd for 3 days, followed by 150 mg PO bid for 8–12 wks. The patient is instructed to quit smoking on day 5–7. Bupropion is contraindicated in patients at risk for seizures. Clonidine (Catapres) at low doses has also been used to decrease the sympathetic-mediated response to nicotine withdrawal.

ASPIRIN

Use of ASA (81–325 mg PO qd) is the standard of care in secondary prevention. In primary prevention, limited data suggest that its use decreases the risk of nonfatal MI, and it is recommended for people with significant risk factors.

SEDENTARY LIFESTYLE

The AHA recommendation is 30 mins of moderate exercise daily, building up from 5–10 mins/day (see Cardiac Rehabilitation).

HORMONE REPLACEMENT THERAPY

The HERS study found no reduction of risk of cardiovascular events in postmenopausal women with CAD taking hormone-replacement therapy (HRT). 1-yr cardiovascular mortality was higher in the HRT group; at 4 yrs, there was no difference. There was a 0.4%/yr increased risk of thromboembolism. Based on results of this and the follow-up HERS II study, initialization of HRT is not recommended for secondary prevention to reduce the risk of events in women with CAD [2,3].

The Women's Health Initiative [3] is a very large trial that assessed primary prevention of multiple outcomes: CAD, breast cancer, stroke, pulmonary embolism, hip fracture, colorectal cancer, and total mortality. The trial was stopped after 5 yrs because the breast cancer rate in the HRT group was unacceptably high. The hazard ratios for the above outcomes are as follows: 1.29, 1.26, 1.41, 2.13, 0.66, 0.63, and 0.98, respectively. The results of this trial raise a specter over the use of HRT in primary prevention of CAD. Further interpretation of these results is forthcoming, and future statements from the ACC/AHA will have high impact on the future use of HRT.

LIPOPROTEIN(A)

Similar in structure to plasminogen, the normal function of Lp(a) is unknown. There is some evidence that Lp(a) levels may correlate with risk of vascular disease. Currently, Lp(a) levels are not recommended as part of routine screening.

HOMOCYSTEINE

Homocystine levels have been linked to rapid progression of CAD. In some studies, reducing levels of homocysteine has been shown to reduce the rate of coronary restenosis after angioplasty. In one study, patients undergoing angioplasty were randomized to receive folic acid (1 mg), vitamin B_{12} (400 μg), and pyridoxine (10 mg) together as folate treatment or to a placebo group. Researchers followed 205 patients for 6 mos after angioplasty to assess restenosis measured by follow-up angiogram as the primary end point. Folate treatment was found to reduce plasma homocystine level, and coronary artery luminal diameters were significantly larger at follow-up in the folate group. There was also significant reduction in the need for target lesion revascularization in the folate group. These results have been cited to suggest treatment of all patients undergoing angioplasty with folic acid, vitamin B_{12}, and pyridoxine [4].

COMMON MISTAKES IN PREVENTIVE CARDIOLOGY

Mistakes commonly made in preventive cardiology include

- Lipid lowering with statins is frequently not started during hospitalization for ACS.
- Patients do not reach published goals for LDL, BP, or blood glucose.
- Failure to initiate smoking cessation counseling during hospitalization.
- Incorrect choice of antihypertensive agents given other risk factors.

CARDIAC REHABILITATION

Cardiac rehabilitation comprises an individualized regimen of physical activity and health education designed to reduce the symptoms of cardiac disease and improve cardiac function for those who have experienced MI and/or those with heart failure. A cardiac rehabilitation program should include medical evaluation, prescribed activity, risk factor modification, and counseling. Given that CAD is the leading cause of death and a major cause of physical disability in the United States, the need for primary and secondary prevention cannot be overemphasized.

Proven Benefits

- The **benefits** of cardiac rehabilitation have been proven in multiple trials. One metaanalysis showed a significant decrease in all-cause mortality and cardiovascular mortality in post-MI patients who were randomized to cardiac rehabilitation programs as compared to controls [5]. The clinical benefits include decreases in symptoms of angina pectoris in patients with coronary disease and in symptoms related to heart failure in those with decreased LV function. This improvement in mortality was thought to be secondary to improved cardiovascular fitness, improved patient surveillance, and risk factor reduction.

- The improvement in patients' **functional status** with cardiac rehabilitation depends on the intensity of exercise. With moderate-intensity exercise, the improvement in cardiovascular status is due to peripheral adaptations. These include increased O_2 extraction by skeletal muscles, with a corresponding decrease in myocardial O_2 demand and requirement for coronary blood flow. In addition, there is decreased systemic vascular resistance and increased vagal tone, resulting in decreased heart rate. With high-intensity exercise, there are also improvements in cardiac function. It has been demonstrated that patients with CAD who undergo exercise training show an improvement in ejection fraction, thallium-perfusion defects, and peak exercise capacity. The mechanism by which cardiac function improves is unclear, however, and likely multifactorial.

- Studies examining why **cardiac function** improves have looked at three major mechanisms: (a) regression of coronary stenoses, (b) formation of collateral vessels, and (c) improved endothelial function. In the SCRIP trial, patients with known coronary disease were randomized to usual care or a risk-reduction and exercise program. Patients in the intervention group had a slowing of coronary artery luminal narrowing and decreased cardiac events compared to controls. In the Lifestyle Heart Trial, patients with known coronary disease were randomized to usual care or an intensive lifestyle change consisting of a low-fat vegetarian diet, smoking cessation, and moderate exercise. Patients in the intervention group demonstrated a regression in coronary atherosclerosis and decreased cardiac events compared to controls. These studies have been criticized, because the changes in luminal diameter were relatively small and could not fully explain the improvement in myocardial perfusion and cardiac-related symptoms. In studies examining the formation of collateral vessels, results have been variable, with only some studies demonstrating angiographically visible collateral vessels. It is thought that intramyocardial as well as epicardial collateral vessels likely form in patients with ischemic coronary disease who receive exercise training. Improved endothelial cell function after exercise rehabilitation has focused on improved nitric oxide–related vasodilation. Other possible mechanisms include improved microcirculation (arteriole) vasodilation and decreased blood viscosity due to a decrease in coagulation factors.

- The benefits of **cardiac rehabilitation** have been shown in multiple special populations. Elderly patients (>65 yrs) account for a large portion of cardiac-related deaths and acute MIs; however, these patients are less likely to be referred for cardiac rehabilitation. Multiple benefits have been shown for elderly patients participating in cardiac rehabilitation programs, including improved exercise capacity, improved cardiac mortality, reduced subsequent hospitalizations, and improved control of other cardiac risk factors. Patients with heart failure and LV systolic dysfunction have been shown to improve functional capacity with exercise training. This improvement is predominantly due to improved oxidative capacity of skeletal muscles, with some improvement in ventricular function.

- Despite the many proven benefits, only 10–47% of eligible patients are referred to a cardiac rehabilitation program. One of the major concerns is the safety of rehabilitation programs. Cardiac rehabilitation is **indicated** for patients with a diagnosis of an acute MI, those who have undergone coronary revascularization, and those with stable angina. Cardiac rehabilitation is also appropriate for elderly patients and those with heart failure or who have undergone a heart transplant. A trial sponsored by the NIH designed to assess the effect on mortality of exercise among patients with heart failure is currently enrolling.

- In **summary,** the improvements related to exercise training include a decrease in activity-related symptoms, including angina, dyspnea, fatigue, and, sometimes, claudication. The mechanisms for these improvements include (a) improved O_2 transport due to increased cardiac output and O_2 consumption and (b) reduced myocardial O_2 requirement due to decreased resting heart rate and systolic BP.

Components of Exercise Training

- **Aerobic and strength (isometric) training** have been shown to have beneficial effects. In aerobic training, an increase in heart rate is the predominant effect and parallels the intensity of the activity. In younger patients, an increase in stroke volume accompanies the increased heart rate, as compared to elderly patients, in whom the increase in heart rate is the dominant effect. Systolic BP also increases with increasing aerobic activity. Isometric training improves endurance and aids in the return to occupational and recreational activities. Strength training has a substantial effect on systolic BP, with less of an effect on heart rate and cardiac output. In unfit individuals, strength training may provoke angina, ventricular dysfunction, and/or arrhythmias. Patients should achieve adequate aerobic capacity before starting strength training.
- Both **arm and leg exercises** should be included in exercise programs, as only trained muscle groups will show improvement in O_2 extraction. Leg training is predominantly preformed with treadmills or stationary bikes, whereas calisthenics, shoulder wheels, rowing machines, and arms ergometers improve arm strength. The workload for arm training is approximately one-half of leg work. Given that most daily activities include arm and leg work, both muscle groups should be included in exercise programs.
- **Prerehabilitation exercise testing** helps to define safe levels of activity and guide the amount of surveillance needed in a rehabilitation program. A graded exercise test is safely performed within several weeks after an acute MI. The test is sign or symptom limited, as opposed to heart rate limited, given that antianginal medications may attenuate the effect on heart rate. Arm testing may be done for patients who are limited by musculoskeletal problems or claudication. A predischarge exercise test also allows for risk stratification. High-risk patients may have low exercise capacity [4–6 metabolic equivalents (METS)], be limited by anginal symptoms or ST changes, and develop exercise-induced hypotension or ventricular arrhythmias. Using a radionuclide with exercise tests helps to define the patient's level of risk. Patients who are identified as low risk during exercise testing may be better suited to an accelerated rehabilitation program and resumption of activities.
- An **exercise prescription** is established and is based on maximal heart rate (220 – age). Initially, 10–20 mins at 50–60% maximum heart rate is the recommended workload, performed at least three times/wk. Gradually, the patient works up to 70–85% maximum. Warm-up and cool-down periods of activity are also used.

Implementation of a Cardiac Rehabilitation Program

- Cardiac rehabilitation should begin in the inpatient setting and continue after discharge from the hospital. Initially, patients undergo an evaluation of base-line risk factors and assessment of psychological and physical disability, which includes graded exercise testing.
- The **inpatient** phase of rehabilitation begins with early in-hospital ambulation. This portion of rehabilitation is designed to minimize the effects of deconditioning, which include reduced physical work capacity, orthostatic intolerance, increased blood viscosity, and reduced pulmonary ventilation. Patients should be started on low-intensity activities (1–2 METS), with a gradual progression. Initially, patients are encouraged to feed themselves, use a bedside commode, and perform other personal-care activities. Sitting in a chair helps to decrease the hypovolemia associated with immobilization. Exposure to gravitational stress helps to limit hypovolemia, decreased cardiac filling, and deteriorating O_2-carrying capacity. Patients should gradually perform arm and leg stretching and exercises to maintain muscle tone and joint mobility. The major inpatient activity is walking, which is gradually increased in length and pace. Most household activities require 2–3 METS of activity, and patients should try to achieve this level of activity before discharge. If patients have steps at home, stair climbing should be practiced while in the hospital. Disproportionate responses to low levels of activity may require activity restriction and/or clinical reevaluation. These concerning responses may be due to (a) symptoms,

including angina, palpitations, or dyspnea; (b) tachycardia or bradycardia; (c) ST changes or arrhythmias; or (d) hypotensive responses to exercise. The latter effect should be interpreted based on a patient's medication regimen. Use the hospital stay to educate patients on their disease, new medications, anticipated tests, activity restrictions, and concerning signs or symptoms. Early ambulation and discharge have not been shown to increase morbidity or mortality and instead are associated with improved functional status and well being.

- The **outpatient** phase depends on the perceived risk of a patient having a recurrent event and his or her overall functional status. For low- or moderate-risk patients, a home-based walking program with periodic exercise counseling and risk-factor assessments may be appropriate. A home regimen should consist of gradually increasing intensity of walking or jogging or use of a stationary bicycle. For low-risk patients, ECG monitoring has not been shown to increase the safety of exercise programs. Once patients have achieved an exercise capacity of 7–8 METS at home, maintaining a regimen can be done independently. For older patients and those with myocardial ischemia, heart failure, or serious arrhythmia, on-site cardiac rehabilitation with greater supervision may be necessary. High-risk patients should initially have ECG-monitored exercise due to the increased risk of adverse effects.

KEY POINTS TO REMEMBER

- Primary and secondary prevention of CAD rank among the first orders of business in a patient with suspected risk factors, known risk factors, or CAD.
- The Framingham database has provided important predictive values of adverse cardiac events by sex, age, total cholesterol, smoking status, HDL cholesterol, and systolic BP.
- Cholesterol and BP should be aggressively treated when elevated, especially in individuals with known other risk factors or target organ damage.
- In general, thiazide diuretics and beta blockers are first line in the treatment of HTN. The recently published ALLHAT trial confirmed this with regard to a thiazide diuretic, showing equivalence compared to a dihydropyridine calcium channel blocker and an ACE inhibitor. Furthermore, thiazide diuretics are inexpensive.
- Certain clinical situations, however, dictate the use of certain classes of antihypertensives.
- Cardiac rehabilitation should be planned for most patients after discharge from the hospital and appropriate assessment.

NOTE ADDED IN PROOF

An update to the JNC 6 criteria, JNC 7, was published during press [6]. The guidelines published therein generally follow JNC 6, but have even lower BP thresholds for treatment, advising careful follow-up of "prehypertensive" patients (systolic BP, 120–139 mm Hg).

SUGGESTED READING

Ades PA. Medical progress: cardiac rehabilitation and secondary prevention of coronary heart disease. *N Engl J Med* 2001;345:892–902.

Alexander JK. Obesity and coronary heart disease. *Am J Med Sci* 2001;321(4):215–224.

Anonymous. Overweight, obesity, and health risk. National Task Force on the Prevention and Treatment of Obesity. *Arch Intern Med* 2000;160(7):898–904.

Expert Panel on Detection, Evaluation, and Treatment of High Blood Cholesterol in Adults. Executive summary of the third report of the National Cholesterol Education Program Expert Panel on Detection, Evaluation, and Treatment of High Blood Cholesterol in Adults (Adult Treatment Panel-III). *JAMA* 2001;285:2486–2497.

Gielen S, Schuler G, Hambrecht R. Exercise training in coronary artery disease and coronary vasomotion. *Circulation* 2001;103(1):E1–E6.

Gotto AM, Whitney E, Stein EA, et al. Relation between baseline and on-treatment lipid parameters and first acute major coronary events in the Air Force/Texas Coronary Atherosclerosis Prevention Study (AFCAPS/TexCAPS). *Circulation* 2000;101:477–484.

Haskell WL, Alderman EL, Fair JM, et al. Effects of intensive multiple risk factor reduction on coronary atherosclerosis and clinical cardiac events in men and women with coronary artery disease: the Stanford Coronary Risk Intervention Project (SCRIP). *Circulation* 1994;89:975–990.

Keteyian SJ, Levine AB, Brawner CA, et al. Exercise training in patients with heart failure: a randomized, controlled trial. *Ann Intern Med* 1996;124:1051–1057.

Kobashigawa JA, Leaf DA, Lee N, et al. A controlled trial of exercise rehabilitation after heart transplantation. *N Engl J Med* 1999;340:272–277.

Lavie CJ, Milani RV. Cardiac rehabilitation and preventive cardiology in the elderly. *Cardiol Clin* 1999;17(1):233–242.

O'Connor GT, Buring JE, Yusuf S, et al. An overview of randomized trials of rehabilitation with exercise after myocardial infarction. *Circulation* 1989;80:234–244.

Rossouw JE, Anderson GL, Prentice RL, et al. Risks and benefits of estrogen plus progestin in healthy postmenopausal women: principal results from the Women's Health Initiative randomized controlled trial. *JAMA* 2002;288:321–333.

Sacks FM, Pfeiffer MA, Moye LA, et al. The effect of pravastatin on coronary events after myocardial infarction in patients with average cholesterol levels. *N Engl J Med* 1996;335:1001–1009.

Scandinavian Simvastatin Survival Study Group. Randomised trial of cholesterol lowering in 4,444 patients with coronary heart disease: the Scandinavian Simvastatin Survival Study (4S). *Lancet* 1994;344:1383–1389.

Sixth report of the Joint National Committee on Prevention, Detection, Evaluation, and Treatment of High Blood Pressure. *Ann Intern Med* 1997;157:2413–2446.

The ALLHAT Officers and Coordinators for the ALLHAT Collaborative Research Group. Major Outcomes in High-Risk Hypertensive Patients Randomized to Angiotensin-Converting Enzyme Inhibitor or Calcium Channel Blocker vs Diuretic: The Antihypertensive and Lipid-Lowering Treatment to Prevent Heart Attack Trial (ALLHAT). *JAMA* 2002;288:2981–2997.

Third report of the Expert Panel on Detection, Evaluation, and Treatment of High Blood Cholesterol in Adults (Adult Treatment Panel III) Executive Summary. NIH Publication No. 01-3305. Bethesda: U.S. Department of Health and Human Services, Public Health Service, National Institutes of Health, National Heart, Lung and Blood Institute, 2001.

REFERENCES

1. Dietary supplementation with *n*-3 polyunsaturated fatty acids and vitamin E after myocardial infarction: results of the GISSI-Prevenzione trial. Gruppo Italiano per lo Studio della Sopravvivenza nell'Infarto miocardico. *Lancet* 1999;354:447.

2. Hulley S, Grady D, Bush T, et al. Randomized trial of estrogen plus progestin for secondary prevention of coronary heart disease in postmenopausal women. *JAMA* 1998;280:605–618.

3. Grady D, Herrington D, Bittner V, et al. Cardiovascular disease outcomes during 6.8 years of hormone therapy. *JAMA* 2002;288:49–57.

4. Schnyder G, Roffi M, Pin R, et al. Decreased rate of coronary restenosis after lowering of plasma homocysteine levels. *N Engl J Med* 2001;345:1593–1600.

5. Oldridge NB, Guyatt GH, Fischer ME, et al. Cardiac rehabilitation after myocardial infarction. Combined experience of randomized clinical trials. *JAMA* 1988;260:945–950.

6. Chobanian AV, Bakris GL, Black HR, et al. The Seventh Report of the Joint National Committee on Prevention, Detection, Evaluation, and Treatment of High Blood Pressure: The JNC 7 Report. *JAMA* 2003;289(19):2560–2571.

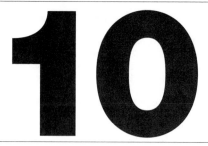

Management of Acute and Chronic Heart Failure

Michael J. Riley and
Peter A. Crawford

INTRODUCTION

Heart failure (HF) is the constellation of symptoms and signs resulting from cardiac dysfunction. HF may occur because of an acute insult on a previously normal heart, or it may be superimposed on chronic cardiac dysfunction. HF must be distinguished semantically from **cardiomyopathy.** HF is a clinical state in which a patient usually exhibits a low cardiac output and is not able to accommodate elevated left- and/or right-sided filling pressures, resulting in a variety of historical and physical exam features. Cardiomyopathy can, and frequently does, occur in the absence of symptoms or clinical HF. Such cardiomyopathic patients are termed **compensated.** One goal of therapy in patients with HF is to render them compensated.

It also is important to classify HF by its cardinal forms of pathogenesis: **systolic dysfunction, diastolic dysfunction, valvular disease, or pericardial disease.** Any of these general processes can lead to HF. The presentations of these forms of HF overlap, but important clinical subtleties distinguish them on history and physical exam, if not with further testing. Moreover, these four forms of pathogenesis often overlap: only one or all four can occur simultaneously in the same patient. Of note, systolic dysfunction is almost always accompanied by at least some degree of diastolic dysfunction. The converse is not true: Diastolic dysfunction commonly occurs in a heart that contracts normally. Therefore, it is important to classify the cause of HF in every patient you assess.

Identify potential **precipitating factors** and address them rapidly, as patients with acute HF have high mortality and may deteriorate quickly. Some inciting factors include acute myocardial ischemia, arrhythmias (e.g., AF), infective endocarditis or various other causes of acute valvular dysfunction, hypertensive crisis, myocardial toxins (e.g., doxorubicin chemotherapy, alcohol, cocaine), various inflammatory processes, and the peripartum state or postcardiac surgery. Acute right HF may develop in the setting of pulmonary embolism. In the context of chronic, compensated pump dysfunction, acute HF may occur secondary to the factors mentioned above or as a result of noncompliance with either the prescribed dietary (e.g., excessive salt intake) or medical regimen. Medical noncompliance includes failure to take cardiac medications as prescribed or use of medications that hinder the effects of appropriate agents (e.g., NSAIDs). **Renal artery stenosis, acute severe mitral regurgitation, and left-main coronary artery occlusion are common factors that lead to dramatic, acute onset HF with "flash" pulmonary edema.**

An important consideration in the differential diagnosis of chronic HF is **high-output failure.** Although the majority of patients with HF exhibit a reduced cardiac output, cardiac output is high with this entity; however, one or both ventricles is unable to accommodate the filling pressures created by the condition. LV systolic function may be normal or abnormal. On Swan-Ganz catheterization, the cardiac output can be as high as 15 L/min, and the pulmonary capillary wedge and right atrial pressures are elevated. The most notable causes for high-output failure include anemia, left-to-right intracardiac or extracardiac (e.g., dialysis shunts, arteriovenous malformations) shunt, hyperthyroidism, and wet beriberi. If the cause is left-to-right shunt, pulmonary HTN is often present. Treatment is similar to low-output failure, but treatment of the underlying cause is mandatory.

ACUTE CARDIOGENIC PULMONARY EDEMA

Acute cardiogenic pulmonary edema is often the most intense and frightening symptom of acute LV dysfunction. As a result of marked elevations of left atrial and pulmonary capillary pressures, fluid rapidly accumulates in the alveolar spaces and pulmonary interstitium, interfering with gas exchange and hindering adequate oxygenation. Patients are usually overtly anxious, tachypneic, and tachycardic. They usually note dyspnea, orthopnea, paroxysmal nocturnal dyspnea, and possibly chest discomfort. Exam findings usually include elevated jugular venous pressure, an S_3 in the setting of systolic dysfunction, or an S_4 in the setting of diastolic dysfunction. The serum brain natriuretic peptide is elevated, because it is liberated by the LV when the end-diastolic pressure is high. The syndrome must be quickly identified and treatment initiated rapidly to prevent progressive hypoxemia, clinical deterioration, and death. Administer supplemental O_2 quickly, and monitor response by continuous pulse oximetry. Rapidly identify and treat precipitating factors. Obtain an ECG to evaluate for ischemia or arrhythmia and check cardiac enzymes serially to rule out infarction. Consider electrical cardioversion in the setting of a precipitating arrhythmia (e.g., AF or VT).

Agents to Treat Pulmonary Edema

Various pharmacologic agents used to treat acute pulmonary edema are discussed below.

Nitrates

Nitroglycerin (NTG) is considered the agent of choice for treating acute pulmonary edema. NTG dilates both arteries (systemic and coronary) and veins, quickly reducing afterload and preload and, as a consequence, relieving pulmonary congestion. It is available in multiple formulations. Sublingual NTG, either in pill or spray form, can be administered quickly without the need for IV access. The usual dose is 0.3–0.6 mg q5mins, not to exceed 1.2 mg in 15 mins. To ensure adequate absorption, spray is preferred over tablets if the patient has dry mucous membranes. IV NTG can be initiated at a rate of 5–10 μg/min and titrated upward every few minutes to the desired effect or to a maximum of 300 μg/min. Nitrate tolerance (i.e., declining effectiveness with continuous administration) can develop quickly (by 24 hrs) but can be avoided with the use of nitrate-free intervals. Because of their delay in onset of action, NTG pastes, ointments, and transdermal patches are not used to treat acute pulmonary edema. Side effects of nitrates include headache, nausea, vomiting, hypotension, and, rarely, bradycardia and methemoglobinemia. Nitrates are contraindicated if the systolic BP is <90 mm Hg, if there is severe aortic stenosis or HCM with an outflow gradient, or if the patient has recently taken sildenafil (Viagra).

Morphine Sulfate

Because of its rapid venodilatory effect and its ability to curb the intense anxiety associated with O_2 starvation, morphine sulfate is useful in the treatment of acute pulmonary edema. It can be administered in doses of 2–5 mg slow IV push, with close observation for potential adverse effects, including hypotension or respiratory depression.

Diuretics

Apart from its ability to reduce total body salt and water, furosemide given as a single dose of 40–80 mg IV is useful in treating acute pulmonary edema. It acts a direct venodilator, thereby reducing preload. A second dose can be administered after 15–20 mins, with close attention to urine output and volume status.

Nitroprusside

A powerful vasodilatory agent, sodium nitroprusside can be used to augment afterload and preload reduction when the aforementioned agents are inadequate, usually in the setting of a hypertensive crisis. Sodium nitroprusside is also used in patients with severe pump failure due to systolic dysfunction to reduce systemic vascular resistance when a Swan-Ganz catheter is in place [see Chap. 24, Procedures in Cardiovascular Critical Care (Intraaortic Balloon Pump, Swan-Ganz Catheterization, Temporary Transvenous Pacemaker)]. It is usually started at a dose of 0.1 μg/kg/min IV and titrated to a maximum dose of 5 μg/kg/min. Given its potency and risk of hypotension, titration of this agent should be guided by arterial catheterization. Besides hypotension, common side effects include nausea, vomiting, and diaphoresis. In the setting of significant hepatic or renal impairment, patients may develop cyanide or thiocyanate toxicity, respectively. Nitroprusside is contraindicated in the setting of acute myocardial ischemia, given its ability to worsen ischemia by precipitating a coronary steal phenomenon. If used >24 hrs, a thiocyanate level must be checked to assess for accumulation.

Bronchodilators
Nebulized albuterol in 2.5-mg doses may be a useful adjunct if significant bronchospasm is present.

Inotropic Agents
If pulmonary edema proves refractory to the previously listed measures, use of inotropic agents such as dobutamine or milrinone (Primacor) may be effective in the setting of severe LV systolic dysfunction. Use these agents and adjust doses with the aid of pulmonary artery catheterization. Inotropic agents are proarrhythmic and may increase myocardial O_2 demand, so they must be used with extreme caution in the setting of active ischemia or arrhythmia. Choose the smallest dose necessary to provide the desired response to avoid side effects. Dobutamine is a relatively beta$_1$-adrenergic receptor–specific sympathomimetic that increases contractility and heart rate. It is initiated at a dose of 2–3 μg/kg/min IV and titrated, according to response, to a maximum of 15 μg/kg/min. Its potency is reduced in the setting of high degrees of beta blockade (in this setting, milrinone may be preferred). Milrinone is a phosphodiesterase inhibitor that inhibits the hydrolysis of cAMP, the second messenger downstream of beta-adrenergic signaling. It has more potent vasodilatory properties than dobutamine, a difference that can be useful (to reduce pulmonary HTN) or harmful (it may cause systemic hypotension). Milrinone is started with a bolus dose of 0.25–0.75 μg/kg IV over 10–15 mins and then infused at a rate of 0.375–0.75 μg/kg/min. Because it is a potent vasodilator, avoid it in the setting of systemic hypotension. It is excreted primarily via the kidney and **requires significant dose reduction, or avoidance, in patients with renal insufficiency.** Inotropic agents are not helpful and may be harmful in the setting of heart failure due to HCM with LV outflow tract obstruction.

Brain Natriuretic Peptide (Nesiritide, Natrecor)
Several demonstrations with a recombinant preparation of brain natriuretic peptide have shown it is quite effective in effecting a natriuresis, lowering filling pressures, improving patient symptoms, and shortening hospitalization length [1,2]. Note that this medication is usually not necessary first-line therapy for patients presenting with acute pulmonary edema, and its expense is an important issue. For patients responding poorly to conventional diuretics and management with NTG, however, particularly in the setting of some degree of renal impairment, this medication can be useful. It is initiated with a 2 μg/kg IV bolus, followed by a 0.01 μg/kg/min continuous drip that can be titrated up to 0.03 μg/kg/min and administered for a maximum of 48 hrs.

CARDIOGENIC SHOCK
Cardiogenic shock is the most severe manifestation of acute cardiac pump failure. Despite available treatment modalities, it carries a short-term mortality rate of 50–80%. The optimal management strategy has yet to be defined through randomized, controlled clinical trials. The most common cause of cardiogenic shock is an extensive

MI, usually with a loss of >40% of functioning myocardium. Other causes include mechanical complications of acute MI (e.g., papillary muscle rupture, VSD or free-wall rupture, or acute valvular incompetence) or RV infarction, tamponade, acute aortic regurgitation, acute pulmonary embolus, arrhythmia, or myocarditis. It consists of a constellation of hemodynamic and clinical findings, including increased ventricular filling pressures, reduced cardiac output (cardiac index <2 L/min/m^2), systemic hypotension (systolic BP <90 mm Hg), tachycardia, increased systemic vascular resistance (>2100 dynes/sec/cm^{-5}), and evidence of end-organ hypoperfusion (e.g., altered mental status, oliguria, metabolic acidosis). Patients are often mildly confused or obtunded, and their extremities are cool. Evaluation should include urgent transthoracic echocardiography to identify any of the aforementioned precipitating events and invasive hemodynamic monitoring with the aid of Swan-Ganz and peripheral arterial catheterization to guide and assess response to treatment. Management in a cardiac ICU is imperative, and early involvement of cardiac surgery is frequently appropriate (see also Chap. 5, Cardiovascular Emergencies).

Initial Supportive Measures

Provide supplemental O_2 to the degree necessary to ensure adequate oxygenation. Rapidly diagnose and treat arrhythmias. Place pulmonary artery and peripheral arterial catheters for close hemodynamic monitoring.

Vasopressors

Vasopressors are vital agents for the initial stabilization of patients in cardiogenic shock to raise BP to an acceptable level. **Dopamine** is usually the first agent administered, starting at 5 μg/kg/min IV and titrating to a maximum of 20 μg/kg/min. If dopamine is inadequate, **norepinephrine** (Levophed), a potent vasoconstrictor, may be used for BP support; it is started at 0.04 μg/kg/min IV and titrated to a maximum dose of 0.4 μg/kg/min (or 50 μg/min). Inotropes, such as dobutamine and milrinone, although never used as monoagents in the setting of severe hypotension, may be added if BP is supported adequately with other agents to augment cardiac output.

Intraaortic Balloon Pump

An intraaortic ballon pump (IABP) may be inserted in patients who are unresponsive to medical management or as a bridge to coronary revascularization or cardiac surgery. It can effectively increase cardiac output by reducing afterload and augment arterial BP [see Chap. 24, Procedures in Cardiovascular Critical Care (Intraaortic Balloon Pump, Swan-Ganz Catheterization, and Temporary Transvenous Pacemaker)]. It is important to note that it can improve coronary perfusion via diastolic pressure augmentation. Complications of IABP insertion may include bleeding, infection, aortic wall damage, peripheral ischemia, hemolysis, thrombocytopenia, and acute renal failure from renal atheroembolism. **Aortic dissection and aortic insufficiency are absolute contraindications to IABP use.**

Revascularization

Numerous studies (e.g., the SHOCK trial [3]) have demonstrated the importance of rapidly restoring blood flow to the infarct-related artery in patients with acute MI complicated by cardiogenic shock. In this setting, mechanical revascularization is more effective than thrombolytic therapy at restoring coronary blood flow. These patients should undergo urgent cardiac catheterization with revascularization of the culprit artery by percutaneous transluminal coronary angioplasty or bypass grafting, depending on the degree and distribution of CAD found. Emergent cardiac surgery may provide the only hope of survival for patients with cardiogenic shock secondary to one of the aforementioned mechanical complications.

CHRONIC HEART FAILURE

Chronic HF affects approximately 2% of the adult population in the United States (4.5 million patients) and accounts for a large percentage of U.S. health care expenditures each year. Asymptomatic LV dysfunction, usually undiagnosed, likely affects millions more. Surprisingly, HF is the only cardiac disease that is increasing in prevalence. As the prevalence of HF increases with aging of the population, management of HF will become an increasingly important and costly issue.

Pathophysiology

The pathophysiology of HF initiates with a structural insult; infarct, HTN, genetics, toxins, metabolic syndromes, and infection are all possible contributing factors. These insults usually lead to activation of the renin-angiotensin, sympathetic nervous, cytokine, and natriuretic peptide systems. With time, the unopposed influence of these hormones yields as process known as *cardiac remodeling*. The ventricle shape changes, with dilation being a common response. The myocardium also changes microscopically, with myocate apoptosis and intercellular fibrosis evident.

History and Physical Exam

Patients with chronic HF present with a variety of classic findings on history and physical exam. They note increased dyspnea on exertion, orthopnea, and paroxysmal nocturnal dyspnea; they may note lower-extremity edema, abdominal distention, and decreased appetite. Risk factors include CAD, history of HTN or diabetes, valvular heart disease risk factors (rheumatic, infectious, anorectic drugs), and prior exposures (chemotherapy: cardiomyopathy; radiation, surgery: constrictive pericarditis); carefully assess these in the history. Exam findings may include elevated neck veins [jugular venous distention (JVD)], the S_3/S_4, a diffuse and displaced apical impulse, crackles in the lungs, lower-extremity edema, hepatojugular reflux, ascites, hepatomegaly, pulsus alternans, a diminished carotid upstroke, and/or muscle wasting (**cardiac cachexia**, especially in the neck, shoulders, and face). Note that patients with chronically developed HF may not exhibit physical or radiographic signs of pulmonary edema, because the pulmonary microvasculature gradually accommodates to the left-sided increased filling pressure. In this setting, the increased jugular venous pressure is the clue to the diagnosis.

Etiology

The first task when presented with a patient who exhibits HF is to determine the **etiology:** systolic, diastolic, valvular, pericardial, or a combination. Detect and treat acute ischemia and arrhythmias appropriately. Diminished carotid upstroke intensity, diminished S_1 intensity, a diffuse and displaced apical pulse, and an S_3 all suggest systolic dysfunction; their absence suggests that a diastolic component may be significant. Note **murmurs** carefully, as they may be entirely causative or merely contributing. Pericardial disease requires a high index of suspicion to detect. Tachycardia in the setting of hypotension should always trigger the possible diagnosis of tamponade. Constrictive pericarditis (see Chap. 16, Disease of the Pericardium) is suggested by JVD, lower-extremity edema, ascites, and absence of lung crackles. Isolated right HF occurs with JVD, lower-extremity edema, hepatomegaly, a right-sided S_3/S_4 (increased intensity with inspiration), and/or ascites in the absence of lung crackles. **The physical exam's importance cannot be underestimated.** As recently as 2001, a primary article demonstrated the prognostic significance of JVD and the S_3, with each being an independent predictor of mortality [4]. Furthermore, in the "days of the giants" of medicine and cardiology, these diagnoses were all made entirely by history and physical exams.

Diagnostic Studies

Diagnostic studies help distinguish the pathophysiology behind HF. **If there is systolic dysfunction, it is of utmost importance in the patient newly presenting with HF to determine if the cause is ischemic or nonischemic.** Initial indicated studies include chest x-ray (assessment of heart size, pulmonary edema with Kerley lines, pulmonary vascular redistribution), ECG, CBC, UA, electrolytes and creatinine, and TSH. Employ transthoracic echocardiography early in the assessment process. Coronary angiography is appropriate in patients with angina or significant ischemic changes on ECG. Noninvasive stress testing is appropriate in patients without angina but who may have coronary disease. Screening for rare causes with tests such as iron studies (hemochromatosis), serum protein electrophoresis (amyloid), and Coxsackie viral PCR (myocarditis) is useful occasionally. Endomyocardial biopsy is rarely useful, as the treatment is usually not impacted. For example, immunosuppressive therapy has been demonstrated not to be useful in patients with viral myocarditis. In rare circumstances, such as giant cell myocarditis, eosinophilic myocarditis, and amyloidosis, treatment will be altered by the result of the biopsy. **Remember that the majority of HF is caused by ischemic heart disease (prior MI), HTN, or idiopathic nonischemic disease whose treatment is not altered by the underlying cause, provided patient is maximally revascularized.**

Management

In stark contrast to acute HF, in which case the major goals of management are to stabilize the patient and reduce short-term morbidity and mortality, the goals of chronic HF management are (a) improving long-term survival, (b) reducing symptoms of HF, (c) increasing functional capacity and thereby reducing the number of hospitalizations for decompensated HF, and (d) preventing—and potentially reversing—cardiac remodeling. Although a large number of pharmacologic agents and nonpharmacologic approaches are used to manage CHF, the most appropriate combination of these different modalities depends to a great extent on the **functional class** of the patient. The **New York Heart Association (NYHA) Functional Classification** is the most widely used.

- I: Patients with cardiac disease but with virtually no limitation of physical activity
- II: Patients with cardiac disease that causes slight reduction of physical activity (dyspnea with overt exertion)
- III: Patients with cardiac disease that causes marked reduction of physical activity (dyspnea with minimal exertion, ordinary activities of daily living)
- IV: Patients with cardiac disease that causes inability to perform any physical activity (dyspnea at rest)

Treatment strategies available for HF are outlined below. They are usually used in combination, depending on the underlying etiology of the HF and the particular patient's symptoms.

Nonpharmacologic Approaches

All patients with HF should adhere to a diet with moderate **salt restriction.** Reducing dietary intake of sodium helps to reduce water retention, thereby reducing symptoms of vascular congestion. Additionally, low-salt diets help reduce the dose of diuretic agent needed to keep a patient's volume status balanced and acceptable. HF patients should avoid alcohol. **Weight reduction** is important for obese patients. **Comorbid conditions,** such as HTN, diabetes mellitus, and hyperlipidemia, should be identified and managed appropriately. **Regular exercise,** including cardiac rehabilitation consisting of mild to moderate amounts of regular aerobic activity, has been shown in numerous studies to improve functional capacity and reduce symptoms (although not mortality) in HF patients and should be encouraged. A trial sponsored by the NIH is under way that further assesses the role of exercise in heart failure. **Close follow-up** with a cardiologist is vital, both to encourage compliance with an often extensive medical regimen and to avoid use of any agents that may reduce the effectiveness of or adversely interact with HF medications.

Pharmacologic Agents

ACE Inhibitors

Numerous studies have demonstrated the ability of ACE inhibitors to substantially reduce morbidity and mortality in patients with HF. These agents are the cornerstone

TABLE 10-1. ACE INHIBITORS USED IN HF

Drug	Initial dose	Usual maximum dose
Captopril	6.25 mg PO tid	50 mg PO tid
Enalapril	2.5 mg PO bid	20 mg PO bid
Fosinopril	5–10 mg PO qd	40 mg PO qd
Lisinopril	2.5–5 mg PO qd	20–40 mg PO qd or divided bid
Quinapril	10 mg PO bid	40 mg PO bid
Ramipril	1.25–2.5 PO qd	10 mg PO qd

From Hunt SA, Baker DW, Chin MH, et al. ACC/AHA Guidelines for the Evaluation and Management of Chronic Heart Failure in the Adult. http://www.acc.org/clinical/guidelines/failure/hf_index.htm, 2001, with permission.

of therapy in patients with systolic dysfunction. In the setting of a recent MI, the SAVE, AIRE, and TRACE trials are classic examples of studies that demonstrated morbidity and mortality benefit with use of ACE inhibitors. Independent of the setting of acute MI, the ATLAS, CONSENSUS, and SOLVD trials also demonstrated morbidity and mortality benefit with use of ACE inhibitors in HF with systolic dysfunction. Thus, they are first-line agents and are considered a mandatory part of the treatment regimen for patients with systolic dysfunction (independent of the presence of HF symptoms), barring any absolute contraindications. In addition, the HOPE study demonstrated that even in patients with **normal** LV function who had risk factors such as CAD or diabetes, the use of ramipril decreased morbidity and mortality. ACE inhibitors reduce afterload and preload, thereby reducing vascular congestion and symptoms. More important, they attenuate the deleterious effect of the renin-angiotensin system on cardiac myocytes, including hypertrophy, apoptosis, remodeling, and progressive dysfunction. Many specific agents exist (Table 10-1), and the dose chosen should be at least equivalent to the dose shown to reduce mortality in various clinical trials. Patients are usually started on a low dose of a specific agent and titrated slowly toward goal, paying careful attention to serum creatinine, potassium, and BP. Side effects include cough (due to an increase in bradykinin levels, whose metabolism is inhibited by ACE inhibitors), angioedema (rare and an absolute contraindication to further ACE-inhibitor therapy), dysgeusia, hyperkalemia, renal insufficiency, hypotension, and teratogenicity. They should not be used in the presence of bilateral renal artery stenosis, because they can abruptly worsen creatinine clearance.

Angiotensin-II Receptor Blockers
Because angiotensin-II receptor blockers (ARBs) (Table 10-2) do not increase bradykinin levels and do not cause cough, they are often used as a substitute for ACE inhibitors in patients who are intolerant to the drugs for these reasons. Similar to ACE inhibitors, they can cause hyperkalemia and worsening renal function. Early studies, such as ELITE-II and RESOLVD, showed promise for ARBs in HF management. Therefore, ARBs should be used in patients intolerant to ACE inhibitors. The recent Val-HeFT study confirmed this and showed nonmortality–derived benefit with ACE inhibitor–ARB combination but no mortality benefit with combination ACE inhibitor/ARB therapy compared to ACE inhibitor alone. In patients who are already being treated with an ACE inhibitor and beta blocker, however, the addition of an ARB appeared to worsen survival. Thus, ACE inhibitors are preferred over ARBs, but ARBs have an important role in ACE inhibitor–intolerant patients.

Beta Blockers
Once thought deleterious in HF management, **beta blockers are now considered first-line treatment in patients with HF** (Table 10-3). Numerous studies, including

TABLE 10-2. ANGIOTENSIN-RECEPTOR ANTAGONISTS USED IN HF

Drug	Initial dose	Usual maximum dose
Candesartan	8 mg PO qd	32 mg PO qd
Irbesartan	75 mg PO qd	300 mg PO qd
Losartan	25 mg PO qd	100 mg PO qd
Valsartan	80 mg PO qd	320 mg PO qd
Telmisartan	20 mg PO qd	80 mg PO qd

From *Tarascon pocket pharmacopeia.* Loma Linda, CA: Tarascon Publishing, 2002, with permission.

MERIT-HF, MOCHA, and CIBIS, have demonstrated the ability of various beta-blocking agents to reduce mortality in HF patients. Metoprolol (beta$_1$ selective) and carvedilol (alpha$_1$/beta$_1$/beta$_2$ nonselective) have emerged as the most studied and effective agents for HF. Their beneficial effect stems from beta-blockers' ability to attenuate deleterious effects of adrenergic stimulation and upregulation present in HF, resulting in stabilization of remodeling or even **reverse remodeling,** an actual improvement of systolic function in some patients. Although most of the previously mentioned studies assessed patients with NYHA class II–III symptoms, the COPERNICUS trial showed significant mortality reduction with beta blockade in class IV patients. The forthcoming COMET trial compares carvedilol and metoprolol. Initiate beta blockers only in patients with well-compensated HF (euvolemic) on optimal doses of standard HF medication (including ACE inhibitors and diuretics). They should be started at low doses and advanced as tolerated to doses shown to be beneficial in clinical trials. Beta blockers should be used with caution in patients with reactive airway disease, cardiac conduction system disease, and bradycardia.

Digoxin
Digitalis glycosides were among the first medications used for the treatment of symptomatic HF. By inhibiting the Na^+/K^+-ATPase enzymes in cardiac myocytes, digoxin increases the velocity of myocyte shortening, effectively increasing the force of ventricular contraction. Although digoxin has not been shown to reduce mortality in HF, multiple trials, including the DIG study, have shown it reduces symptoms of HF and improves functional status, thereby reducing hospitalizations and improving quality of life. It is the drug of choice in controlling ventricular rate in AF among patients with HF. Studies, including PROVED and RADIANCE, showed worsening of symp-

TABLE 10-3. BETA-ADRENERGIC RECEPTOR ANTAGONISTS USED IN HF

Drug	Initial dose	Usual maximum dose
Bisoprolol	1.25 mg PO qd	10 mg PO qd
Carvedilol	3.125 mg PO bid	25 mg PO bid (50 mg bid if >85 kg)
Metoprolol tartrate (Lopressor)	6.25 mg PO bid	75 mg PO bid
Metoprolol succinate (Toprol XL)	12.5 mg PO qd	200 mg PO qd

From Hunt SA, Baker DW, Chin MH, et al. ACC/AHA Guidelines for the Evaluation and Management of Chronic Heart Failure in the Adult. http://www.acc.org/clinical/guidelines/failure/hf_index.htm, 2001, with permission.

toms and increased hospitalizations after withdrawing digoxin from the regimen of HF patients who were previously tolerating the drug.

Historically in HF, digoxin was loaded IV ("digitalization"), and subsequent doses of 0.25–0.375 mg PO qd were given. However, increasing evidence is mounting that demonstrates adequate symptom improvement with a lower-dose regimen, 0.125 mg PO qd, extended to qod if there is renal impairment. Not only is this dosing effective, but it also reduces the likelihood of development of digoxin-related toxicity, a significantly morbid event that is in part created by **digoxin's small therapeutic window,** particularly in women. Serum levels between 0.5–2.0 mg/dL have been historically deemed "therapeutic," **but toxicity may occur despite a therapeutic level,** and achievement of these levels is not required for symptomatic improvement. One exception to the avoidance of IV digoxin loading is in the setting of HF with AF with rapid ventricular response, in which case it often is loaded. Toxicity is enhanced in the setting of renal failure (particularly relevant in HF patients who have tenuous hemodynamics that lead to renal failure), hypokalemia, hypomagnesemia, and in the presence of other agents that effectively increase serum digoxin levels (e.g., amiodarone). Toxic side effects include GI upset, visual disturbances (scotomas, halos around lights), and arrhythmias (including AV nodal and other conduction blocks, supraventricular and ventricular arrhythmias). Digoxin-associated tachyarrhythmias are classically treated with IV phenytoin. See Chap. 14, Bradycardia and Permanent Pacemakers, for management of bradyarrhythmias in the setting of digoxin toxicity.

Diuretics

Increased intravascular volume in chronic HF causes symptoms of fluid overload, including dyspnea, orthopnea, paroxysmal nocturnal dyspnea, fatigue, etc. In addition, data suggest that volume overload also leads to increased ventricular wall stress with remodeling and hypertrophy. Diuretics control volume overload and, thus, are important agents in the treatment regimen for HF (Table 10-4). Several types of diuretics exist and can be classified according to site of action in the nephron. These include loop diuretics (e.g., furosemide, the most commonly used diuretic in chronic HF), thiazide diuretics, and potassium-sparing diuretics. With the exception of spironolactone [see Spironolactone (Aldactone)], however, no diuretic has been shown to reduce mortality in HF. Use the lowest dose of diuretic that will keep the patient euvolemic to reduce the incidence of side effects. Ideally, an HF regimen including optimal doses of ACE inhibitors should allow the diuretic dose to be reduced substantially. Diuretic resistance is a common problem with prolonged use. Often, the underlying factor leading to resistance is failure to adhere to a low-salt diet or the use of medications that interfere with diuretics' mechanism of action (e.g., NSAIDs, probenecid). Sometimes, the dose and/or dosing frequency must be increased or a second diuretic must be added for synergy (e.g., metolazone to furosemide). Side effects include hypokalemia (usually requiring potassium supplementation), hyponatremia, alkalosis, and hyperglycemia. Particular to thiazide diuretics, hyperuricemia, hyperlipidemia, and hypercalcemia may result. Use IV diuretics early in a patient's presentation with congestive HF, as absorption of PO diuretic is reduced due to bowel wall edema.

TABLE 10-4. LOOP DIURETICS USED IN HF

Drug	Initial dose	Usual maximum dose
Bumetanide	0.5–1 mg PO qd–bid	Up to 10 mg PO qd
Furosemide	20–40 mg PO qd–bid	Up to 400 mg PO qd
Torsemide	10–20 mg PO qd–bid	Up to 400 mg PO qd

From Hunt SA, Baker DW, Chin MH, et al. ACC/AHA Guidelines for the Evaluation and Management of Chronic Heart Failure in the Adult. http://www.acc.org/clinical/guidelines/failure/hf_index.htm, 2001, with permission.

Combination Therapy: Hydralazine and Nitrates

In patients who absolutely cannot tolerate ACE inhibitors or ARBs due to cough, angioedema, or renal dysfunction, the combination of hydralazine (Apresoline) and nitrates is an acceptable alternative. The VheFT-I trial showed some symptomatic relief in HF patients treated with this regimen and even some reduction in mortality (although not to the same extent as ACE inhibitors). Hydralazine at a dose of 75–100 mg PO tid-qid is usually combined with isosorbide dinitrate at a dose of 10–30 mg PO tid. Side effects of this regimen include hypotension and a lupus-like syndrome (hydralazine). This regimen also does not foster compliance because of this complicated dosing.

Spironolactone (Aldactone)

Because of the results of the RALES study, which showed a 30% reduction in mortality in patients with NYHA class III–IV HF treated with Aldactone, in addition to substantial reductions in HF symptoms and hospitalizations, Aldactone is recommended in the treatment of patients with severe HF. The recommended dose is 25 mg PO daily. Possible side effects include hyperkalemia (thus, patients on loop diuretics and Aldactone may need reduction or discontinuation of K^+ supplements) and gynecomastia.

Anticoagulation

Chronic anticoagulation is indicated if there is concomitant AF, a prior cardioembolic event, a recent large (particularly anterior) MI, or a demonstrated intracardiac thrombus. Anticoagulation is controversial in the setting of reduced ejection fraction alone.

Inotropic Therapy

Home dobutamine and milrinone (see Inotropic Agents above for description and dosing) frequently are used in patients who have severe LV dysfunction refractory to maximum PO medications. Such patients usually exhibit tenuous hemodynamics, with systolic BPs in the 90–100 mm Hg range, and are frequently in acute renal failure when overdiuresed. The hemodynamic window in which they live is very narrow, and their symptoms are usually improved on inotropes. There are no adequately sized randomized controlled trials that assess the morbidity and mortality of patients who are on chronic inotropes, although one must be aware of the higher theoretical risk of ventricular arrhythmias in the presence of inotropes. There is no supported role of routine intermittent inotrope use (the "dobutamine holiday"). One note on the selection of an inotrope is that unlike dobutamine, milrinone (if not contraindicated) permits the concomitant administration of beta blockers, which are of tremendous benefit in HF. A distinct disadvantage with IV inotropic therapy is the requirement for an indwelling IV line, which predisposes to risk of infection and thrombosis.

DIASTOLIC DYSFUNCTION

A special note should be made with regard to therapy for patients with isolated diastolic dysfunction. The condition is diagnosed by physical exam and echocardiography. With isolated diastolic function, physical exam features of HF are present, including JVD, and possibly pulmonary edema. The apical pulse may be pronounced, and the S_4 is present on auscultation. On echocardiography, systolic function may be normal, but diastolic filling patterns are typically abnormal on spectral Doppler [see Chap. 22, Imaging and Diagnostic Testing Modalities (Nuclear Imaging, Echocardiography, and Cardiac Catheterization)]. This condition is common among those with diabetes mellitus, those with chronic, poorly treated HTN, often in the setting of concentric LVH, and in the elderly: It accounts for >50% of HF in persons >75 yrs, compared with <10% in those <65 yrs, and is more common in women [5–7]. To understand treatment, one must appreciate that diastolic dysfunction is a disorder of both **relaxation** (a calcium-dependent physiologic process) and **stiffness** (structural property), and available therapies target one or both of these problems. Relaxation is an energy-dependent process that occurs early in diastole. Stiffness, which plays more of a role in the diastasis and atrial filling, is determined in part by compliance and is more passive.

Practically speaking, the most important features of **management** include control of diabetes and HTN, ventricular rate if AF is present, volume status, and ischemia. Coronary revascularization, if appropriate, may improve diastolic function. To date, no large trials of a specific therapy for diastolic dysfunction have been completed. With angiotensin therapy (ARBs, ACE inhibitors), it is possible that the sarcomeric, cellular, and interstitial remodeling that underlies both poor relaxation and stiffness may be reversible. At this point, pharmacologic management is empiric and should be guided by prevailing comorbidities and symptomatic relief. Diuretics and nitrates can be used to relieve congestion and orthopnea, but cautious attention for overdiuresis and declining renal function are essential. Often, seemingly minor increases in the dose of a diuretic can overwhelm the delicate volume status of older patients with diastolic dysfunction. ACE inhibitors and beta blockers should be used in patients who have vascular disease or have had an MI, although specific improvement in diastolic dysfunction has not been demonstrated [8,9]. Calcium channel blockers and ARBs are effective antihypertensive agents in elderly patients and may provide symptomatic relief in some patients with diastolic chronic HF. The beneficial effects of digoxin on chronic HF symptoms and rehospitalization also extend to patients with diastolic dysfunction and are an alternative when other therapies are ineffective [10]. Ultimately, a trial of different medications may be the best way of managing pharmacotherapy in older patients with diastolic dysfunction.

DEVICE THERAPY

For patients with severe HF refractory to maximal medical management, device therapy has been designed and is used in patients who usually exhibit severe systolic dysfunction (ejection fraction $\leq 25\%$).

Biventricular Pacemaker

Among patients with HF, there commonly is intraventricular conduction delay (QRS duration >130 msecs) found on ECG. This conduction abnormality can lead to poorly coordinated ventricular contraction and, therefore, may significantly impair LV function. Biventricular (BiV) pacemakers usually consist of pacing leads in the right atrium, the RV, and a cardiac vein draining the LV (juxtaposed against the lateral LV wall). The device electronically restores coordinated contraction of the two ventricles, "resynchronizing" ventricular contraction. AV timing can also be specified to optimize hemodynamics. The MUSTIC investigators evaluated this treatment modality in a series of patients with severe HF and prolonged QRS intervals on ECG and showed that BiV pacing increases exercise tolerance and improves other quality-of-life measures. The MIRACLE investigators [11] demonstrated in patients with symptomatic HF improvements in distance walked in 6 mins, functional class, quality of life, time on the treadmill during exercise testing, ejection fraction, required hospitalizations, and use of IV medications for the treatment of HF. There was no mortality benefit.

Implantable Cardioverter-Defibrillator

Patients with severe HF, particularly those with CAD, are at significant risk for malignant ventricular arrhythmias and sudden cardiac death. Implantable cardioverter-defibrillators (ICDs) are similar in design to pacemakers except that they are programmed to detect and terminate potentially lethal arrhythmias. The AVID trial established ICD therapy as superior to antiarrhythmic pharmacotherapy in patients with LV systolic dysfunction (ejection fraction <40%) and a history of sustained ventricular arrhythmia, showing a significant reduction in sudden death with ICD placement. The MADIT and MUSTT trials showed a survival benefit in patients with LV dysfunction, prior MI, and nonsustained VT with prophylactic ICD placement compared to drug therapy. The MADIT2 trial showed mortality benefit in prophylactic implantation in patients with a prior MI and LV ejection fraction <30% alone. See Chap. 15, Tachyarrhythmias, Sudden Cardiac Death, and Implantable Cardioverter-Defibrillators, for further discussion. The combination of ICDs with BiV pacemakers was investigated in the COMPANION trial, whose preliminarily released results reveal benefit of BiV-ICD implantation for appropriate patients.

Ventricular Assist Device

Ventricular assist devices (VADs) are mechanical pumps that unload the RV or LV and support the associated circulation (pulmonary or systemic, respectively), restoring normal hemodynamics and end-organ function. The RVAD withdraws blood from the right atrium and returns it to the main pulmonary artery; the LVAD pumps blood from the implanted left atrium or LV apex and returns it to the ascending aorta; the BiVAD supports both circulations. A variety of technologic advances have yielded portability and improved long-term outcomes: 90% of patients implanted are discharged from the hospital, and approximately 60% survive to transplant. Traditionally, the goal of VADs has been to "bridge" patients to transplant, providing patients with chronic HF who are too sick to survive to transplant with some form of support. The shortage of donor hearts available has increased the use of these devices, which in some patients are implanted for years. Such patients exhibit signs and symptoms of organ hypoperfusion. A small subset of patients, such as those with postcardiotomy shock, a large MI, or fulminant myocarditis, receive VADs as a "bridge to recovery," merely allowing time for the heart to recover in the setting of cardiogenic shock. The contraindications to VAD therapy traditionally are those of cardiac transplantation (see Cardiac Transplantation).

There has been interest in using VADs as destination therapy in patients who are not transplant candidates. The REMATCH trial [12] demonstrated some reduction in mortality for patients compared to maximal medical management. Mortality was very high in both groups, however. The INTrEPID trial is ongoing and evaluates this issue with a different device from that used in the REMATCH trial, with hope that the number of strokes is reduced. The most common complications of VAD implantation are bleeding, thromboembolism (cerebrovascular accident), and infection.

The modern total artificial heart has been implanted in several people in the United States over the last few years and remains experimental. In future generations, the total artificial heart may be a solution to the shortage of donor hearts available.

CARDIAC TRANSPLANTATION

The definitive therapy for the failing heart is cardiac transplantation. Candidates have failed maximal medical therapy and often have evidence of organ hypoperfusion. Maximal O_2 consumption ($\dot{V}O_2$max, in mL/kg/m^2) is assessed in potential candidates by measuring O_2 uptake during treadmill exercise. A $\dot{V}O_2$max <14 (or <50% predicted for age and size) is considered predictive of a poorer 1-yr survival with medical therapy than with cardiac transplantation.

Transplantation has been very successful. In the 1980s, the number of cardiac transplants increased dramatically because of the presence of cyclosporin immunosuppressant. The 1-yr survival after transplant is 85%, with 5-yr survivals of 70%. Success depends on careful selection of patients and vigorous follow-up posttransplant. **Transplantation is not a cure** but replaces one medical condition with another. **Contraindications** include severe pulmonary HTN, moderate to severe renal insufficiency, active infection, severe COPD or reactive airway disease, primary hepatic dysfunction with coagulopathy, morbid obesity, recent stroke, severe nontreatable neurologic or psychiatric dysfunction, severe peripheral vascular or carotid artery disease, advanced age (>70), and disseminated malignancy. Patients who are ventilator dependent fare very poorly. Despite the exclusion criteria, approximately 30% of patients who are listed die while waiting for a donor heart; as a result, VADs have filled an important niche.

Transplantation **complications** include acute rejection, infection (common infections as well as those of the immunocompromised, such as CMV and pneumocystis), increased risk for the development of malignancy, and chronic rejection (transplant CAD or allograft vasculopathy). Aggressive immunosuppression, infection prophylaxis, endomyocardial biopsy surveys, assessment for allograft vasculopathy, control of HTN, tumor surveillance, and use of a statin are all required to promote increased survival. A high suspicion for acute rejection must be maintained for all transplant patients presenting to the hospital with virtually **any** chief complaint.

KEY POINTS TO REMEMBER

- HF is a very common entity in Western civilization, resulting in a high degree of morbidity and mortality.
- The underlying cause of acute HF should be determined to limit morbidity and mortality and to prevent future recurrence.
- The first order of business in the assessment of a newly diagnosed cardiomyopathy with systolic dysfunction is to determine the contribution of CAD to the condition.
- Cardiomyopathy with chronic symptoms of HF should be aggressively treated with nonpharmacologic and pharmacologic therapy.
- In the absence of contraindication, ACE inhibitors form the cornerstone of appropriate medical therapy for acute and chronic HF. Furthermore, beta blockers should be administered as soon as a patient has been rendered euvolemic with diuresis. Each is started at a low dose and titrated up.
- Ideally, the beta blocker is titrated to reach maximum dose, a feature that is less important than with ACE inhibitors.
- Digoxin is associated with an improvement in HF symptoms and reduced hospitalizations but is not associated with improved survival.
- Acute and chronic HF not responsive to PO therapy may require IV inotropy, mechanical therapy, or even heart transplantation in appropriate patients.

ACKNOWLEDGMENT

We thank Roger Kerzner for his research and input on diastolic dysfunction.

SUGGESTED READING

Antiarrhythmics versus Implantable Defibrillators (AVID) Investigators. A comparison of antiarrhythmic drug therapy with implantable defibrillators in patients resuscitated from near-fatal ventricular arrhythmias. *N Engl J Med* 1997;337:1576–1583.

Braunwald E, Zipes DP, Libby P. Treatment of heart failure: pharmacological methods. In: Braunwald E, ed. *Heart disease: a textbook of cardiovascular medicine*. Philadelphia: WB Saunders, 2001.

Brown NJ, Vaughan DE. Angiotensin-converting enzyme inhibitors. *Circulation* 1998; 97:1411–1420.

CIBIS Investigators and Committees. A randomized trial of beta-blockade in heart failure: the Cardiac Insufficiency Bisoprolol Study (CIBIS). *Circulation* 1994;90:1765–1773.

Cohn JN, Archibald DG, Ziesche S, et al. Effect of vasodilator therapy on mortality in chronic congestive heart failure. Results of a Veterans Administration Cooperative Study. *N Engl J Med* 1986;314:1547–1552.

CONSENSUS Trial Study Group. Effects of enalapril on mortality in severe congestive heart failure: results of the Cooperative North Scandinavian Enalapril Survival Study (CONSENSUS). *N Engl J Med* 1987;316:1429–1435.

COPERNICUS Trial Study Group. Effect of carvedilol on survival in severe chronic heart failure: results of the Carvedilol Prospective Randomized Cumulative Survival (COPERNICUS) Study Group. *N Engl J Med* 2001;22:1651–1658.

Hunt SA, Baker DW, Chin MH, et al. ACC/AHA guidelines for the evaluation and management of chronic heart failure in the adult. A report of the American College of Cardiology/American Heart Association Task Force on Practice Guidelines (Committee to Revise the 1995 Guidelines for the Evaluation and Management of Heart Failure), 2001. Available at http://www.acc.org/clinical/guidelines/failure/hf_index.htm.

Hunt SA, Baker DW, Chin MH, et al. ACC/AHA guidelines for the evaluation and management of chronic heart failure in the adult: executive summary. A report of the American College of Cardiology/American Heart Association Task Force on Practice Guidelines (Committee to Revise the 1995 Guidelines for the Evaluation and Management of Heart Failure). *Circulation* 2001;104:2996–3007.

Jessup M, Brozena S. Heart failure. *N Engl J Med* 2003;348(20):2007–2018.
Multicenter Automatic Defibrillator Implantation Trial (MADIT) Investigators. Improved survival with an implanted defibrillator in patients with coronary disease at high risk for ventricular arrhythmia. *N Engl J Med* 1996;335:1933–1940.
Multisite Stimulation in Cardiomyopathies (MUSTIC) Study Investigators. Effects of multisite biventricular pacing in patients with heart failure and intraventricular conduction delay. *N Engl J Med* 2001;344:873–880.
Packer M, Gheorghiade M, Young JB, et al., for the RADIENCE Study. Withdrawal of digoxin from patients with chronic heart failure treated with angiotensin-converting enzyme inhibitors. *N Engl J Med* 1993;329:1–7.
Pitt B, Poole-Wilson PA, Segal R, et al. Effect of losartan compared with captopril on mortality of patients with symptomatic heart failure: randomised trial. The Losartan Heart Failure Survival Study (ELITE II). *Lancet* 2000;355:1582–1587.
Pitt B, Zannad F, Remme WJ, et al. The effect of spironolactone on morbidity and mortality in patients with severe heart failure. Randomized Aldactone Evaluation Study (RALES) Investigators. *N Engl J Med* 1999;341:709–717.
RESOLVD Pilot Study Investigators. Comparison of candesartan, enalapril, and their combination in congestive heart failure. *Circulation* 1999;100:1056–1064.
SHOCK Investigators. Early revascularization in acute myocardial infarction complicated by cardiogenic shock. *N Engl J Med* 1999;9:625–634.
Valsartan Heart Failure Trial (Val-HeFT) Investigators. A randomised trial of the angiotensin-receptor blocker valsartan in chronic heart failure. *N Engl J Med* 2001;345:1667–1675.

REFERENCES

1. Intravenous nesiritide vs nitroglycerin for treatment of decompensated congestive heart failure: a randomized controlled trial. *JAMA* 2002;287(12):1531–1540.
2. Colucci WS, Elkayam U, Horton DP, et al. Intravenous nesiritide, a natriuretic peptide, in the treatment of decompensated congestive heart failure. Nesiritide Study Group. *N Engl J Med* 2000;343(4):246–253.
3. Hochman JS, Sleeper LA, Webb JG, et al. Early revascularization in acute myocardial infarction complicated by cardiogenic shock. SHOCK Investigators. Should We Emergently Revascularize Occluded Coronaries for Cardiogenic Shock. *N Engl J Med* 1999;341(9):625–634.
4. Drazner MH, Rame JE, Stevenson LW, et al. Prognostic importance of elevated jugular venous pressure and a third heart sound in patients with heart failure. *N Engl J Med* 2001;345:574–581.
5. Vasan RS, Larson MG, Benjamin EJ, et al. Congestive heart failure in subjects with normal versus reduced left ventricular ejection fraction: prevalence and mortality in a population-based cohort. *J Am Coll Cardiol* 1999;33:1948.
6. Wong WF, Gold S, Fukuyama O, et al. Diastolic dysfunction in elderly patients with congestive heart failure. *Am J Cardiol* 1989;63:1526.
7. Kitzman DW, Gardin JM, Gottdiener JS, et al. Importance of heart failure with preserved systolic function in patients > or = 65 years of age. CHS Research Group. Cardiovascular Health Study. *Am J Cardiol* 2001;87:413.
8. Yusuf S, Sleight P, Pogue J, et al. Effects of an angiotensin-converting-enzyme inhibitor, ramipril, on cardiovascular events in high-risk patients. The Heart Outcomes Prevention Evaluation Study Investigators. *N Engl J Med* 2000;342:145–153.
9. Aronow WS. Management of older persons after myocardial infarction. *J Am Geriatr Soc* 1998;46:1459–1468.
10. The effect of digoxin on mortality and morbidity in patients with heart failure. The Digitalis Investigation Group. *N Engl J Med* 1997;336:525.
11. Abraham WT, Fisher WG, Smith AL, et al. Cardiac resynchronization in chronic heart failure. *N Engl J Med* 2002;346(24):1845–1853.
12. Rose EA, Gelijns AC, Moskowitz AJ, et al. Long-term mechanical left ventricular assistance for end-stage heart failure. *N Engl J Med* 2001;345:1435–1443.

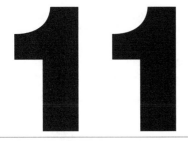

Atrial Fibrillation

Michael J. Riley and
Peter A. Crawford

INTRODUCTION

Epidemiology

Atrial fibrillation (AF) is the most common sustained arrhythmia seen in clinical practice and accounts for significant morbidity and mortality worldwide. Epidemiologic data derived from the Framingham Study, among others, suggest that AF affects up to 1% of the general population, with a cumulative incidence slightly higher in men than in women. The prevalence of AF increases dramatically with the presence of structural heart disease and with age. Specifically, data indicate a prevalence of 0.5% in the population subgroup aged 50–59, increasing steadily for each decade to almost 10% for those in their ninth decade of life. The importance of AF as a clinical entity cannot be overemphasized, as its presence portends a mortality rate twice that of the general population. Most important, AF accounts for up to a fivefold increase in the risk of stroke, particularly in the setting of rheumatic heart disease. And because analysis of Framingham data also indicates that the age-adjusted prevalence of AF is increasing, the actual impact of AF on overall morbidity and mortality may be much greater than initially realized.

CAUSES

Pathophysiology

- Although there are many theories to explain the mechanism of **AF**, the one most widely accepted cites **atrial reentry** as the underlying electrophysiologic abnormality. According to this theory, multiple reentrant impulses propagate throughout the atria in a chaotic fashion, producing an atrial rate in excess of 400 bpm. Except in cases in which an accessory pathway is present (see Fig. 15-8), conduction travels through the AV node to trigger ventricular contraction. Because the excitability of the AV node is considerably less than that of atrial tissue, conduction slows and usually produces a ventricular rate of 110–170 bpm (in the absence of intrinsic conduction system disease or concomitant drug therapy). Mounting evidence suggests that persistent AF promotes atrial remodeling, thus making recurrent or chronic AF more likely.
- **Atrial flutter (AFl)** is a common atrial arrhythmia that results from atrial reentry, usually after a single circuit in the right atrium that circles the annulus of the tricuspid valve. It classically presents as a sawtooth pattern of atrial activity on ECG (particularly seen as inverted F waves in II, III, and aVF and upright waves in V_1). The general principles of management of AFl are very similar to AF (see Management) but are often more difficult to rate-control than AF.

Associated Conditions

Common conditions that lead to or are associated with AF include valvular heart disease [including mitral stenosis, mitral valve prolapse (MVP), mitral annular calcifica-

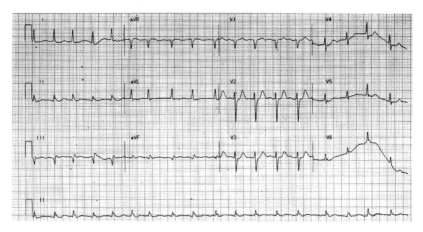

FIG. 11-1. AF.

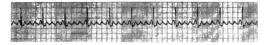

FIG. 11-2. Atrial flutter. Note that conduction is regular at 4:1. Conduction through the AV node can also be variable in atrial flutter, yielding variable RR intervals and an irregular rhythm.

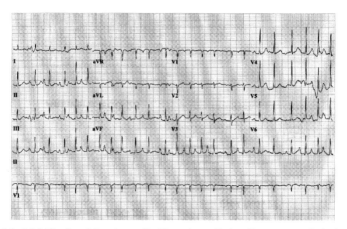

FIG. 11-3. Multifocal atrial tachycardia. Note three distinct P wave morphologies with three distinct PR intervals. The rhythm is irregular but clearly not AF.

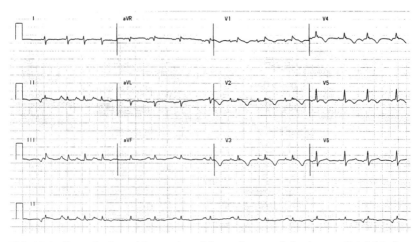

FIG. 11-4. Sinus rhythm with ectopic atrial complexes and short runs of atrial tachycardia. The overall rhythm is irregular.

tion], HCM or dilated cardiomyopathy, CAD, HTN, diabetes mellitus, sick sinus syndrome, Wolff-Parkinson-White (WPW) syndrome (discussed in Rate Control), and hyperthyroidism or hypothyroidism. AF commonly occurs in the setting of acute MI, pulmonary embolism, pericarditis, acute alcohol intoxication ("holiday heart"), cardiac surgery, infections, and use of cholinergic drugs or theophylline. Echocardiographic correlates include LVH, left atrial enlargement, reduced LV function, and mitral valve abnormalities. Seek evidence for any of the above conditions during the history and physical exam. **Vagally mediated AF** occurs in highly trained athletes, commonly while sleeping or after a meal. This form is particularly responsive to disopyramide (Norpace; see Table 11-4). Approximately 10–15% of patients will present with lone AF, having no identifiable risk factors or cardiac structural abnormality.

Differential Diagnosis

AF (Fig. 11-1) should be differentiated from other rhythms that may appear similar to it, because approaches to management of various arrhythmias may vary widely. These include AFl (Fig. 11-2), multifocal atrial tachycardia (Fig. 11-3), frequent premature atrial complexes (Fig. 11-4), and other supraventricular arrhythmias (see Chap. 15, Tachyarrhythmias, Sudden Cardiac Death, and Implantable Cardioverter-Defibrillators).

PRESENTATION

History

Patients with AF can present with a wide variety of symptoms, determined to a large extent by underlying cardiac function, comorbidities, and patient perception, or they may be asymptomatic. Common complaints include palpitations, dizziness, fatigue, chest pain, dyspnea, or presyncope. Patients may present with unstable angina in the setting of significant CAD, heart failure (HF) with pulmonary edema (with underlying LV dysfunction, mitral stenosis, or a tachycardia-induced cardiomyopathy), focal neurologic deficits (in the setting of an embolic stroke), severe abdominal or extremity pain (in the setting of peripheral embolization with mesenteric or limb ischemia), or frank syncope.

Physical Exam

Physical exam usually reveals a rapid heart rate with an irregularly irregular rhythm, an S_1 that can vary in intensity from beat to beat, and absence of an S_4 or a waves. If HF is present, exam may reveal an S_3, jugular venous distention (JVD), or rales. A goiter may be present (thyrotoxicosis). Other possible findings include focal neurologic deficits or evidence of peripheral embolization.

ECG

ECG reveals absence of P waves and an often coarse, undulating baseline (see Fig. 11-1). The ventricular rhythm is irregularly irregular at a rate usually between 110 and 170 bpm. QRS complexes are narrow, except in the setting of an underlying bundle-branch block, **Ashman's phenomenon** (aberrant conduction of the atrial impulses due to a difference in refractory period between the right- and left-bundle branches), or with concomitant ventricular ectopy.

MANAGEMENT

Initial Diagnostic Testing

Besides a 12-lead ECG, initial workup should include echocardiography to evaluate for valvular or other cardiac structural abnormality, thyroid function tests, and pulse oximetry. Perform other testing as history and physical exam dictate (e.g., serial cardiac enzymes if acute MI suspected, known CAD, or multiple CAD risk factors; ABG sampling and $\dot{V}/\dot{Q}$ scan if acute pulmonary embolism suspected; brain imaging with neurologic deficits; theophylline level).

Treatment

The therapeutic approach to AF is best divided into three broad areas: (a) regulation of the ventricular rate, (b) reduction of the risk of thromboembolic complications (anticoagulation), and (c) restoration and maintenance of sinus rhythm. Ultimately, the specific approach to management of AF will vary for individual patients and will depend, to a large extent, on concomitant illnesses or conditions, patient preferences, and severity of symptoms or complications. Management considerations fall into the classes outlined by the ACC and the AHA (see http://www.ahajournals.org/misc/sci-stmts_topindex.shtml and the preface for an outline of the classes) [1]. Fig. 11-5 provides an overview of the general management of chronic AF.

Rate Control
AF usually produces a ventricular rate of 110–170 bpm in the absence of drug therapy or intrinsic conduction system disease. The rapid ventricular response to AF typically accounts for most symptoms that patients experience. This rapid rate can lead to decreased diastolic filling and impairment of LV function, ACS in the setting of significant CAD, and acute pulmonary edema, particularly in the setting of diastolic dysfunction or valvular heart disease (e.g., mitral stenosis). If this rapid rate persists for several weeks or more, patients may develop a tachycardia-induced cardiomyopathy with accompanying LV dysfunction (often, this cardiomyopathy is reversible once rate is controlled).
- **General approach:** Rate control can be viewed as having two distinct phases: **acute** control, in which the ventricular rate is reduced to an acceptable level within a few minutes [best accomplished by IV preparations of medications used to control rate (Table 11-1)] and **long-term** control, typically accomplished with PO agents (Table 11-2). In the absence of significant symptoms secondary to the rapid rate, IV medications are unnecessary and best avoided in favor of PO preparations, given the added risk of hypotension and/or symptomatic bradycardia with IV agents. If symptoms are severe or if the patient is hemodynamically unstable, the treatment of choice is immediate direct-current cardioversion (see Chap. 5, Cardiovascular

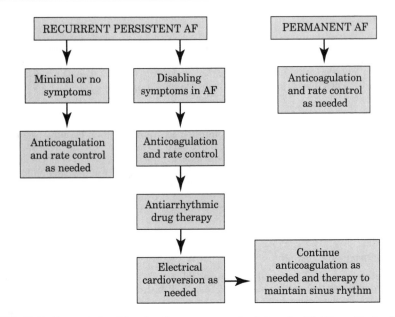

FIG. 11-5. General algorithm for the management of chronic AF. (From Fuster V, Ryden LE, Asinger RW, et al. ACC/AHA/ESC Guidelines for the management of patients with atrial fibrillation: executive summary. *Circulation* 2001;104:2118–2150, with permission.)

Emergencies). Treatment of AF with a preexcited ventricular response in the setting of WPW syndrome is drastically different and is covered in Chap. 15, Tachyarrhythmias, Sudden Cardiac Death, and Implantable Cardioverter-Defibrillators.

• **Pharmacologic rate control:** Three main types of drugs are used to control the ventricular response to AF: (a) beta-adrenergic blocking agents, (b) calcium channel blockers, and (c) digitalis glycosides. **Beta blockers** are available in IV and PO formulations and are effective agents for blunting AV nodal conduction and, thus, the rapid ventricular response to AF. They are the agents of choice in AF associated with thyrotoxicosis, acute MI, or the postop state, in which case beta blockers have been shown to improve mortality. They should be used cautiously in patients with relative contraindications, including reactive airway disease or bronchospasm and acute HF. **Calcium channel blockers** are available in IV (Table 11-1) and PO (Table 11-2) preparations; they are classified into two main types: dihydropyridines [e.g., felodipine (Plendil), nifedipine (Adalat, Procardia)] and nondihydropyridines [e.g., diltiazem (Cardizem, Cardia XT, Dilacor XR, Diltia XT, Tiazac), verapamil (Calan, Isoptin, Verelan)]. Dihydropyridines have minimal, if any, effect on AV nodal conduction and, thus, are not useful for rate control in AF. Both diltiazem and verapamil are effective rate-control agents and are available in immediate- or sustained-release forms. Similar to beta blockers, these agents have negative inotropic effects and, thus, can exacerbate HF, so they should be used cautiously in patients with concomitant LV dysfunction. **Digoxin** is available in IV and PO forms. It slows the ventricular rate in AF through a mechanism different from that of beta blockers or calcium channel blockers. Specifically, it blunts AV nodal conduction by increasing vagal tone. Its onset of action is significantly delayed compared to other agents, and although effective in patients at rest, it loses its effect with exercise or in other situations producing excess sympathetic tone. Evidence suggests that digoxin may even

TABLE 11-1. STANDARD IV MEDICATIONS COMMONLY USED FOR RATE CONTROL IN AF

Drug[a]	Loading dose	Onset	Maintenance dose	Major side effects	Class recommendation
Diltiazem	0.25 mg/kg IV over 2 mins	2–7 mins	5–15 mg/hr infusion	Hypotension, heart block, HF	I[b]
Esmolol[c]	0.5 mg/kg over 1 min	5 mins	0.05–0.2 mg/kg^{-1}/min^{-1}	Hypotension, heart block, bradycardia, asthma, HF	I
Metoprolol[c]	2.5–5 mg IV bolus over 2 mins; up to three doses	5 mins	NA	Hypotension, heart block, bradycardia, asthma, HF	I[b]
Propanolol[c]	0.15 mg/kg IV	5 mins	NA	Hypotension, heart block, bradycardia, asthma, HF	I[b]
Verapamil	0.075–0.15 mg/kg IV over 2 mins	3–5 mins	NA	Hypotension, heart block, HF	I[b]
Digoxin	0.25 mg IV every 2 hrs, up to 1.5 mg	2 hrs	0.125–0.25 mg/day	Digitalis toxicity, heart block, bradycardia	IIb[d]

NA, not applicable.
[a]Drugs are listed alphabetically within each class of recommendation.
[b]Class IIb in congestive HF.
[c]Only representative members of the type of beta-adrenergic antagonist drugs are included in the table, but other similar agents could be used for this indication in appropriate doses.
[d]Class I in congestive HF.
From Fuster V, Ryden LE, Asinger RW, et al. ACC/AHA/ESC guidelines for the management of patients with atrial fibrillation: executive summary. *Circulation* 2001;104:2118–2150, with permission.

TABLE 11-2. STANDARD PO MEDICATIONS COMMONLY USED FOR RATE CONTROL IN AF

Drug[a]	Loading dose	Onset	Usual maintenance dose[b]	Major side effects	Recommendation
Digoxin	0.25 mg PO q2h; up to 1.5 mg	2 hrs	0.125–0.375 mg/day	Digitalis toxicity, heart block, bradycardia	I
Diltiazem	NA	2–4 hrs	120–360 mg/day in divided doses; slow release available	Hypotension, heart block, HF	I
Metoprolol[c]	NA	4–6 hrs	25–100 mg bid	Hypotension, heart block, bradycardia, asthma, HF	I
Propranolol[c]	NA	60–90 mins	80–240 mg/day in divided doses	Hypotension, heart block, bradycardia, asthma, HF	I
Verapamil	NA	1–2 hrs	120–360 mg/day in divided doses; slow release available	Hypotension, heart block, HF; digoxin interaction	I
Amiodarone	800 mg/day for 1 wk 600 mg/day for 1 wk 400 mg/day for 4–6 wks	1–3 wks	200 mg/day	Pulmonary toxicity, skin discoloration, hypothyroidism, corneal deposits, optic neuropathy, warfarin interaction, proarrhythmia, digoxin interaction	IIb

NA, not applicable.

[a]Drugs are listed alphabetically within each class of recommendation.

[b]Recommended maintenance dosages are the usual ones necessary, but higher doses may be appropriate in some patients.

[c]The table includes representative members of the type of beta-blocker drugs, but other, similar agents could be used for this indication in appropriate doses.

From Fuster V, Ryden LE, Asinger RW, et al. ACC/AHA/ESC guidelines for the management of patients with atrial fibrillation: executive summary. *Circulation* 2001;104:2118–2150, with permission.

prolong episodes in patients with paroxysmal AF. Digoxin is best suited for patients with coexisting LV dysfunction (given its positive inotropic effect), as an adjunct to beta-blocker or calcium channel–blocker therapy, or as the primary rate-control agent in patients intolerant of calcium channel blockers and beta blockers. Digoxin can cause serious adverse effects, including GI toxicity and symptomatic bradycardia. The optimal dose depends, to a large extent, on a patient's renal function. A significant disadvantage is that it can take up to 10 hrs to reach peak effect. Avoid use in patients with acute renal failure or end-stage renal disease.
* Finally, **amiodarone** (Cordarone) can be used for refractory rate control in acute circumstances in which a patient's BP will not tolerate beta blockers or calcium channel blockers (i.e., systolic BP <90 mm Hg). In addition to its properties as a class III antiarrhythmic (see Table 11-4), amiodarone also has AV nodal–blocking activity. IV amiodarone may also lower BP, particularly if given quickly, due to its solvent. The caveat to using amiodarone in this setting is the small chance that it will cardiovert AF to sinus rhythm and thereby increase the risk of thromboembolism in patients not known with certainty to have had AF for <48 hrs (see Thromboembolic Risk Reduction). Occasionally, this will be the last resort in patients who are becoming hemodynamically unstable, before electrical cardioversion. **Note that amiodarone and digoxin have a strong metabolic interaction, resulting in much higher serum digoxin levels.**
* **Nonpharmacologic rate control (chronic AF):** In patients who are persistently tachycardic or who remain symptomatic despite treatment with pharmacologic agents, or for whom serious contraindications to drug therapy exist, rate control can be accomplished by ablation of the AV node and implantation of a permanent pacemaker. Although several methods of AV nodal ablation are available, the most widely used is radiofrequency ablation (RFA). In this procedure, a catheter is percutaneously introduced under fluoroscopic guidance to the heart in the vicinity if the His bundle, and radiofrequency energy is delivered in a precise fashion to ablate the AV node, thus controlling the ventricular rate by producing complete heart block. A permanent pacemaker is implanted, and the most appropriate mode is selected, based on the nature of the AF (VVIR mode for chronic AF and dual-chamber pacemaker with mode-switching capability for paroxysmal AF; see Chap. 14, Bradycardia and Permanent Pacemakers). A major disadvantage of this procedure is its irreversibility. **Patients who undergo AV nodal ablation carry the same risk of thromboembolic complications and still require anticoagulation.**

Thromboembolic Risk Reduction
* **Anticoagulation** has a central role in the management of AF. With AF, the overall stroke risk without anticoagulation is 6% per yr. With ASA, the risk is 3% per yr, and with Coumadin and an INR of 2–3, the rate is 1% per yr [2]. As a result of these data, guidelines for anticoagulation in the setting of AF have been established. For example, patients with AF as a consequence of rheumatic heart disease should receive long-term therapy with warfarin at a goal INR of 2–3, barring absolute contraindications to anticoagulation. These patients experience an extraordinarily high rate of stroke and other thromboembolic events without anticoagulation, as demonstrated by Framingham data. For patients without rheumatic heart disease, there are certain risk factors for thromboembolism that, if present, necessitate long-term anticoagulation. Obviously, patients with permanent AF or paroxysmal AF need long-term anticoagulation to reduce the stroke risk. Clinical risk factors include advanced age (>65 yrs), previous stroke or TIA, HTN, diabetes mellitus, congestive HF, presence of a prosthetic heart valve, and thyrotoxicosis. Additionally, echocardiographic findings increasing the risk of thromboembolism include left-atrial enlargement and a reduced LV ejection fraction (Table 11-3). Patients <65 yrs and without any of the risk factors mentioned above can safely be treated with ASA alone. For patients >65 yrs or with risk factors, long-term treatment with warfarin (INR, 2–3) is necessary. Particularly close monitoring of INR is needed in patients >75 yrs, given the increased risk of bleeding. Other factors (e.g., fall risk or intracranial lesions) may preclude warfarin, making ASA the only acceptable method of anticoagulation.

TABLE 11-3. APPROPRIATE ANTICOAGULATION IN VARIOUS AF POPULATIONS

Patient features	Antithrombotic therapy	Grade of recommendation
Age <60 yrs; no heart disease (lone AF)	ASA (325 mg PO/day) or no therapy	I
Age <60 yrs; heart disease but no risk factors[a]	ASA (325 mg PO/day)	I
Age ≥ 60 yrs; no risk factors[a]	ASA (325 mg PO/day)	I
Age ≥ 60 yrs, with diabetes mellitus or CAD	PO anticoagulation (INR, 2–3)	I
	Addition of ASA, 81–162 mg/day, is optional	IIb
Age ≥ 75 yrs, especially women	PO anticoagulation (INR, ~ 2)	I
HF; LV ejection fraction ≤ 0.35; thyrotoxicosis; HTN	PO anticoagulation (INR, 2–3)	I
Rheumatic heart disease (mitral stenosis); prosthetic heart valves; prior thromboembolism; persistent atrial thrombus on TEE	PO anticoagulation (INR, 2.5–3.5 or higher may be appropriate)	—

[a]Risk factors for thromboembolism include HF, LV ejection fraction <0.35, and history of HTN.
From Fuster V, Ryden LE, Asinger RW, et al. ACC/AHA/ESC guidelines for the management of patients with atrial fibrillation: executive summary. *Circulation* 2001;104:2118–2150, with permission.

- Early studies of patients who underwent cardioversion for AF without anticoagulation revealed an unacceptably large (7%) overall incidence of thromboembolism. With anticoagulation, the incidence dropped to <1%. For this reason, **the AHA recommends that patients undergoing cardioversion for AF, whether electric or pharmacologic, receive systemic anticoagulation with warfarin for 3–4 wks before and at least 4 wks after restoration of sinus rhythm, unless an absolute contraindication exists.**
- Although few data exist about the thromboembolic risk within the first 48 hrs of onset of AF, it is generally accepted as safe to cardiovert without anticoagulation during this period. For AF >48 hrs in duration, it is recommended that patients be treated with warfarin, with a goal INR of 2–3 for 3 wks before and at least 4 wks after cardioversion. The purpose of treatment after cardioversion is to protect from thromboembolism during the period of atrial electromechanical dyssynchrony, in which normal electrical activity is restored, but normal atrial contraction (particularly of the left atrial appendage, where thrombi often form) lags.
- Emerging data are lending credit to an alternate approach to thromboembolic risk reduction surrounding cardioversion for AF. In this new approach, patients who are to be cardioverted are systemically anticoagulated with heparin and then undergo TEE to evaluate for the presence of intraatrial thrombus, particularly in the left atrial appendage. If the TEE demonstrates the absence of thrombi, then patients may be safely electrically cardioverted, followed by at least 4 wks of warfarin therapy. This eliminates the need for weeks of preprocedural anticoagulation and any attendant risk of bleeding during this period. The ACUTE Investigators Study has demonstrated the safety and efficacy of this approach compared to the more traditional method [3].

TABLE 11-4. VAUGHAN WILLIAMS CLASSIFICATION OF ANTIARRHYTHMIC MEDICATIONS AND SOME COMMON ADVERSE REACTIONS

Class IA	Quinidine
	GI side effects
	Cinchonism (tinnitus, hearing loss, vision change, delirium)
	Prolonged QTc and torsades de pointes
	Hemolytic anemia and idiopathic thrombocytopenic purpura
	Proarrhythmia: distal conduction defects but AV nodal enhancement
	Disopyramide (also strong anticholinergic)
	Congestive HF
	Anticholinergic side effects, including glaucoma and urinary retention
	Thrombocytopenia and agranulocytosis
	Procainamide
	Lupus-like syndrome (spares kidneys)
	Proarrhythmia: distal conduction defects but AV nodal enhancement
Class IB (not useful in atrial arrhythmias)	Lidocaine
	CNS disturbance
	Augmented AV conduction: rapid ventricular response with AF
	Mexiletine
	CNS disturbance
	GI disturbance
	Tocainide (rarely used)
	Phenytoin
	Hypotension
Class IC	Flecainide
	Proarrhythmia; conversion of AF to AFl with 1:1 ventricular response
	Congestive HF
	Propafenone
	Proarrhythmia; conversion of AF to AFl with 1:1 ventricular response
	Bronchospasm (beta-blocking activity)
	Congestive HF
Class II	Beta blockers
	Bradycardia
	Bronchospasm
	Congestive HF
Class III	Amiodarone (also AV nodal–blocking properties)
	Pulmonary fibrosis
	Hypo- or hyperthyroidism
	Transaminase elevation

(*continued*)

TABLE 11-4. CONTINUED

	Photosensitivity
	Skin and corneal deposition
	Bradycardia
	Warfarin and digoxin interations
	Dofetilide
	Prolonged QTc and torsades de pointes (up to 8%)
	Sotalol (also beta-blocking properties)
	Prolonged QTc and torsades de pointes
	Bradycardia
	Congestive HF
	Ibutilide
	Prolonged QTc and torsades de pointes
	Bretylium (not useful in atrial arrhythmias)
	Proarrhythmia (initial catecholamine liberation)
	Hypotension
Class IV	Calcium channel blockers (dihydropyridine and nondihydropyridine)

Restoration and Maintenance of Sinus Rhythm

- Much debate exists regarding the importance of restoring and maintaining normal sinus rhythm in patients with AF. No studies have demonstrated a survival benefit or a reduction in thromboembolic events with chronic rhythm control over the alternate strategy of ventricular rate control and long-term anticoagulation. Restoration of sinus rhythm does, however, reduce symptoms and improve cardiac performance. The recently published Atrial Fibrillation Follow-up Investigation of Rhythm Management (AFFIRM) trial [4] asked whether rhythm control or rate control was preferable for long-term outcomes. This prospective, randomized trial revealed that, among patients who were symptomatically and hemodynamically able to tolerate AF, no significant differences in overall survival exist between rhythm and rate control. In fact, rhythm control groups tended toward higher incidence of death and ischemic strokes, likely due to lower use of Coumadin in this group. Thus, particularly in patients prone to persistent or chronic AF, rate control and anticoagulation are sufficient, assuming the patient tolerates the rhythm.
- **Direct current cardioversion** (DCC) is the preferred method of restoring sinus rhythm in patients with AF. In the absence of hemodynamic instability (in which case DCC should be carried out emergently), DCC should be performed in a controlled environment with insurance of adequate anticoagulation duration and extent (or TEE clearance), hemodynamic monitoring, and the assistance of anesthesia personnel, if necessary, for airway protection. For AF, 200 J are delivered initially, followed by increasing joules if the first countershock proves unsuccessful. The electrical shock should be synchronized to avoid precipitation of VF.
- A variety of **pharmacologic agents** exist for the restoration and maintenance of sinus rhythm (Tables 11-4 and 11-5; Fig. 11-6). Although the conversion rate with drugs is much lower than with electrical cardioversion, these agents are commonly used as alternatives to DCC, adjuncts to DCC, or as salvage therapy in case of failed DCC. Many of these medications maintain sinus rhythm with much greater efficacy (collectively, approximately 50% at 1 yr) than their rate of cardioversion. Ibutilide (Vaughan Williams class III agent) is the only antiarrhythmic approved for acute IV

TABLE 11-5. ANTIARRHYTHMIC MEDICATIONS USED IN AF

Drug[a]	Route of administration	Dosage[b]		Potential acute adverse effects
Amiodarone	PO	Inpatient: 1.2–1.8 g/day in divided dose until 10 g total, then 200–400 mg/day maintenance or 30 mg/kg as single dose		Hypotension, bradycardia, QT prolongation, torsades de pointes (rare), GI upset, constipation, phlebitis (IV), photosensitivity, pulmonary toxicity, polyneuropathy, hepatic toxicity, thyroid dysfunction, warfarin and digoxin interations
		Outpatient: 600–800 mg/day divided dose until 10 g total, then 200–400 mg/day maintenance		
	IV/PO	5–7 mg/kg over 30–60 mins, then 1.2–1.8 g/day continuous IV or in divided PO doses until 10 g total, then 200–400 mg/day maintenance		
Disopyramide	PO	400–750 mg, divided bid or tid		QT prolongation, torsades de pointes, heart failure, glaucoma, urinary retention, dry mouth
Dofetilide	PO	Creatinine clearance (mL/min)	Dose (µg bid)	QT prolongation, torsades de pointes; adjust dose for renal function, body size, and age
		>60	500	Contraindicated if QTc>440 msec at baseline
		40–60	250	
		20–40	125	
		<20	Contraindicated	
Flecainide	PO	200–300 mg, divided bid[c]		Hypotension, rapidly conducting atrial flutter
	IV	1.5–3.0 mg/kg over 10–20 mins[c]		
Ibutilide	IV	1 mg over 10 mins; repeat 1 mg when necessary		QT prolongation, torsades de pointes

(continued)

TABLE 11-5. CONTINUED

Drug[a]	Route of administration	Dosage[b]	Potential acute adverse effects
Procainamide	PO	1–4 g in divided doses	Torsades de pointes, lupus-like syndrome, GI intolerance
Propafenone	PO	450–600 mg	Hypotension, rapidly conducting atrial flutter
	IV	1.5–2.0 mg/kg over 10–20 mins[c]	
Quinidine[d]	PO	0.75–1.5 g in divided doses over 6–12 hrs, usually given with a rate-slowing drug	QT prolongation, torsades de pointes, GI upset, hypotension
Sotalol[e]	PO	160–320 mg PO, divided bid	QT prolongation, torsades de pointes, bradycardia, congestive HF if IV dysfunction, bronchospasm, and contraindicated in renal insufficiency

[a]Drugs are listed alphabetically.
[b]Dosages given in the table may differ from those recommended by the manufacturers.
[c]Insufficient data are available on which to base specific recommendations for the use of one loading regimen over another for patients with ischemic heart disease or impaired LV function, and these drugs should be used cautiously or not at all in such patients. IV flecainide is not available in the United States. Flecainide and propafenone are usually given with a rate-slowing drug.
[d]Use of quinidine to achieve pharmacologic conversion of AF is controversial, and safer methods are available with the alternative agents listed in the table. Quinidine should be used with caution.
[e]Not effective for cardioversion but has success in maintaining sinus rhythm after cardioversion.
Adapted from Fuster V, Ryden LE, Asinger RW, et al. ACC/AHA/ESC guidelines for the management of patients with atrial fibrillation: executive summary. *Circulation* 2001;104:2118–2150, with permission.

use for cardioversion. The risk of QTc prolongation, however, is significant in patients with underlying structural heart disease, which predisposes to torsades de pointes. Unfortunately, proarrhythmia is a common adverse reaction seen with many of these agents, and several trials—including the CAST study [5]—have shown an increase in mortality with long-term use of these agents. Therefore, extreme caution must be used in initiating pharmacologic therapy, with close monitoring (usually inpatient) for ECG abnormalities and proarrhythmia. As demonstrated in Fig. 11-6, the use of each antiarrhythmic is specified by the underlying cardiac pathology, with potentially catastrophic consequences if not noted. In addition, each antiarrhythmic carries specific common adverse reactions when used chronically (see Tables 11-4 and 11-5).

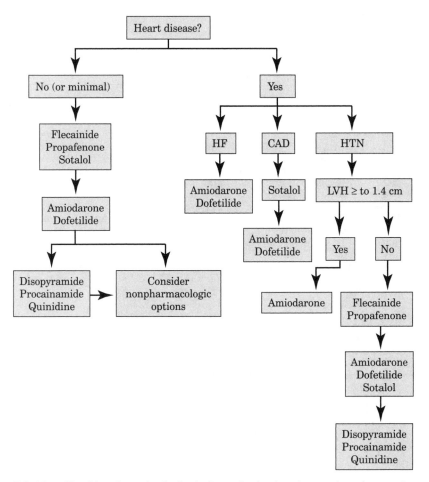

FIG. 11-6. Algorithm for antiarrhythmic drug selection based on patient characteristics. (From Fuster V, Ryden LE, Asinger RW, et al. ACC/AHA/ESC guidelines for the management of patients with atrial fibrillation: executive summary. *Circulation* 2001;104:2118–2150, with permission.)

- Other, **nonpharmacologic** methods of restoring and maintaining sinus rhythm exist or are in developmental stages. The **Maze** procedure is a cardiac operation in which a sternotomy is performed and a series of carefully placed incisions or RFA burns are made in the atria to channel the erratic electrical activity to the AV node. Percutaneous approaches, including **pulmonary vein isolation and ablation,** are used in specialized settings. Other experimental approaches include implantable atrial defibrillators and rapid atrial pacemakers. With regard to maintenance of sinus rhythm with isolated AFl, percutaneous approaches are widely used. Because AFl propagates along a single reentrant circuit (unlike AF), it can often be ablated with radiofrequency energy (RFA). In fact, RFA successfully eliminates AFl in >90% of cases. Because the AV node remains intact, pacemaker implantation is not needed, and patients usually convert from AFl to normal sinus rhythm with RFA. Therefore, 3 wks of anticoagulation or TEE is required before this procedure, as well as at least 4 wks after the procedure. AFl commonly coexists with AF, rendering RFA less useful in those cases.

KEY POINTS TO REMEMBER

- The three components of the management of AF are **anticoagulation** (thromboembolism risk reduction), **rate control** (to alleviate symptoms and to prevent the development of tachycardia-mediated cardiomyopathy), and **rhythm control** (required in a sizable subset of AF patients because of symptoms).
- Whether paroxysmal, persistent, or permanent, most patients should be given some form of anticoagulation long term (unless contraindicated).
- Patients who are **known** to have recent (<48 hrs) onset of AF can be safely cardioverted chemically or electrically (or given medicines such as amiodarone) without TEE assessment of the left atrial appendage. **Initially,** however, a brief trial of rate control and observation is appropriate to assess if the patient will convert spontaneously. Such patients most commonly are already in the hospital when AF initiates, as they have been monitored. Anticoagulation is still strongly recommended **after** cardioversion (unless contraindicated) for at least 1 mo (long term if the rhythm is likely to recur).
- It is **not advisable** to cardiovert (i.e., electrically or via antiarrhythmic medication) patients who present to the office or ER in AF (because the duration of the arrhythmia cannot be definitively determined) without TEE clearance or at least 3 wks of anticoagulation with warfarin. The **exception** is hemodynamically unstable patients.
- Any hemodynamically stable patient undergoing electrical or pharmacologic cardioversion requires at least 3 wks of warfarin or a TEE before cardioversion, and at least 4 wks of warfarin after cardioversion. Therefore, TEE does not eliminate the need for anticoagulation.
- Postop AF (e.g., after coronary artery bypass grafting) requires anticoagulation but often resolves spontaneously or with cardioversion. 1 mo after the last episode of AF, anticoagulation with Coumadin usually can be stopped.
- Patients who tolerate AF (paroxysmally or chronically) fare no worse with rate control and anticoagulation alone than patients who are given antiarrhythmics to maintain normal sinus rhythm. The decision to use antiarrhythmics should be made very carefully because of the associated adverse effects.
- AFl can be more difficult to rate-control than AF. Thromboembolism protection with anticoagulation is still required. The reentrant circuit responsible for the rhythm can often be ablated, but many patients who exhibit AFl will also demonstrate AF.
- Never say, "...cardioverted **with** digoxin" or beta blockers or calcium channel blockers. One should say "converted spontaneously after rate-control with..." (digoxin, beta blocker, or calcium channel blockers).

SUGGESTED READING

Faddis MN. Cardiac arrhythmias. In: Ahya S, Flood K, Paranjothi S, eds. *The Washington manual of medical therapeutics*, 30th ed. Philadelphia: Lippincott Williams & Wilkins, 2001:153–180.

Mason JW. A comparison of seven antiarrhythmic drugs in patients with ventricular tachyarrhythmias. Electrophysiologic Study vs. Electrocardiographic Monitoring Investigators. *N Engl J Med* 1993;329:452–458.

Preliminary resport of the Stroke Prevention in Atrial Fibrillation Study. *N Engl J Med* 1990;322:863–868.

Prytowsky EN, Benson DW, Fuster V, et al. Management of patients with atrial fibrillation. A statement for health care professionals. From the Subcommittee on Electrocardiography and Electrophysiology, American Heart Association. *Circulation* 1996;93:1262–1277.

Stroke Prevention in Atrial Fibrillation Investigators. Warfarin vs. aspirin for prevention of thromboembolism in atrial fibrillation: Stroke Prevention in Atrial Fibrillation II Study. *Lancet* 1994;343:687–691.

REFERENCES

1. Fuster V, Ryden LE, Asinger RW, et al. ACC/AHA/ESC guidelines for the management of patients with atrial fibrillation: executive summary. *Circulation* 2001; 104:2118–2150.

2. Stroke Prevention in Atrial Fibrillation Investigators. Stroke Prevention in Atrial Fibrillation Study. Final results. *Circulation* 1991;84:527–539.

3. Assessment of Cardioversion Using Transesophageal Echocardiography (ACUTE) Investigators. Use of transesophageal echocardiography to guide cardioversion in patients with atrial fibrillation. *N Engl J Med* 2001;344:1411–1420.

4. Van Gelder IC, Hagens VE, Bosker HA. A comparison of rate control and rhythm control in patients with recurrent persistent atrial fibrillation. *N Engl J Med* 2002;347:1834–1840.

5. Cardiac Arrhythmia Suppression Trial (CAST) Investigators. Preliminary report on effect of encainide and flecainide on mortality in a randomized trial of arrhythmia suppression after myocardial infarction. *N Engl J Med* 1989;321: 406–412.

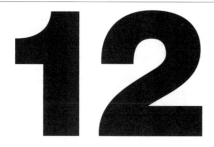

Assessment and Management of the Dilated, Restrictive, and Hypertrophic Cardiomyopathies

J. Mauricio Sánchez,
Martin S. Maron,
and Peter A. Crawford

INTRODUCTION

Heart failure (HF) is the final common pathway in a myriad of varying cardiac disease processes. It may result from any of several causes, most commonly ischemic heart disease; however, other causes account for almost one-half of reported cases. These causes are distinctive because they are not the result of pericardial, hypertensive, congenital, or valvular disease. Identifying the cause of HF can be important to guide the appropriate therapy. These diseases may be grouped by their morphologic type and clinical mechanism of dysfunction for greater ease of diagnosis and management. This chapter discusses these entities.

DILATED CARDIOMYOPATHY

Dilated cardiomyopathy is the most common form of nonischemic cardiomyopathy. It is characterized by ventricular dilatation, contractile dysfunction, and symptoms of HF.

Idiopathic Dilated Cardiomyopathy

Idiopathic dilated cardiomyopathy is a primary myocardial disease of unknown cause characterized by LV or biventricular dilatation and impaired myocardial contractility [1]. Incidence is thought to be approximately 6 in 100,000 persons per yr [2]; this is thought to be an underestimation of true incidence based on asymptomatic cases [3]. It is the most common cause of cardiomyopathy in young patients. It is important to differentiate idiopathic disease from secondary disease, as these may be potentially reversible causes requiring tailored treatment. Patients commonly present initially with symptoms of HF, with left-sided symptoms predominating. Symptoms include progressive dyspnea on exertion, orthopnea, paroxysmal nocturnal dyspnea, and fatigue. Approximately 90% of patients had symptoms of New York Heart Association class III or IV disease at the time of diagnosis [4]. The natural history of the disease is difficult to determine, given the unknown length of asymptomatic disease. Symptomatic patients generally have a poor prognosis. 5-yr mortality rates in recent studies average approximately 20% [5,6]. The underlying cause of HF has prognostic value in patients with unexplained cardiomyopathy [5]. Pathogenesis of this disease is thought to be due to one of four mechanisms: (a) familial disease, (b) viral myocarditis, (c) immune abnormalities, and (d) metabolic abnormalities. Familial dilated cardiomyopathy is occasionally associated with mutations to genes encoding sarcomeric proteins [27]. The mechanism of one does not preclude the other, and these may occur together. The major histologic features include hypertrophy and degeneration of myocytes, varying degrees of interstitial fibrosis, and occasional small clusters of lymphocytes [6]. Clinical management is that of standard management for HF (see Chap. 10, Management of Acute and Chronic Heart Failure).

Toxin-Induced Cardiomyopathy

Toxin-induced cardiomyopathy, primarily **alcohol cardiomyopathy,** is a major cause of HF. Alcoholic cardiomyopathy accounts for more than one-third of cases of dilated cardiomyopathy. Alcohol consumption may affect myocytes by (a) direct toxicity of alcohol or metabolites, such as aldehyde; (b) nutritional defects, most commonly thiamine deficiency; and rarely, (c) additives (i.e., cobalt, which was used in the 1960s as a foam stabilizer). Alcoholic cardiomyopathy most commonly occurs in men 30–55. Patients present in biventricular failure, with left-sided symptoms predominating. Concomitant skeletal muscle myopathy involving shoulders and pelvic girdle is common. Patients may also present with "holiday heart syndrome," with HF in association with tachyarrhythmia-like AF. The key to long-term treatment is complete abstinence as soon as possible. This may result in reversal of myocardial depression [7]. Prognosis of patients who do not cease drinking is poor, with 5-yr mortality of 50%. Management of acute episodes is otherwise unchanged from other forms of dilated cardiomyopathy. **Cocaine,** when used chronically, can have similar effects on the myocardium, although by different mechanisms.

Other cardiac toxins, including **anthracyclines,** particularly doxorubicin hydrochloride, are well known to result in a dilated cardiomyopathy. Total cumulative dose is important in determining risk [8]. Patients who receive <400 mg/m^2 are at low risk, whereas patients who receive >700 mg/m^2 have a 20% increased likelihood of developing this syndrome. The exact mechanism is unknown. Therapy with monoclonal antibody against Her2/erbB [trastuzumab (Herceptin)] increases the likelihood of developing cardiomyopathy. Carefully evaluate patients, especially those with known heart disease, before beginning and during use of such chemotherapeutic agents, particularly for breast cancer patients.

Peripartum Cardiomyopathy

Peripartum cardiomyopathy is a rare form of cardiomyopathy of unknown cause occurring during the last trimester of pregnancy and up to 6 mos postpartum. Patients manifest symptoms most commonly in the second month postpartum. Approximately 20% of women with this disorder either die or survive only due to heart transplantation [9]. The remaining majority recover partially or completely. The risk of recurrence in women during a subsequent pregnancy is high and associated with a significant decrease in LV function and even death [10].

High-Output Cardiomyopathy

High-output cardiomyopathy may result from anemia, hyperthyroidism, left-to-right shunts, thiamine deficiencies (wet beriberi), and other diseases (i.e., Paget's, Albright's). In all conditions, there is a constant need to maintain a high cardiac output due to some other underlying abnormality; although uncommon, these do occur and may be corrected by addressing the underlying abnormality. These patients may present with symptoms of HF; they are tachycardic, with an increased pulse pressure. Physical exam reveals a hyperdynamic apical impulse and warm extremities. A systolic flow murmur may be heard due to increased flow across the aortic valve. A bruit or thrill over an extremity or site of injury may be appreciated if the patient has a fistula; this may aid in diagnosis. Right-heart catheterization shows high cardiac output, with high filling pressures [pulmonary capillary wedge pressure (PCWP) and right atrial pressure]. Left-to-right shunts are caused by intracardiac or extracardiac communications between high pressure, high-O$_2$-content blood and lower-pressure, lower-O$_2$-content blood. Intracardiac communications include VSD, atrial septal defects, patent ductus arteriosus, or ruptured sinus of Valsalva into the right atrium or ventricle. Extracardiac communications may be iatrogenic (dialysis fistula), genetic (hereditary hemorrhagic telangiectasias, Osler-Weber-Rendu disease) or secondary to trauma (penetrating injury). Compression of the fistula should result in decrease in heart rate in a substantial shunt. A bruit over the thyroid or the presence of a goiter may suggest hyperthyroidism. High-output cardiomyopathy patients may also present in AF and have other stigmata of this disease. Thiamine deficiency should be suspected in patients with a history of alcoholism and malnutrition. These patients may have marked edema, peripheral vasodilatation, and pulmonary congestion (wet beriberi). They may also experience peripheral neuropathy, hyperkeratosis, and glossitis (dry beriberi).

HIV-Associated Cardiomyopathy

HIV-associated cardiomyopathy is increasingly recognized as a common cause of dilated cardiomyopathy. Although pathogenesis of this particular etiology is unclear, various hypotheses explain it as due to infection of myocytes by HIV-1 or a coinfection of a cardiotropic virus, or as a result of cardiotoxicity of medical treatment, particularly the nucleoside analogs [11].

RESTRICTIVE CARDIOMYOPATHY

Restrictive cardiomyopathy is heart disease that results from impairment of ventricular filling, normal to decreased diastolic volume, and normal or increased wall thickness. Systolic function may be normal or impaired depending on the underlying etiology and the point in pathogenesis [12]. Patients present with symptoms of dyspnea, orthopnea, paroxysmal nocturnal dyspnea, peripheral edema, ascites, and weakness. Angina does not occur except in amyloidosis (small vessel disease). Initial evaluation should attempt to differentiate from constrictive pericarditis, which presents with similar symptoms (see Chap. 16, Disease of the Pericardium). Patients do not have cardiomegaly (except for bilateral atrial enlargement, **which at times is massive**) and have a nondisplaced point of maximal impulse on physical exam. **Kussmaul's sign** may be present on exam but is more commonly seen in constrictive pericarditis. An S_4 is commonly present. On heart catheterization, diastolic filling in the RV and LV occurs with a "dip-and-plateau," or "square root sign" in restrictive cardiomyopathy, as in constrictive pericarditis. In restrictive cardiomyopathy, classically, LV end-diastolic pressure is greater than RV end-diastolic pressure by approximately 5 mm Hg, unlike constrictive pericarditis, in which they are equal. Note that the influence of respiratory variation seen in constrictive pericarditis is absent in restrictive cardiomyopathy. **Distinguish restrictive cardiomyopathy from a restrictive diastolic filling pattern, as the latter can be exhibited in any progressed cardiomyopathy** [See Chap. 22, Imaging and Diagnostic Testing Modalities (Nuclear Imaging, Echocardiography, and Cardiac Catheterization)].

Myocardial Restrictive Cardiomyopathy

Noninfiltrative
Idiopathic restrictive cardiomyopathy is characterized by a mild to moderate increase in cardiac weight, with biatrial enlargement occurring commonly. Atrial appendage thrombi are present in approximately 10% of cases. Patchy endocardial fibrosis is present and may extend into the conduction system, resulting in complete heart block. This may be familial and associated with or without a distal myopathy. A familial nonhypertrophic restrictive cardiomyopathy with autosomal-dominant inheritance and variable penetrance has also been described in association with Noonan's syndrome [13].

   Diabetic cardiomyopathy can result in systolic and diastolic dysfunction in the absence of large-vessel abnormalities or disruption in myocardial capillary basal lamina. The restrictive component stems from interstitial fibrosis in the myocardium with atrophy of myocytes. The severity of dysfunction is related to the degree of metabolic derangement. This may even be seen in children with poorly controlled disease.

Infiltrative
Amyloidosis can result in the infiltration of amyloid into the heart, causing a restrictive cardiomyopathy. Injury to cardiac tissue results from the replacement of normal myocardial contractile elements with interstitial deposits. There are many types of amy-

loidosis. Cardiac involvement is seen most commonly in **primary amyloidosis** (AL amyloidosis) caused by the production of light-chain immunoglobulins by plasma cells. Primary amyloidosis is also associated with the nephrotic syndrome and renal failure; intestinal malabsorption and pseudo-obstruction; liver and endocrine organ infiltration and dysfunction; Howell-Jolly body formation due to hyposplenism, and macroglossia; peripheral neuropathy; carpal tunnel syndrome; and ecchymoses due to capillary damage. The peripheral neuropathies can cause autonomic dysfunction (orthostasis, dysphagia), as well as somatic nerve dysfunction. **Secondary amyloidosis** (AA) is due to acute phase–reactant apolipoprotein precursors and more commonly is limited to the liver, spleen, and adrenals. Amyloidosis can also be due to deposition of beta$_2$-microglobulin in chronic hemodialysis patients. Amyloid infiltration is also common in the elderly. This particular form of amyloidosis is known as **senile amyloidosis,** which results from the deposition of normal **transthyretin** into myocardium. Mutations in the transthyretin gene may also result in cardiac disease and are associated with **familial amyloidosis,** which differs clinically from other forms of amyloidosis with more common neuropathies, less renal involvement, no macroglossia, and less serious cardiac involvement, although it does affect the conduction system more frequently.

Amyloid deposition in the heart results in eventual **impairment of diastolic filling** due to the decreased compliance and firm nature of the myocardium. Amyloid deposits are seen histologically as insoluble amyloid fibrils in all chambers of the heart as apple-green birefringence on Congo red histologic stain. Deposition results in increased wall thickness without cavity dilatation. The degree of wall thickness prognosticates survival, with a 2.4-yr survival for patients with normal wall thickness to 0.4-yr survival in patients with markedly increased wall thickness. Amyloid deposits may also be found in the conduction system, resulting in a variety of cardiac arrhythmias. ECG classically shows low volts with poor R wave progression. Two-dimensional echocardiograph findings characteristic of cardiac amyloidosis include a granular, sparkling appearance. In the absence of these findings, severe diastolic impairment may still exist.

The **workup** starts with a serum protein electrophoresis and urine protein electrophoresis. Fat-pad biopsy and congophilic staining have an 80% sensitivity, and gingival biopsy is used also. Endomyocardial biopsy is also performed but is unnecessary if the clinical presentation and hemodynamics suggest the diagnosis, especially in the setting of another tissue source for biopsy.

Treatment is that of diastolic dysfunction with salt restriction and diuretics (see Chap. 10, Management of Acute and Chronic Heart Failure). **Digoxin is particularly contraindicated in amyloidosis.** Treat the underlying cause if possible. Prognosis is often poor. Chemotherapy for AL amyloidosis may extend patient survival.

SARCOIDOSIS. **Sarcoidosis** may cause interstitial inflammation resulting in subsequent diastolic impairment with intact systolic function. Cardiac involvement occurs in 5% of cases of sarcoidosis. **The most common manifestation of cardiac sarcoid disease is conduction system disease.** Myocardial restriction results from patchy scar formation around infiltrating, noncaseating granulomas in the myocardium. Diffuse hypokinesis may be seen, as well as focal wall-motion abnormalities. A posterobasal aneurysm may also be present. Disease course is variable, with the most dramatic presentations being sudden cardiac death due to ventricular tachyaurrhythmias or high-degree heart block [14].

Gaucher's and Hurler's cardiomyopathy are rare genetic disorders that may be associated with an infiltrative cardiomyopathy. Gaucher's cardiomyopathy is an autosomal-recessive disease produced by mutations of the glucocerebrosidase gene that result in the accumulation of the lipid glucocerebroside in differing tissue beds, including the heart. Hurler's cardiomyopathy is a genetic disorder caused by a mutation in the chromosome pair responsible for producing alpha-L-iduronidase. This results in a mucopolysaccharidosis accumulation in various tissues, including the heart. These diseases are usually diagnosed during childhood due to other more pronounced manifestations, such as neurologic and musculoskeletal abnormalities.

Hemochromatosis may result in restrictive cardiomyopathy secondary to abnormal iron metabolism and subsequent deposition into myocardium. Hemochromatosis may be primary, due to an autosomal-recessive genetic abnormality, or secondary, due to iron overload. Primary hemochromatosis results in iron deposition into the myocardium, testes, pancreas, liver, and joints. Patients may present with diabetes, skin discoloration, and signs of diastolic dysfunction. Workup starts with iron studies, with an elevated **transferrin saturation** being most suggestive, followed by biopsy of an accessible organ (often liver). Treatment of underlying disease is of utmost importance to prevent progression of disease; this may involve phlebotomy and chelation therapy. In the presence of diastolic dysfunction, standard therapy may be started.

Glycogen storage diseases, such as Pompe's type II, have also been implicated in restrictive cardiomyopathies. This autosomal-recessive disorder results from the deficiency of the acid alpha-glucosidase, a lysosomal hydrolase, and produces cardiomyopathy usually only in the infantile form.

Endomyocardial Restrictive Cardiomyopathy

Hypereosinophilic Syndrome
Hypereosinophilic syndrome (Löffler's endocarditis, parietalis fibroblastica) is an obliterative, restrictive cardiomyopathy thought to result from toxic damage of intracytoplasmic granular content of activated eosinophils [15]. It occurs mainly in **temperate** climates and is associated with a hypereosinophilic syndrome consisting of modest eosinophilia, arteritis, and thromboembolism. Patients have endocardial thickening and obliteration of the cardiac apex. It is usually an aggressive disease that is rapidly progressive. It is more common in men than women. Use of corticosteroids and cytotoxic drugs in the early phase of disease may improve symptoms and survival [16].

Endomyocardial Fibrosis
Endomyocardial fibrosis (EMF) is a restrictive cardiomyopathy that also may be associated with eosinophilia [17]. It affects mainly children and occurs commonly in equatorial Africa (**tropical** climates). Patients experience EMF and obliteration of the cardiac apex. Fibrotic involvement may be localized or diffuse. Presentation is often insidious, with presentation of worsening biventricular failure. Prognosis is poor but depends on the degree and location of involvement. Surgical excision of fibrotic endocardium and valve replacement may help symptoms in the fibrotic stage but are palliative. Mortality for such procedures is 15–25% [18].

Carcinoid Heart Disease
Carcinoid heart disease is the result of prolonged and untreated carcinoid syndrome. It occurs in approximately one-half of all cases with tricuspid insufficiency as the predominant lesion. Lesion formation is correlated directly to the concentration of circulating and urinary levels of serotonin and 5-hydroxyindoleacetic acid [19]. Lesions are seen predominantly on the RV endocardium. Tricuspid stenosis and regurgitation, as well as pulmonic stenosis, are commonly seen.

Radiation-Induced Heart Disease
Radiation-induced heart disease may result in a restrictive cardiomyopathy due to increased interstitial fibrosis, particularly of the RV. Usually, however, radiation induces constrictive pericarditis. Radiation can also accelerate CAD.

Treatment
Restrictive cardiomyopathies usually impair diastolic function selectively, but as the disease progresses and intercellular fibrosis occurs, systolic function becomes compromised as well. Details on the treatment of congestive HF (including isolated diastolic dysfunction) are presented in Chap. 10, Management of Acute and Chronic Heart Failure.

HYPERTROPHIC CARDIOMYOPATHY

HCM is defined as myocardial hypertrophy in the absence of an identifiable cause or underlying etiology. This disease has been known by several names in the past, including *hypertrophic obstructive cardiomyopathy* (HOCM) and *idiopathic hypertrophic subaortic stenosis* (IHSS). There are varying types of HCM, including one associated with increased risk of sudden death in the young and a benign form of HCM associated with HTN in the elderly. Prevalence is approximately 1 in 500 [20]. It is the most common genetically transmitted cardiac disease. It is transmitted in an autosomal-dominant fashion, but variable penetrance and severity is the rule. The disease can be caused by a mutation in genes that encode proteins of the cardiac sarcomere, such as beta-myosin heavy chain, cardiac troponin T, alpha-tropomyosin, and myosin-binding protein C genes [21]. Obstruction occurs in only 25% of cases, with varying phenotypic and clinical expression. Histologic exam reveals disarray of cell arrangement and architecture most commonly found in the LV outflow tract, septum, apex, and midventricle. Small-vessel coronary disease, with arteriolar wall thickening, is also characteristic. **Importantly, it is the leading cause of sudden death in athletes <35.**

History

Many patients are asymptomatic, whereas others present with dyspnea, paroxysmal nocturnal dyspnea, fatigue, syncope, or even sudden cardiac death. Symptoms largely result from elevated LV pressure caused by lack of compliance secondary to hypertrophy of the myocardium. Subendocardial myocardial ischemia may also occur and has been demonstrated on thallium perfusion studies. The exact mechanism is undetermined, but it is thought most likely to be secondary to supply-demand mismatch.

Symptoms of syncope and presyncope are the result of impaired cerebral blood flow. In HCM, this may be due to tachyarrhythmia or obstruction resulting in inadequate cardiac output. Such symptoms in older adults are not necessarily as worrisome as in children and younger adults. The annual mortality rate for HCM is between 1% and 6%, with most deaths occurring suddenly.

Physical Exam

Patients with the presence of an LV outflow tract gradient can manifest several findings on physical exam, including a systolic ejection murmur at the left lower sternal border. This murmur is preload dependent and **intensifies with maneuvers that decrease preload,** such as standing and the Valsalva maneuver. The only other systolic murmur that intensifies with decreased preload is the mitral regurgitation (MR) murmur associated with mitral valve prolase (actually, it lengthens). Conversely, the systolic ejection murmur of HCM **decreases** with squatting (which increases preload and afterload) and handgrip (which increases afterload). Amyl nitrite decreases systemic vascular resistance and decreases LV volume, which increases the murmur of HCM. As only one-third of HCM patients manifest obstruction, the majority of patients will not have a murmur on exam. Other findings include **bisferiens** (bifid) carotid pulse and a large *a* wave on jugular venous pulse associated with an S_4.

Diagnostic Testing

Echocardiography
The easiest and most useful test for diagnosing HCM is echocardiography. The diagnosis of HCM can be made by identifying a hypertrophied, nondilated LV in the absence of another cause capable of producing hypertrophy. LV wall thickness >15 mm in any segment satisfies criteria for the diagnosis. Wall thickness is often asymmetric within the septum, and when this asymmetry biases the septum, the term **asymmetric septal hypertrophy (ASH)** is applied. Echocardiography can also identify other morphologic characteristics of HCM, including the presence and quantification of an LV outflow tract gradient, MR, and estimation of diastolic dysfunction (with Doppler flow recordings). MR in HCM is in part due to the Venturi effect created by turbulent flow through the LV outflow tract. This causes **systolic anterior motion (SAM) of the mitral valve,** which in turn posteriorly directs the jet of MR. Provocation with inhaled amyl nitrite increases the out-

flow gradient and, thus, the velocity of the spectral Doppler jet. Amyl can, therefore, provoke a latent outflow tract obstruction as well, roughly corresponding to a gradient that may be unveiled with activity, creating dyspnea on exertion.

ECG
Close to 95% of all HCM patients have an abnormal ECG. These abnormalities are diverse and include LVH pattern, with ST–T wave abnormalities, deep Q waves involving inferior and precordial leads (not indicative of transmural infarct), and left atrial enlargement. Prominent T-wave inversions in the precordial leads are characteristic of apical HCM (seen in patients of Japanese descent).

Chest X-Ray
Cardiomegaly may be noted on chest x-ray, along with left atrial enlargement and, occasionally, intersitial edema.

Cardiac Catheterization
Left- and right-heart catheterization are primarily reserved for those patients referred for invasive intervention, or if the question of epicardial coronary disease warrants evaluation. On coronary angiography, one classically sees systolic compression of the septal perforator branches of the left anterior descending artery **(septal milking)**. Hemodynamic assessment is also very important. In the setting of a resting gradient, the intraventricular systolic pressure is greater than that in the aorta (normally these are equal). This can be measured with a catheter within the LV lumen and one within the aorta. As the intraventricular pressure catheter is withdrawn out of the LV and into the aorta, the measured systolic pressure equalizes with that of the aorta, as the tip of the catheter is pulled past the outflow tract obstruction (Fig. 12-1A). Furthermore, an important diagnostic maneuver should be mentioned. In any heart, the creation of a PVC by the manipulation of a catheter placed into the LV causes a compensatory pause, and the following beat will occur with greater contractility. In normal hearts, the aortic pulse pressure increases with this post-PVC beat, and there is no pressure gradient (difference) between the aorta and LV. However, in HCM, the post-PVC aortic pulse pressure will remain the same, or decrease, and the pressure gradient between the LV and aorta will increase. This is known as the **Brockenbrough-Braunwald sign** and is considered the most specific sign of **dynamic LV outflow tract obstruction,** which is seen in many patients with HCM (Fig. 12-1B).

Pathology

LVH
There is diverse heterogeneity among the phenotypic expression of LVH. There is no pathognomonic pattern of LVH in HCM; however, in HCM, the majority of patients have involvement of the interventricular septum and anterolateral wall. Other areas of hypertrophy include the posterior septum, posterobasal free wall, and even concentric patterns of wall thickness. One variant of HCM is Yamaguchi's apical HCM, which accounts for 25% of HCM in Japan but only 1% of cases outside of Japan. It is distinguished by a localized apical hypertrophy in the distal LV, resulting in a spade-like configuration.

Of note, recent genetic data have shown occurrence of patients who are genotype-positive but have delayed penetrance of the phenotype (LVH) until later decades of life. The prognosis and clinical course of these patients remain undefined.

Cellular
The cellular substrate of HCM is defined by a unique cellular architecture characterized by **hypertrophied myocytes arranged in a chaotic pattern** at oblique and perpendicular angles. There is also an increased volume of interstitial collagen matrix.

Intramural coronary arteries also are abnormal in approximately 80% of patients. They exhibit thickened walls and a narrow lumen. This form of "small vessel disease" leads to microvascular ischemia which, through time, promotes replacement fibrosis.

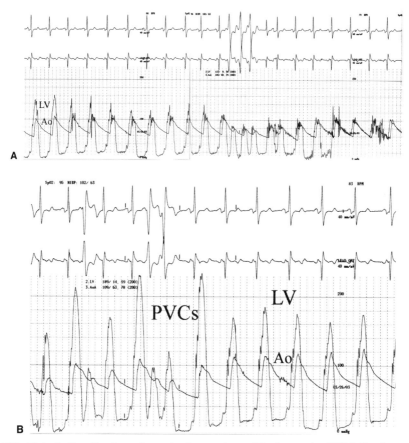

FIG. 12-1. A: Baseline hemodynamics in a patient with obstructive HCM. On the x axis of this tracing (time), the LV catheter is gradually pulled back from the LV to the aorta. Note that as the LV catheter is withdrawn past the obstruction, the LV systolic pressure equalizes with that of the aorta. As the catheter is pulled past the aortic valve, the waveform becomes aortic in nature. **B:** The Brockenbrough-Braun-wald sign. A series of PVCs is created by manipulation of the LV catheter. Note that on the post-PVC beat, the gradient (pressure difference) between the LV and aorta increases. *The finding specific to obstructive HCM is the constant aortic pulse pressure (systolic – diastolic) in this beat compared to non–post-PVC beats.* Ao, aortic pressure catheter; LV, left ventricular pressure catheter.

These morphologic characteristics (LVH, interstitial collagen matrix, microvascular ischemia, and replacement fibrosis) contribute to an LV chamber that is morphologically abnormal and can lead to diastolic dysfunction and congestive HF. It can also create a substrate for malignant arrhythmias and sudden death.

Clinical Presentation

HCM has a wide spectrum of clinical presentations. Most patients have mild or no symptoms. The two most common symptoms are dyspnea and chest pain, although palpitations, dizziness, syncope, orthopnea, and paroxysmal nocturnal dyspnea may also occur. The mechanism for dyspnea is a result of elevated left atrial pressure from impaired relaxation. Chest pain can be multifactorial in origin. Myocardial O_2 mismatch resulting from increased myocardial mass, "small vessel disease," increased wall stress, and epicardial coronary disease are all mechanisms for the manifestation of chest pain. Of note, patients with HCM often have reversible defects on radionuclide scanning, even in the absence of epicardial coronary disease; however, up to 20% of patients with HCM also have concurrent CAD. As a result, patients with HCM presenting with classic anginal symptoms and in whom the etiology of the chest pain is unclear should be considered for coronary angiography.

Clinical Course

Due to the heterogenous nature of HCM, the disease can follow several discrete clinical courses. These include (a) high risk for sudden cardiac death (recent unselected data have put annual mortality rates at 1%); (b) development of congestive symptoms requiring drug treatment or surgery (or alternatives to surgery); (c) development of AF and its consequences, including stroke; and (d) development of no or mild symptoms in many patients.

The specific genetic mutation can help predict the severity of the outflow gradient, the risk of sudden cardiac death, both, or neither. The role of routine genetic testing for individual patients to establish a diagnosis is extremely limited, but genetic testing can be useful in familial cohorts to assess prognosis, as well as in genetic counseling.

Risk Profile and Treatment Strategies

Sudden Death

HCM is the most common cause of cardiovascular sudden death in young people. This aspect of the disease has attracted enormous attention and has been the focus of intense debate regarding proper methods of risk stratification. Sudden death in HCM has a higher prevalence in young patients (<30), may not be preceded by other manifestations of the disease, and although most patients die while sedentary, vigorous physical exertion can be a trigger mechanism for a lethal event. **Patients considered to be at high risk for sudden death are associated with the following markers: prior cardiac arrest or spontaneous sustained VT, family history of premature HCM-related sudden death, repetitive or exertional syncope, multiple runs of nonsustained VT on Holter monitoring, LVH >30 mm, and hypotensive response to exercise testing [24,25,28].** Note that electrophysiologic study does not have diagnostic utility.

Limited data exist on the efficacy of antiarrhythmic drugs in the prevention of sudden death, rendering this treatment strategy a limited role. In addition, the relatively young age of most patients at risk for sudden death brings into question the long-term tolerability of most antiarrhythmic agents. **Currently, the standard of care supports the implantation of an ICD for secondary prevention of sudden death.** The selection of patients for **primary prevention** with ICD implantation should be based on the presence of the previously described high-risk clinical features and the clinical judgment of the treating physician.

Due to the fact that intense physical exertion can be a trigger for sudden death, the current recommendation [29] is to disqualify patients with HCM from participation in organized competitive athletics.

Heart Failure

Drug treatment of congestive symptoms in HCM relies on the use of **negative** inotropic agents, as these decrease the gradient across the LV outflow tract. Atenolol and verapamil are the most common agents used to alleviate congestive symptoms. The severity of SAM and MR can be reduced as well. Beta blockers help reduce symptoms of dyspnea and angina, as well as aid in reducing the provocable gradient. Beta blockers work by slowing heart rate and thereby reducing myocardial O_2 demand and improving diastolic filling. Up to one-third of patients have a clinical response to beta blockers. For patients not responding to a beta blocker, the calcium channel blocker verapamil may be used. Usually, one class of drug is administered at a time, as combining both agents offers no known advantage. However, patients presenting with HF due to HCM should not receive verapamil, as some series have shown poor outcomes in this setting. Some centers have found a role for the use of disopyramide (Norpace) (particularly in patients with obstruction) when other agents have been unsuccessful. The use of ACE inhibitors is **not recommended unless there is significant HTN,** as these drugs can worsen the gradient by peripheral vasodilation. There is also **no role for digoxin,** as this agent acts as a positive inotrope and can increase the outflow obstruction. **Nitrates are contraindicated,** because they decrease preload and thereby increase the gradient across the LV outflow tract. Likewise, **inotropes, such as dobutamine, are ineffective** and sometimes harmful, as the positive inotropy also increases the gradient across the LV outflow tract and can yield significant hypotension. Pacemakers are useful in some populations (see Refractory Symptoms). Diuretics, prudently used, can be useful for patients with HF secondary to HCM.

Atrial Fibrillation

AF can occur in up to 25% of patients with HCM. It often is poorly tolerated, as patients normally depend on the atrial contribution to ventricular filling. Rate control can be achieved through the use of beta blockers or verapamil. Although it is unclear how effective antiarrhythmic therapy with amiodarone is in maintaining sinus rhythm after electrical or pharmacologic cardioversion, it is currently the agent of choice for this indication. Anticoagulation with Coumadin should be administered to patients with paroxysmal or chronic AF to prevent thromboembolic complications.

Refractory Symptoms

When patients develop congestive symptoms that are refractory to maximum drug treatment and have basal outflow obstruction, several therapeutic options exist.

Septal myotomy-myectomy (Morrow procedure) is the gold standard for relief of obstructive symptoms in such patients. In this procedure, the surgeon uses a transaortic approach to resect a small amount of septal muscle to relieve the subaortic obstruction. In experienced centers, operative mortality is 1–2%, and long-term data have shown a reduction in congestive symptoms and increase in exercise capacity in most patients. Concomitant mitral valve replacement may be necessary if there is no relief of SAM with myectomy alone.

Alcohol septal ablation has been developed more recently and may be appropriate for many patients. It is performed by injecting 2–5 cc of 95–100% alcohol into the first major septal perforator branch of the left anterior descending artery, thereby producing an infarct in the ventricular septum. As a result, localized wall thinning occurs, thereby enlarging the outflow tract and reducing the intraventricular gradient. Current data have shown that septal ablation can substantially reduce the gradient and relieve symptoms in many patients. AV block requiring a permanent pacemaker occurs approximately 30% of the time. In addition, the long-term risk of sudden death with the addition of a myocardial scar on a cardiac substrate already predisposed to arrhythmogenesis is an unresolved issue. Many of these patients already have or are candidates for an implanted defibrillator.

After some initial enthusiasm for the role of the **dual-chamber pacemaker** for the relief of obstructive symptoms in HCM, there is now consensus that its role is limited. Pacing in HCM appears to provide symptomatic benefit largely as a result of the placebo effect, but one study did show objective improvement in symptoms for patients >65 yrs [26]. Its implantation may eliminate concern for drug-associated bradycardia and consequently allow maximization of dosing.

Heart Transplantation

In patients with nonobstructive HCM who are symptomatic despite maximal medical therapy, heart transplantation is a viable option. Furthermore, some patients evolve to a dilated cardiomyopathy, requiring assessment for heart transplantation for refractory symptoms and limitations on survival.

KEY POINTS TO REMEMBER

- A wide variety of pathologic processes can afflict the heart. These processes yield anatomic and pathologic features that can be loosely organized into dilated, restrictive, and hypertrophic cardiomyopathies.
- Determination of the underlying cause of dilated cardiomyopathy usually does not strongly impact the nature of its treatment. The role of endomyocardial biopsy is very limited in this setting.
- Assessment for the cause of a restrictive cardiomyopathy can be important, because a systemic disease process may be secondarily affecting the heart. Distinguish restrictive cardiomyopathy from a restrictive diastolic filling pattern [see Chap. 22, Imaging and Diagnostic Testing Modalities (Nuclear Imaging, Echocardiography, and Cardiac Catheterization)], as the latter can be exhibited in any progressed cardiomyopathy.
- HCM is a relatively common condition characterized by a number of pathologic and clinical features, each of which is present variably in affected patients.
- Treatment of obstructive symptoms, such as dyspnea, and stratifying for risk of sudden cardiac death, particularly in the young, are the most important features in caring for patients with HCM.

SUGGESTED READING

Fuster V, Alexander W, O'Rourke R. *Hurst's the heart,* 10th ed. New York: McGraw-Hill, 1987.

REFERENCES

1. Report of the WHO/ISFC task force on the definition and classification of cardiomyopathies. *Br Heart J* 1980;44:672–673.
2. Codd MB, Sugrue DD, Gersh BJ, et al. Epidemiology of idiopathic dilated and hypertrophic cardiomyopathy: a population-based study in Olmsted County, Minnesota, 1975–1984. *Circulation* 1989;80:564–572.
3. Dec GW, Fuster V. Idiopathic dilated cardiomyopathy. *N Engl J Med* 1994;331:1564–1575.
4. Sugrue DD, Rodeheffer RJ, Codd MB, et al. The clinical course of idiopathic dilated cardiomyopathy: a population-based study. *Ann Intern Med* 1992;117:117–123.
5. Felker GM, Thompson RE, Hare JM, et al. Underlying causes and long-term survival in patients with initially unexplained cardiomyopathy. *N Engl J Med* 2000;342:1077–1083.
6. Tazelaar HD, Billingham ME. Leukocytic infiltrates in idiopathic dilated cardiomyopathy: a source of confusion with active myocarditis. *Am J Surg Pathol* 1986;10:405–412.
7. Obrador D, Ballester M, Carrio I, et al. Presence, evolving changes, and prognostic implications of myocardial damage detected in idiopathic and alcoholic dilated cardiomyopathy by ^{111}In monoclonal antimyosin antibodies. *Circulation* 1994;89:2054.
8. Von Hoff DD, Layard MW, Basa P, et al. Risk factors in doxorubicin-induced congestive heart failure. *Ann Intern Med* 1979;91:710.
9. Heider AL, Kuller JA, Strauss RA, et al. Peripartum cardiomyopathy: review of the literature. *Obstet Gynecol Surv* 1999;54:526–531.
10. Elkayam U, Tummala PP, Rao K, et al. Maternal and fetal outcomes of subsequent pregnancies in women with peripartum cardiomyopathy. *N Engl J Med* 2001;344(21):1567–1571.
11. Acierno LJ. Cardiac complications in acquired immunodeficiency syndrome (AIDS): a review. *J Am Coll Cardiol* 1989;13:1144–1154.
12. Richardson P, McKenna W, Bristow M, et al. Report of the 1995 World Health Organization/International Society and Federation of Cardiology Task Force on the definition and classification of cardiomyopathies. *Circulation* 1996;93:841–842.

13. Cooke RA, Chambers JB, Curry PV. Noonan's cardiomyopathy: a non-hypertrophic variant. *Br Heart J* 1994;71:561–565.
14. Kushwaha SS, Fallon JT, Fuster V. Restrictive cardiomyopathy. *N Engl J Med* 1997;336:267–276.
15. Tai PC, Ackerman SJ, Spry CJ, et al. Deposits of eosinophil granule proteins in cardiac tissues of patients with eosinophilic endomyocardial disease. *Lancet* 1987;1:643–647.
16. Kim CH, Vlietstra RE, Edwards WD, et al. Steroid-responsive eosinophilic myocarditis: diagnosis by endomyocardial biopsy. *Am J Cardiol* 1984;53:1472–1473.
17. Fauci AS, Harley JB, Roberts WC, et al. The idiopathic hypereosinophilic syndrome: clinical pathophysiologic, and therapeutic considerations. *Ann Intern Med* 1982;97:78–92.
18. Metras D, Coulibaly AO, Ouattara K. The surgical treatment of endomyocardial fibrosis: results in 55 patients. *Circulation* 1985;72[Suppl II]:II274–II279.
19. Robiolio PA, Rigolin VH, Wilson JS, et al. Carcinoid heart disease: correlation of high serotonin levels with valvular abnormalities detected by cardiac catheterization and echocardiography. *Circulation* 1995;92:790–795.
20. Maron BJ, Gardin JM, Flack JM, et al. Prevalence of hypertrophic cardiomyopathy in a general population of young adults: echocardiographic analysis of 4111 subjects in the CARDIA Study. *Circulation* 1995;92:785–789.
21. Spirito P, Seidman CE, McKenna WJ, et al. The management of hypertrophic cardiomyopathy. *N Engl J Med* 1997;336(11):775.
22. Maron BJ. Hypertrophic cardiomyopathy. *Lancet* 1997;350:127–133.
23. Spirito P, Seidman CE, McKenna WJ, et al. Management of hypertrophic cardiomyopathy. *N Engl J Med* 1997;30:775–785.
24. Spirito P, Bellone P, Harris K, et al. Magnitude of left ventricular hypertrophy and risk of sudden death in hypertrophic cardiomyopathy. *N Engl J Med* 2000; 342:1778–1785.
25. Maron B, Shen WK, Link M, et al. Efficacy of implantable cardioverter-defibrillators for the prevention of sudden death in patients with hypertrophic cardiomyopathy. *N Engl J Med* 2000;342:365–373.
26. Maron B, Nishimura RA, McKenna W, et al. Assessment of permanent dual-chamber pacing as a treatment for drug-refractory symptomatic patients with obstructive hypertrophic cardiomyopathy: a randomized, double-blind cross-over study (M-PATHY). *Circulation* 1999;83:903–907.
27. Kamisago M, Sharma SD, DePalma SR, et al. Mutations in sarcomere protein genes as a cause of dilated cardiomyopathy. *N Engl J Med* 2000;343(23):1688–1696.
28. Maron BJ. Hypertrophic cardiomyopathy: a systematic review. *JAMA* 2002; 287:1308–1320.
29. Thompson PD, Klocke FJ, Levine BD, et al. 26th Bethesda conference: recommendations for determining eligibility for competition in athletes with cardiovascular abnormalities. Task Force 5: coronary artery disease. *Med Sci Sports Exerc* 1994;[10 Suppl]:S271–S275.

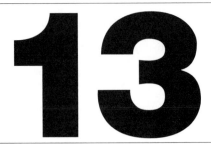

Valvular Heart Disease

Alan Zajarias and
Peter A. Crawford

INTRODUCTION

The group of diseases affecting the mobility and closure of heart valves is termed **valvular heart disease.** It can be categorized as congenital or acquired and can affect any of the four valves.

AORTIC VALVE

Aortic Stenosis

Epidemiology

The obstruction of the LV outflow tract yields a gradient (systolic pressure difference between the LV outflow tract and ascending aorta). The etiologies can be divided into three categories:

- **Supravalvular:** This etiology is most rare and is considered a form of congenital heart disease associated with elphin facies, hypercalcemia, and pulmonary stenosis (Williams syndrome).
- **Subvalvular:** This etiology is seen in 10% of patients with aortic stenosis (AS) and is caused by fixed membranous ridge or fibrous tunnel in the LV outflow tract or dynamic obstruction associated with HCM. The membranous ridge form eventually causes aortic insufficiency due to damage to the AV from the chronically diverted jet of blood flow caused by the membrane.
- **Valvular:** This category can be further divided by etiology and age of presentation.
- **Rheumatic:** Presents in patients between 40 and 60 yrs and must be accompanied by mitral valve disease. Pathologically, AV commissures are fused. It is seen infrequently in the United States.
- **Congenital:**
  - **Unicuspid:** Presenting in the first three decades of life.
  - **Bicuspid:** Presenting between 40–60 yrs, with an estimated prevalence of 1–2% of population. Abnormal valve anatomy causes turbulent flow, promoting calcification and degeneration of the aortic valve. This is commonly associated with aortic insufficiency. A subset of bicuspid AV is associated with coarctation of the aorta.
- **Calcific/degenerative:** This is the most common cause of AS in the United States. It is encountered at >70 and produces calcification of the valve from the base to the leaflets without commissural fusion. It is exacerbated by abnormal calcium metabolism (i.e., chronic renal insufficiency, Paget's disease, etc.) and carries the same risk factors as atherosclerosis.

Natural History

AS is a progressive disease characterized by an asymptomatic progression until the valvular area reaches a minimal threshold. Although difficult to predict in individual cases, it is estimated that the aortic valve gradient increases 7–15 mm Hg/yr, and the aortic area decreases an average of 0.12 cm^2/yr [1]. Asymptomatic patients have a similar life expectancy as people without AS. Symptoms generally begin once the valvular area is <1 cm^2. It is estimated that once patients experience **angina, syncope, and signs of CHF** (the three classic signs of progressive AS), their 50% survival rate is 5, 3, and 2 yrs, respectively. Symptomatic patients experience arrhythmia-associated sudden death due to ischemia or hypertrophy-induced ventricular dysfunction.

Pathophysiology

Progressive AS generates an increase in intraventricular pressure to maintain adequate cardiac output. In response to chronic pressure overload, ventricular walls hypertrophy to reduce wall stress (law of Laplace). Ventricular hypertrophy causes decrease in ventricular compliance, which impairs passive filling and increases preload dependence on atrial contraction. Concentric hypertrophy increases the LV end-diastolic pressure (LVEDP), which decreases myocardial perfusion pressure and compresses subendocardial vessels, generating subendocardial ischemia. Diastolic dysfunction, evidenced by decreased compliance and a prolonged relaxation phase, is due to ischemia and ventricular hypertrophy and is symptomatically expressed as dyspnea. LV outflow tract obstruction decreases the coronary and systemic blood flow, augmenting myocardial O_2 demand/supply mismatch. Increasing wall stress, elevated LV mass, and systolic pressure increase the myocardial O_2 demand, which further promotes myocardial ischemia. Syncope is thought to be secondary to arrhythmia, a decrease in systemic flow due to fixed valvular obstruction, or an abnormal vasodepressor reflex.

As the disease progresses, myocardial fibrosis develops. The ventricle cannot overcome the wall stress and dilates. Once ventricular dilation occurs, end-stage AS begins. Ventricular dilation and systolic dysfunction cause a fall in the transvalvular gradient (TVG) and cardiac output, causing hypotension and worsening coronary perfusion.

History

Classic symptoms include **angina, syncope, and exertional dyspnea.** Patients with a history of rheumatic fever will have multivalvular disease.

Physical Exam

Physical exam findings include the following:

- Classically, a harsh systolic ejection murmur heard best at the right upper sternal border radiating to both carotid arteries. Its time to peak correlates with severity; **mid- or late systolic peaking indicates more severe AS.**
- S_2 may be **paradoxically split** due to increased ejection time (and later A_2) of the LV or may be decreased in intensity due to loss of the A_2. **Loss of A_2 (soft S_2) also indicates severe AS.**
- S_1 has a normal or a reduced intensity as LV function worsens due to premature closure.
- An opening snap heard best in the left parasternal line may be suggestive of congenital AS. S_3 is a late finding and indicative of systolic dysfunction and heart failure (HF). S_4 reflects atrial contraction on a poorly compliant ventricle.
- Point of maximal impulse (PMI) is sustained and diffuse and not displaced (unless ventricle has dilated).
- **Pulsus parvus et tardus.** Late-peaking and diminished carotid upstroke is seen in severe AS, although it is also seen in elderly patients with generalized atherosclerosis or in systolic dysfunction.
- Systolic thrill in the carotid artery and in the second right intercostal space in the parasternal line.
- In a young patient, look for differential BP in both arms and legs (coarctation and bicuspid AV).
- Other murmurs:
  - Be aware of concomitant mitral stenosis (MS) and/or mitral regurgitation (MR) in patients with rheumatic heart disease.
  - **Gallavardin phenomenon** is an AS murmur heard best at the apex and is easily confused with MR.
  - The presence of aortic insufficiency may be suggestive of a calcified aortic valve that is poorly mobile.

Lab Studies

Lab studies should include the following:

- **ECG:** 80% of patients have left atrial enlargement, and 85% have LVH. AF may suggest concomitant mitral valve disease.
- **Chest x-ray:** Look for evidence of LVH, cardiomegaly, and calcification of the aorta, aortic valve, or coronary arteries. In the lateral film, be aware of poststenotic dilation of the ascending aorta. Rib-notching is seen in coarctation and would lead one to suspect a bicuspid aortic valve.
- **Transthoracic echocardiography:** All patients with suspected AS should undergo echocardiographic evaluation with Doppler interrogation to determine the thickness of the leaflets, number of aortic leaflets, concomitant aortic regurgitation or mitral valve disease, aortic valvular area (AVA), and TVG. TEE is used to determine valvular area and morphology in patients with congenital heart disease for surgery planning. The **continuity equation** is used to calculate the AVA. The principle of continuity states that flow (velocity × area) is equal on both sides of an obstruction. Blood velocity, which can be measured with spectral Doppler, is higher distal to the obstruction. Therefore,

$$(AVA) \times (\text{aortic blood velocity}) = (\text{LV outflow tract area}) \times (\text{LV outflow tract velocity})$$

Normal AVA measures 2–4 cm^2. Disease severity is classified as

- Mild: AVA of >1.5 cm^2 or TVG of 0–20 mm Hg
- Moderate: AVA = 1–1.5 cm^2 and TVG is 20–40 mm Hg
- Severe: AVA <1 cm^2 and TVG >40 mm Hg
- Critical: AVA <0.75 cm^2 and TVG >50 mm Hg

The finding of **aortic sclerosis** is thickening of the AV leaflets, causing turbulent flow and a murmur but no gradient and, thus, no stenosis.

- **Stress testing:** Stress testing is occasionally used in patients with asymptomatic severe AS. It is used as a symptom-limited test and is performed to determine true exercise capacity to time surgery.
- **Dobutamine echocardiography:** Dobutamine echocardiography is used to assess patients with poor LV systolic function and a small aortic transvalvular gradient to determine if the degree of stenosis is fixed or if it can be improved by enhancing LV systolic function. If the calculated valve area increases by ≥ 0.3 cm^2, the AV disorder is often called *aortic pseudostenosis*.
- **Cardiac catheterization:** In the setting of severe AS, many cardiologists recommend cardiac catheterization for all male patients >40 yrs and females >50 yrs to determine presence of CAD and need for concomitant bypass. In addition, if the symptoms and echocardiographic-determined valve area and gradients are discordant, cardiac catheterization with determination of transvalvular pressure gradient, valve area, and cardiac function may be performed. One measuring catheter is within the LV, and the other is within the aorta.
  - Complication rates of cardiac catheterization are increased in patients with AS. Fig. 13-1 demonstrates the hemodynamics observed in AS.
  - The **Gorlin formula** is used to calculate AVA by cardiac catheterization. Right- and left-heart catheterization are required, so that cardiac output and gradient, respectively, can be measured. The Gorlin formula holds that

$$AVA(cm^2) \alpha \frac{\text{cardiac output}}{\sqrt{\text{mean gradient}}}$$

Treatment

- Therapeutic decisions are based primarily on the presence or absence of symptoms, **not** on valvular area or transvalvular gradient. Treatment of severe AS is almost

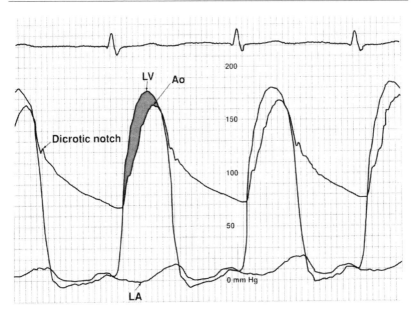

FIG. 13-1. Hemodynamics observed in aortic stenosis. The x axis is time; the y axis is pressure in mm Hg. Ao, aorta; LA, left atrium; LV, left ventricle. (From Murphy JG. *Mayo Clinic cardiology review,* 2nd ed. Philadelphia: Lippincott Williams & Wilkins, 2000, with permission.)

exclusively with **surgical aortic valve replacement (AVR).** Operative mortality is calculated as <3% in young individuals and can be as high as 30% in patients >80 yrs. Consider surgery in symptomatic patients with severe AS, patients with severe AS undergoing coronary artery bypass surgery, and patients with severe AS undergoing ascending aortic or other valvular surgery. If patients are asymptomatic and have a calculated area <1 cm, focus treatment on CAD prevention, maintenance of normal sinus rhythm, and BP control, and instruct them to notify their physicians with the first appearance of symptoms. Some cardiologists use a symptom-limited stress test for asymptomatic patients with severe AS.

- **The choice of AVR type** depends on the patient, surgeon, and cardiologist. The first decision is mechanical prosthetic or bioprosthetic. Bioprosthetic valves (e.g., Carpentier-Edwards, Hancock) are appropriate for patients receiving surgery for emergent aortic insufficiency, as well as poor long-term anticoagulation candidates. These valves can be expected to last approximately 10 yrs. Mechanical valves are further divided into bileaflet (e.g., St. Jude, CarboMedics, or Duromedics) or single-tilting disk (e.g., Medtronic-Hall, Björk-Shiley). Mechanical valves require permanent anticoagulation and can last the life of the patient in the absence of prosthetic-valve endocarditis. The Starr-Edwards caged ball is rarely implanted today, but it is seen in elderly patients who underwent AVR in the past. See p. 267 for anticoagulation guidelines.

- An intraaortic balloon pump (IABP) can be used as a bridge to surgery in unstable patients without aortic insufficiency. Percutaneous valvuloplasty has only been shown to be effective in the pediatric population. In adults, its restenosis rate is >60% at 6 mos and nearly 100% after 2 yrs, without a decrease in mortality. It is only recommended for use as a bridge to surgery for AVR, as a palliative measure in patients with serious comorbid conditions who are not candidates for AVR, or if urgent noncardiac surgery is needed in patients with severe AS. Sodium nitroprusside has also been shown to be useful for patients with critical AS and decompensated HF, while planning definitive therapy.

- **Medical Therapy:** Severe AS is a surgical disease. Nevertheless, there are guidelines for nonsurgical candidates, as well as those waiting for surgery. Treat patients with CHF and AS with gentle diuresis to avoid preload loss. **The use of nitrates is contraindicated in severe AS, because they can precipitate severe hypotension.**
- Vasodilators are only recommended when there is concomitant AS and aortic insufficiency, or AS and CAD. Vasodilators should be short acting, used only in the ICU setting and only as a bridge to surgery. Some evidence has emerged regarding the use of hydroxymethylglutaryl coenzyme A reductase inhibitors (statins) in AS, as they have been shown to slow the progression of the gradient. This intriguing finding requires further substantiation. **Antibiotic prophylaxis is required before surgical procedures** (see p. 218).

Aortic Insufficiency

Etiology
Aortic insufficiency results from involvement of the aortic root or **aortic valve**. Those etiologies precipitating aortic valve involvement include those listed below.

- **Acute rheumatic fever** may induce mild regurgitation, which later degenerates to AS after calcification and fusion of the aortic valve leaflets. It most commonly is seen with concomitant mitral disease.
- **Bicuspid aortic valve** causes malcoaptation of the valvular cusps, generating aortic insufficiency.
- **Congenital abnormalities:**

  - Bicuspid aortic valve is the most common congenital cause of aortic insufficiency.
  - Supracristal VSDs are associated with progressive aortic insufficiency secondary to loss of support of the valvular annulus and/or formation of a sinus of Valsalva aneurysm through the VSD.

- **Infective endocarditis** leads to tissue destruction or formation of vegetations that interrupt adequate valve closure.
- **Senile degeneration** is accompanied by AS.
- **Collagen vascular diseases,** such as, ankylosing spondylitis, rheumatoid arthritis, Reiter's syndrome, giant-cell arteritis, and Whipple's disease
- Progressive dilatation of the ascending aorta causes aortic insufficiency. Etiologies of **aortic root** involvement include
- **Marfan syndrome**
- **Ehlers-Danlos syndrome**
- **Cystic medial necrosis** secondary to HTN
- **Aortic aneurysm**
- **Aortic dissection**
- **Trauma**
- **Tertiary syphilis**
- **Collagen vascular disease**

Natural History and Pathophysiology
Chronic aortic insufficiency is a silently progressive disease, whereas acute aortic insufficiency is a true surgical emergency (see Chap. 5, Cardiovascular Emergencies).

- **Acute aortic insufficiency** causes acute volume overload into a noncompliant LV, causing sudden elevation of the LVEDP and progressive pulmonary venous distention, leading to pulmonary edema. The pulse pressure is often as high as 150 mm Hg.
- **Chronic aortic insufficiency** has two phases: In **compensated** aortic insufficiency, the LV gradually compensates for the volume overload by muscle-fiber stretching, sarcomere replication, and eccentric hypertrophy of the ventricular walls. The ejec-

tion fraction is maintained by Frank-Starling mechanisms at a higher-than-normal preload state. Asymptomatic aortic insufficiency with normal LV function has a 0.2% incidence of sudden death. Asymptomatic individuals with normal LV function may develop asymptomatic LV dysfunction at a rate of 3.5%/yr; patients with asymptomatic aortic insufficiency with normal LV function develop symptomatic LV dysfunction at a rate of 6.5%/yr [2,3].

- In **decompensated** aortic insufficiency, as the ventricle gradually enlarges, the preload reserve is exhausted, and further ventricular dilation occurs. The ejection fraction begins to fall, and the end-systolic dimension of the ventricle increases. Further dilation of the ventricle causes an increase in the LVEDP, resulting in dyspnea. During exercise, a fall in the vascular resistances and a shorter diastole promote forward cardiac output. The subsequent increase in venous return promotes volume overload to the LV, causing fatigue or dyspnea due to increase in the LVEDP and a decrease in the relative cardiac output. Angina is experienced in the presence of normal coronary arteries due to an increase in the myocardial O_2 consumption (high myocardial mass and wall tension), fall of the coronary perfusion pressure (low diastolic pressure), and subendocardial ischemia.
- Age, end-systolic dimension, and ejection fraction are the most important markers of cardiovascular death, symptoms, and LV dysfunction. In one study, end-systolic dimension >50 mm carried a risk of death, symptoms, or LV dysfunction of 19% per yr [4]. Patients with asymptomatic aortic insufficiency with LV dysfunction become symptomatic at a rate of >25% per yr. Patients with symptomatic aortic insufficiency have a mortality rate in excess of 10% per yr [3].

History
ACUTE. Patients with acute aortic insufficiency present with pulmonary edema manifested by severe dyspnea. **Aortic dissection and endocarditis should be high in the differential diagnosis.**

CHRONIC. Symptoms depend on the presence of LV dysfunction and the stage of aortic insufficiency (compensated vs decompensated). Decompensated patients complain of decreased exercise tolerance, fatigue, angina, and persistent palpitations or a hyperdynamic precordium or "neck palpitations." Ask about a family history of Marfan syndrome or aortic dissection, as well as a history of rheumatologic disease.

Physical Exam
ACUTE. On general exam, evaluate for the presence of elongated facies, a highly arched palate, arachnodactyly, pectus excavatum, ectopia lentis, or other marfanoid characteristics. Pulsus paradoxus may evidence cardiac tamponade secondary to aortic dissection. Measure BP in both arms and note the pulse pressure. Look for splinter hemorrhages, Roth's spots, Janeway lesions, or Osler's nodes, which are suggestive of bacterial endocarditis (see Chap. 17, Infective Endocarditis and Acute Rheumatic Fever). Palpate the precordium for an LV heave and PMI displacement. Physical findings may be limited to the presence of a soft diastolic murmur heard best at the third left intercostals space in the parasternal line while the patient is sitting upright.

CHRONIC. A widened pulse pressure >100 mm Hg with a low diastolic pressure is present. Korotkoff sounds may be heard until 0 mm Hg; in this case, the muffling of phase IV correlates with the diastolic BP. The classic "pimp" signs of aortic insufficiency should be familiar: **Musset's sign** (head bobbing with each cardiac cycle), **Corrigan's pulse** (rapid carotid upstroke followed by arterial collapse), **Müller's sign** (pulsation of the uvula), **Traube's sign** (pistol-shot murmur heard on the femoral artery), **Duroziez's sign** (to-and-fro murmur over the femoral artery when partially compressed), **Hill's sign** (>30 mm Hg pressure difference between the popliteal and brachial arterial pressure; greater in lower extremity); and **Quincke's pulse** (visible capillary pulsation in the nail bed after holding the tip of the nail).

Cardiac Exam
Palpate for an LV heave and lateral PMI displacement. Look for a soft S_1 secondary to early closure of the mitral valve and soft systolic ejection murmur at the

base of the heart secondary to volume overload. **Austin Flint murmur** is present; this is a diastolic murmur heard best at the apex and caused by regurgitant aortic flow, generating vibration of the anterior mitral leaflet. It is differentiated from MS murmur by the absence of the opening snap. Patients also have a diastolic murmur heard best at the third left intercostal space in the parasternal line while sitting. Severity of the disease correlates with the duration of the murmur, not the intensity. Wide-open aortic insufficiency exhibits no audible murmur, as there is no diastolic gradient between aorta and LV. Tachycardia is a marker of disease progression.

Diagnostic and Laboratory Studies

- **Chest x-ray** may show pulmonary edema, widened mediastinum, and enlarged heart (cor bovinum).
- Patients may be persistently tachycardic. **ECG** may show evidence of left atrial enlargement or LV hypertrophy. A new conduction block is suggestive of a myocardial abscess in the presence of acute infective endocarditis.
- **Transthoracic echocardiogram** is used to evaluate LV systolic function, end-systolic dimension, aortic annulus, ascending aorta, and sinus of Valsalva. Severity of aortic insufficiency is quantified by the pressure half-time of the regurgitant jet, jet height to LV outflow tract height, jet area to LV outflow tract area, premature closure of the mitral valve, and presence of diastolic flow reversal in the ascending aorta. Table 13-1 reviews the severity of aortic insufficiency as determined by echocardiography.
- **TEE** is used to rule out the presence of vegetations, congenital abnormalities, and aortic root abscesses.
- **Cardiac catheterization** is used when planning surgery; the procedure may be complicated due to widened aortic root. Take care with manipulation to avoid unnecessary endothelial strain, leading to dissection enlargement. Left-heart catheterization is used to document reduced diastolic gradient across AV. An aortogram is often performed to assess the severity of regurgitation. A coronary angiogram in men >40 yrs or women >50 yrs is often performed to plan surgical intervention. Right-heart catheterization is also performed to document pulmonary capillary wedge pressure (PCWP).

Treatment

The basis for adequate treatment is determining the etiology of aortic insufficiency, ensuring hemodynamic stability, and defining the time for surgery. For acute aortic insufficiency, surgical treatment is the mainstay of therapy. Beta blockade or vasodilators (nitroprusside) are indicated to prevent progression of dissection. Treatment with antibiotics is indicated if endocarditis is suspected. Rapid ventricular pacing may be considered to decrease diastole and improve forward cardiac output in the

TABLE 13-1. SEVERITY OF AORTIC INSUFFICIENCY DETERMINED BY ECHOCARDIOGRAPHY

Severity	Pressure half-time (m/sec)	Continuous Doppler slope (m/sec)	AI jet/LVOT area (%)
Mild	>400	<2	<4
Moderate	300–400	2–3	4–25
Moderate–severe	300–400	2–3	25–59
Severe	<300	>3	>60

AI, aortic insufficiency; LVOT, LV outflow tract.
From Marso SP, Griffin BP, Topol EJ, eds. *Manual of cardiovascular medicine.* Philadelphia: Lippincott Williams & Wilkins, 2000, with permission.

absence of dissection. PO vasodilators can be used if the patient is not critically ill. Note that **IABP use is contraindicated** in patients with moderate or severe aortic insufficiency.

For chronic aortic insufficiency, medical therapy is an important aspect of treatment. **Vasodilators** are used in symptomatic severe aortic insufficiency with LV dysfunction in patients who are not surgical candidates. Asymptomatic patients with aortic insufficiency, normal LV function, and HTN also benefit from vasodilators. In asymptomatic patients with severe aortic insufficiency and LV dilation with normal systolic function, **nifedipine** decreases progression and time to surgery by 1–2 yrs [5]. ACE inhibitors may be better tolerated. Patients should be advised against strenuous physical activity.

Initiate preprocedural antibiotic prophylaxis in all patients with aortic insufficiency (see p. 218).

With regard to surgical therapy in aortic insufficiency, controversy exists about the optimal timing of surgery in patients without symptoms and normal LV function. In acute aortic insufficiency, all patients should be considered surgical candidates. If the source of acute aortic insufficiency is endocarditis, the following are all indications for urgent surgical intervention: previous stroke and valvular vegetation, vegetation after remobilization, vegetations persisting after 4 wks of adequate antibiotic treatment, acute valvular dysfunction, or new evidence of heart block indicating aortic root abscess.

In chronic aortic insufficiency, guidelines have been established. Patients who meet the **rule of 55** [i.e., asymptomatic patients with ejection fraction <55% and end-systolic dimension >55 mm, New York Heart Association (NYHA) class II or higher (see Chap. 10, Management of Acute and Chronic Heart Failure), or an aortic root >5.5–6 cm (4.5–5 cm in patients with Marfan syndrome)] should undergo AVR. See the Treatment section under Aortic Stenosis above for types of aortic valves. If the aortic root is aneurysmal, then repair, often with a patch, is also required. Severe preoperative symptoms, reduced exercise tolerance, severely depressed ejection fraction, and duration of LV systolic dysfunction are markers of poor postop outcome.

MITRAL VALVE

The mitral valve permits unidirectional flow from the left atrium (LA) to the LV. It is composed of an annulus, two leaflets, posteromedial and anterolateral papillary muscles, and chordae tendinea. The latter two are considered the mitral subvalvular apparatus. Together with the LV, the interaction between these parts is necessary for the adequate function of the mitral valve.

Incompetence of the mitral valve causes regurgitation of the LV contents in the LA during systole and is known as MR. Incomplete opening of the mitral valve during diastole limits the anterograde flow from the LA to the LV and is known as MS.

Mitral Regurgitation

Etiology

ORGANIC. The organic etiology of MR is due to direct involvement of the mitral valve and mitral subvalvular apparatus.

- **Mitral valve prolapse (MVP)** is characterized by systolic bowing of the posterior leaflet into the LA; it is the most common cause of MR in the United States. It may be associated with Marfan syndrome, Ehlers-Danlos syndrome, or other thoracic-skeletal abnormalities. Myxoid degeneration of the valve occurs and is associated with redundancy of the leaflet.
- Once the most common cause of MR, **rheumatic heart disease** is decreasing in incidence. It can be pure MR or associated with MS.
- Preferentially an age-related ailment, **mitral annular calcification** is associated with diabetes mellitus, chronic renal insufficiency, HCM, and AS.

- **Infective endocarditis** is related to vegetation-induced inappropriate leaflet coaptation or valvular perforation.
- **Chordae tendineae rupture/flail leaflet** occurs secondary to trauma, endocarditis, or may be idiopathic or ischemic.
- **Papillary muscle dysfunction** may be ischemic or caused by myocarditis.
- **Congenital** causes include cleft of the anterior mitral leaflet, which may be seen with ostium primum atrial septal defects or AV canal (in the setting of trisomy 21).
- Drugs include Phentermine-fenfluramine (phen-fen) and ergots.
- **Systemic etiologies** include Libman-Sacks endocarditis, rheumatoid arthritis, and carcinoid syndrome.

FUNCTIONAL.   Related to dilatation of the LV causing elongation of the mitral valve annulus and impeding the mitral valve leaflets from fully coapting.

Pathophysiology
MR is characterized by three stages: acute, chronic compensated, and chronic decompensated. The progression between stages depends on the etiology and severity of MR and individual factors. In the **acute phase,** new-onset mitral valve incompetence **(often due to posteromedial papillary muscle rupture approximately 3 days after inferior MI, leaflet perforation due to endocarditis, or chordal rupture)** causes a decrease in the effective (forward) stroke volume and an increase in blood pooling in the LA. The regurgitated volume and the blood emptying in the LA from the pulmonary veins then enter the LV during diastole, leading to diastolic volume overload and sarcomere stretch. Sarcomere stretch increases LV stroke volume due to the law of Frank-Starling. Increase in the end-diastolic volume causes the LVEDP to rise and subsequently elevate the LA pressure (LAP), because the LA compliance is normal. Elevation of the LAP causes pulmonary congestion and is manifested as dyspnea. Patients develop CHF in the presence of normal or high ejection fraction. MR causes a decrease in the LV afterload by opening a path of less resistance and decreases forward (effective) stroke volume. If the MR is not severe, the LV and LA adapt, and the patients enter the asymptomatic chronic phase.

In the chronic compensated phase, volume overload causes eccentric hypertrophy and LV dilatation, increasing LVEDP. Wall stress increases as the LV radius increases, yet the afterload is unchanged due to LA enlargement. The dilated LV and LA accommodate larger volumes and decrease the LAP and pulmonary congestion. Eccentric hypertrophy, increased preload, normal afterload, and normal contractile function cause an elevated stroke volume, which compensates for the regurgitant flow. As this progresses, a chronic decompensated phase occurs, in which excessive LV dilatation eventually produces a fall in the LV systolic function, decreasing the LV stroke volume and increasing the LV end-systolic volume. Increase in the LV end-systolic volume causes an increase in the LVEDP and LAP, causing pulmonary congestion and CHF. It is postulated that the fall in systolic function is due to loss of myofibrillar elements and calcium-handling abnormalities in the myocytes.

Natural History
The natural history and progression of MR are difficult to characterize due to its different etiologies and changing epidemiology and the use of surgical treatment. Calcification of the mitral annular protects against worsening MR by preventing annulus dilatation. Disease progression is characterized by the following:

- **MVP:** Progresses to severe MR in 10–15% of patients. Men are twice as likely to develop MR as women, and its incidence increases with age (1:200 at age 50 vs 1:25 at age 70). Effective regurgitation orifice increases at a rate of 8.6 mm^2 in 1.5 yrs due to dilation of the mitral valve annulus. Patients may develop anxiety attacks, substernal chest pain, and palpitations.
- **Flail leaflet:** Due to the rupture of chordae tendinea or papillary muscle secondary to trauma, infection, or ischemia, or may be idiopathic. It is associated with

a 6.3% mortality rate per yr, 30% incidence of AF, and 63% incidence of CHF in 10 yrs. By 10 yrs, 90% of the people studied by Lieng [6] had either died or undergone surgical repair. All had an elevated mortality rate: 4.1% per yr and 34% per yr if experiencing NYHA class I–II and NYHA class III–IV symptoms, respectively. Sudden death begins to occur in patients with symptoms of NYHA class II at a rate of 3.1% per yr and 12.7% per yr if ejection fraction <50%. Administer surgical treatment early.

- **Ischemic MR:** Result of myocardial or papillary muscle dysfunction secondary to an ischemic event in the inferior/inferolateral distribution. It is caused by loss of annular contraction and tenting of the mitral valve secondary to apical and posterior displacement of the posteromedial papillary muscle. In one series, patients with MI who developed MR had a 29% mortality rate at 5 yrs when compared to controls (12%) who were matched for age, ejection fraction, and MI [7].
- **Rheumatic:** Compared to the previous three cases, rheumatic MR is relatively stable. Because it is accompanied by mitral annular and subvalvular apparatus calcification, it does not worsen with time. It can be accompanied by MS and other valvular involvement.

History and Physical Exam

- In **acute MR,** symptoms are associated with severity. Patients complain of symptoms of CHF: dyspnea on exertion, cough productive of clear sputum, fatigue, lower-extremity edema. Findings on physical exam may be limited to a short apical systolic murmur with radiation to the axilla. Murmur may be absent or low volume due to the nonincreased compliance of the LA wall, which reduces the pressure difference between the LV and LA.
- In **chronic MR,** take a drug history, family history, and medical illness history. Symptoms only become prominent once decompensation begins. Patients with MVP may complain of anxiety and palpitations. Physical exam in all forms of chronic MR may be notable for LA lift, displaced PMI, and evidence of pulmonary HTN (loud P_2, pulmonary artery tap). The S_2 is widely split due to an early A_2. Auscultation demonstrates an apical holosystolic murmur that radiates to the axilla. **It may radiate to the anterior chest wall if the posterior papillary muscle is involved and toward the back if the anterior papillary muscle (or leaflet) is involved.** In MVP, evidence of a systolic click exists, and there may be a postclick systolic murmur that increases in duration with Valsalva and standing (the click occurs earlier) and decreases in duration (click occurs later) with handgrip. The systolic ejection murmur of HCM is the only other systolic murmur that increases with these maneuvers.

Diagnostic Studies

ECG. ECG may show LA enlargement, LVH, AF, or pathologic Q waves indicating an inferior MI.

CHEST X-RAY. Chest x-ray may show dilatation of the LA (in chronic MR).

TRANSTHORACIC ECHOCARDIOGRAM. Obtain with Doppler interrogation to determine LA and LV dimensions and function and degree of MR. Because the mitral valve annulus is saddle shaped, diagnosis of MVP should only be made if the mitral valve prolapses in the parasternal long-axis view. In patients with chronic MR due to primary valvular disease, the appropriate frequency of echocardiograms depends on the severity of the MR, LV ejection fraction, and LV end-systolic dimension. The severity of MR can be evaluated through several mechanisms:

- Color-flow mapping (regurgitant jet relative to LA size)
- Proximal isovelocity surface area
- Vena contracta
- Effective regurgitant orifice
- Pressure half-time
- Pulmonary vein systolic flow reversal

TABLE 13-2. ASSESSMENT OF MR SEVERITY

Indicators of MR Severity:

Color jet >8 cm^2

Regurgitant volume >60 mL

Regurgitant fraction >55%

Effective regurgitant orifice >0.35 cm^2

3$^+$ MR by left ventriculogram

Pulmonary vein systolic flow reversal

These tools yield echocardiographic criteria for quantifying the severity of MR, some of which are provided in Table 13-2.

Right-Heart Catheterization
Right-heart catheterization is indicated in presurgical assessment. The mean PCWP (corresponding to the LA pressure) and amplitude of v waves on the PCW tracing may reflect severity of MR (the "giant v wave"). Increased amplitude reflects higher LA filling pressures; however, increased v waves may not be seen if MR develops slowly and the LA dilates appropriately, after afterload reduction, with sedation, or in dehydration. Therefore, absent giant v waves do not exclude the presence of MR.

Left Ventriculogram
A left ventriculogram can be used to quantify the severity of MR and is recommended only if there is a discrepancy between the severity obtained by clinical or echocardiographic determination. **1+ contrast** paints the LA incompletely and is cleared after every beat. **2+ contrast** paints the entire LA and is cleared in more than one beat. **3+ contrast** completely opacifies the LA with the same intensity as the ventricle. **4+ contrast** coats the entire LA and the pulmonary veins partially.

Coronary Angiogram
Perform a coronary angiogram when contemplating mitral valve surgery in patients with a history of angina, >1 risk factor for CAD, or if ischemia is the postulated mechanism of MR.

Treatment
In acute MR, patients should be stabilized with adequate aggressive afterload reduction with IV nitroprusside or nitroglycerin if BP is adequate. IABP may aid in management of pulmonary edema and cardiogenic shock, acting as a bridge to surgery. If surgery is not immediately indicated, afterload reduction with ACE inhibitors or hydralazine can be used. Surgery is indicated for **severe acute MR or any flail leaflet or valvular rupture.**

In chronic MR, symptomatic patients with moderate to severe MR should undergo elective surgical repair. Treatment for asymptomatic patients with severe MR is controversial. Treatment type depends on the possibility of mitral valve repair and LV function. Current general guidelines for referral to surgery in the setting of chronic severe MR are as follows:

- NYHA functional class I with ejection fraction >60%, end-systolic dimension <45 mm without AF, or pulmonary HTN: Evaluate clinically q6mos and echocardiographically q12mos.
- NYHA functional class I or II with ejection fraction <60%, end-systolic dimension >45 mm, or with AF or pulmonary HTN: Perform mitral valve repair or replacement.

- NYHA functional class II with ejection fraction >60%, end-systolic dimension <45 mm, or class III–IV regardless of LV function who are likely mitral valve repair candidates: Perform mitral valve repair.
- NYHA functional class II with normal LV function (ejection fraction >60%, end-systolic dimension <45 mm) with low likelihood of mitral valve repair or class III–IV with low likelihood of mitral valve repair with ejection fraction >30%: Perform mitral valve replacement.
- NYHA functional class III–IV with ejection fraction <30% and low likelihood of mitral valve repair: Treat medically due to the high risk of surgery. Candidacy for heart transplantation should be assessed.

Surgical treatment is characterized by mitral valve repair with annuloplasty ring or replacement using one of the prosthetic valves described in Aortic Stenosis. Regarding the decision of repair vs replacement, mitral valve repair is preferred if possible. In any surgery, the subvalvular apparatus should be maintained so that the LV keeps an elliptical shape and preserves adequate function. MV repair is the preferred surgery because of its decreased mortality (2–5% compared to 5–10%), ability to preserve ejection fraction, and avoidance of risk of perpetual anticoagulation; it also has the same incidence for reoperation as mitral valve replacement. The ability to perform mitral valve repair depends on the etiology of MR, characteristics of the mitral valve, and subvalvular apparatus. Postop residual MR is the most common complication of mitral valve surgery and may merit immediate repair if severe. Markers of poor surgical outcome include AF, ejection fraction <60%, end-systolic volume >45 mm, mean pulmonary artery pressure >20 mm Hg, and LVEDP >12 mm Hg.

Medical treatment can be divided into treatment directed toward patients with primary valve abnormalities with normal LV function and treatment directed toward patients with MR with LV dysfunction (usually, MR is secondary to LV dysfunction with dilatation). Symptoms from MR due to cardiomyopathy may be relieved by treating the underlying cardiomyopathy. Diuretics and nitrates ease pulmonary congestion. Rate control and anticoagulation for AF, as well as maintenance of normal sinus rhythm, can also reduce symptoms. Afterload reduction with ACE inhibitors or hydralazine is used to minimize the regurgitant fraction and is thought to be helpful. Revascularization (percutaneously or surgically) for ischemic MR may be helpful. On the other hand, **medical treatment in asymptomatic primary valvular disease is not known to prevent or delay ventricular dysfunction, and it is unknown whether it can improve outcomes among patients with asymptomatic disease progression.** In fact, some experts believe that afterload reduction could actually worsen MR due to MVP and thereby promote disease progression. **Attempts at medical therapy should not delay surgical intervention in the setting of severe MR and/or the onset of LV dysfunction.** Trials are underway to assess the role of ACE inhibitors and beta blockers in chronic MR. Use **antibiotic prophylaxis** in patients with structural valvular abnormalities (see p. 218). Patients with MVP should only receive prophylaxis if they exhibit MR or if the leaflets are thickened. Initiate ASA therapy in patients with MVP only after a TIA.

Mitral Stenosis

Etiology

MS is due primarily to rheumatic heart disease and can be isolated or accompanied by MR or other valvular heart disease. Rheumatic carditis provokes mitral valvulitis, which is manifested by vegetation formation in the mitral commissures and chordae. Repetitive episodes of valvulitis with subsequent healing cause fibrous tissue deposition in the mitral valve, which eventually causes commissural fusion, contracture and thickening of the leaflets, and shortening of the chordae tendinea, resulting in MS. Congenital MS is extremely rare (**Lutembacher syndrome:** rheumatic MS accompanied by an atrial septal defect). Other rare causes of MS include rheumatoid arthritis, healed endocarditis, and mucopolysaccharidosis. Functional MS can be caused by atrial myxoma, ball thrombus, and cor triatriatum.

Pathophysiology

As the mitral valvular area decreases, LV inflow is impaired, and a diastolic pressure gradient between the LA and LV develops. The gradient depends on the stroke volume, diastolic filling time, and LV diastolic pressure. The presence of the LA gradient causes an elevation of the LAP and slowly causes LA enlargement. Increase in LAP is transmitted retrograde to the pulmonary venous circulation, which passively causes pulmonary HTN and an increase in pulmonary vascular resistance. High LAP promotes the development of AF. Pulmonary vascular resistance is reversible at first and responds to valvotomy or replacement, but due to fibrosis, pulmonary vascular resistance eventually becomes fixed and does not decrease with treatment. This resistance is transmitted to the RV, which compensates via hypertrophy and enlargement. RV enlargement augments the amount of tricuspid regurgitation (TR) due to annular dilation. As the RV fails, systemic venous congestion is apparent. In the pulmonary vasculature, capillary wall and alveolar thickening occur in response to the pulmonary HTN and protect against the development of pulmonary edema. Physiologic states (fever, hyperthyroidism, and pregnancy) that increase the stroke volume worsen MS and the LA/LV gradient.

History and Physical Exam

Patients with MS are initially asymptomatic for 10–20 yrs, after their symptoms progress as the mitral valve area (MVA) approaches 2.5 cm^2. Progression of rheumatic MS varies depending on the severity of the original rheumatic insult or due to repeated episodes of carditis. Asymptomatic patients have a >80% survival at 10 yrs. Patients with limiting symptoms have a <15% survival at 10 yrs. Once severe pulmonary HTN develops, survival is estimated at <3 yrs. MS is asymptomatic until the MVA is <1.5 cm^2. Patients experience a gradual decrease in exercise tolerance or physical activity and may change their lifestyles to minimize symptoms. In other cases, a situation that increases the stroke volume generates symptoms, such as pregnancy, hyperthyroidism, and exercise. Patients initially complain of dyspnea, orthopnea, or paroxysmal nocturnal dyspnea, but as the MVA is reduced, patients feel fatigued. Palpitations are common, and 50% may have AF. **Hemoptysis,** hoarseness, exercise-induced angina, and a new systemic embolism may be the presenting symptoms of MS.

On exam, pulse may be irregular due to AF. Malar erythema is a rare finding and is associated with a poor cardiac output and cyanosis. The cardiac exam is remarkable for an irregular rhythm occasionally; normal LV size and function results in a normal PMI; an RV heave and PA tap may be seen in cases of pulmonary HTN. A **loud S$_1$** may be heard. The **opening snap,** heard best at the apex with the diaphragm, occurs after P$_2$. The time from the P$_2$ to the opening snap is an indicator of severity (the earlier the opening snap, the more severe the MS). The **diastolic rumble,** heard best with the bell at the apex, increases after exercise or amyl nitrate infusion. The duration of the rumble is proportional to the severity of MS. A thrill is occasionally present with the patient in the left lateral decubitus position.

Diagnostic Studies

- **Chest x-ray** may be remarkable for redistribution of flow to the upper lung fields, Kerley A and B lines, double atrial shadow, elevation of the left mainstem bronchus, and prominence of the LA appendage between the pulmonary artery and LV.
- **ECG** may detect rhythm abnormalities (AF), RV hypertrophy, right-axis deviation, and P mitrale (large P wave measuring >0.08 secs, LA enlargement).

- **Transthoracic echocardiogram** is fundamental in characterizing and grading the severity of MS. Obtain a transthoracic echocardiogram on diagnosis, after any therapeutic intervention, and if symptomatology worsens. Doppler interrogation of mitral valvular flows for gradient, presence and severity of concomitant MR, determination of LV size and function, and pulmonary artery pressure are all important. Furthermore, mitral valve calcification, leaflet mobility, subvalvular thickening, and leaflet thickening are all critical components. In fact, these four components are each graded in severity and contribute to the **mitral valve score.**

MVA is estimated by

- Direct planimetry with the caveat of being extremely operator dependent.
- Pressure half-time is the amount of time it takes for the diastolic pressure to decrease by 50%. It corresponds to decreasing the velocity by 70% and is dependent on ventricular compliance and the absence of significant aortic insufficiency.
- Continuity equation if no significant aortic insufficiency or MR.
- Proximal isovelocity surface area.

TEE is indicated to determine the presence of an LA appendage thrombus.

Stress echocardiogram is used to quantify changes in the mitral valve gradient and pulmonary HTN with exercise. This is useful if symptoms are out of proportion to apparently mild MS or if symptoms are denied in the presence of apparently significant MS.

Severity is graded as presented in Table 13-3.

- **Cardiac catheterization** is indicated to quantify severity of MS when clinical and echocardiographic parameters are discordant. The Gorlin equation is used to calculate MVA. Remember that right- and left-heart catheterization are necessary. Fig. 13-2 demonstrates the hemodynamics seen in MS.

Treatment

Treatment of MS depends on patient symptoms and a few objective criteria. Medical therapy, percutaneous interventional therapy, and surgical therapy are available. **Medical therapy** is aimed at slowing progression of pulmonary HTN, preventing endocarditis, reducing the risk of thromboembolism, and reducing HF symptoms. For HF, diuretics and a low-salt diet are often adequate to decrease evidence of fluid overload. For AF (which commonly complicates MS), rate control of ventricular response with beta blockade or digoxin is effective. Electric cardioversion has a higher thromboembolic risk with MS, almost always requiring >3 wks of adequate anticoagulation or TEE assessment of the LA. Persistent anticoagulation postcardioversion is required for 4 wks to avoid risk of systemic embolism. Long-term anticoagulation with warfarin is performed if the patient has paroxysmal or sustained AF or had a previous embolic event or in patients with LA >55 mm in diameter (also see Chap. 11, Atrial Fibrillation). **Antibiotic prophylaxis** against endocarditis and recurrent rheumatic fever is also very important (see p. 218).

TABLE 13-3. MITRAL VALVE STENOSIS SEVERITY

Severity	Mitral valve area (cm²)	Mitral valve gradient (mm Hg)
Normal	4–5	0
Mild	1.5–4	<5
Moderate	1.0–1.5	5–12
Severe	<1.0	>12

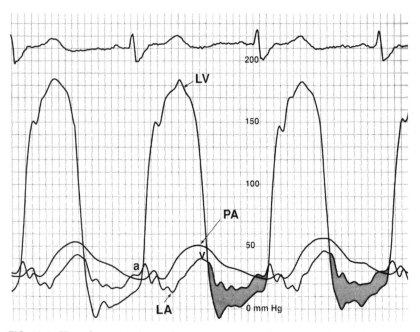

FIG. 13-2. Hemodynamics observed in mitral stenosis. The gray-shaded region corresponds to the diastolic-filling gradient between the left atrium (LA) and left ventricle (LV). PA, pulmonary artery. (From Murphy JG. *Mayo Clinic cardiology review,* 2nd ed. Philadelphia: Lippincott Williams & Wilkins, 2000, with permission.)

Percutaneous balloon valvotomy increases MVA by 1–2 cm² and is accompanied by an 84% 4-yr survival rate and a 6–21% restenosis rate [8]. Mitral valve leaflet mobility, cusp thickening, subvalvular thickening, and calcification are graded to generate a mitral valve score and thereby predict procedural success. Balloon valvotomy is contraindicated in patients with MR and LA thrombus, and it may be complicated by MR, cardiac perforation, embolization, or residual atrial septal defect (the approach is via the right atrium interatrial septum).

Patients with mild MS should be followed, as they are usually stable for many years. Patients with MVA <1.5 cm² with pulmonary artery systolic pressure >50 mm Hg should be considered for percutaneous intervention in the presence or absence of symptoms. Such a procedure should similarly be considered if activity provokes a gradient >15 mm Hg or a pulmonary artery systolic pressure >60 mm Hg. Therefore, in general, percutaneous valvotomy should be the first procedural approach considered. However, **if concomitant MR is moderate to severe, if there is evidence of LA thrombus, or if the mitral valve score is high, the mitral valve is not amenable to balloon valvotomy, and surgical treatment should be considered.**

Surgical mitral valve repair with commissurotomy may be performed in patients meeting criteria for percutaneous intervention but who have a persistent LA thrombus despite adequate anticoagulation. **Surgical replacement** is required for people with moderate to severe MS and significant functional limitation and/or severe pulmonary HTN who are not candidates for percutaneous therapy (because of one or more of the exclusion criteria above) or surgical repair. Replacement is also indicated in the presence of multivalvular disease or recurrent disease after percutaneous therapy.

TRICUSPID VALVE

The tricuspid valve lies between the right atrium and RV. It has three cusps: anterior, posterior, and septal. Primary tricuspid valve disease is relatively uncommon.

Tricuspid Regurgitation

Mild TR is found in up to 70% of normal patients. It is clinically unremarkable in a majority of patients.

Etiology

Secondary TR is caused by RV dilatation and RV failure, most commonly secondary to LV failure or valvular disease, which causes pulmonary HTN, or pulmonary HTN independent of the cardiac disease. Anomalies of the tricuspid valve per se range from

- Infective endocarditis, the most common anomaly and frequently associated with IV drug abuse
- Carcinoid heart disease, commonly presenting as TR but also associated with tricuspid stenosis
- Right-sided MI, causing papillary muscle dysfunction
- Trauma
- Rheumatoid arthritis
- Rheumatic heart disease, indicating severe aortic or mitral valve disease
- Marfan syndrome
- Radiation-induced valvulitis
- Others

History and Physical Exam

Generally, TR is clinically insignificant and well tolerated. Patients may complain of fatigue, early satiety, or loss of appetite depending on the degree of hepatic congestion and lower-extremity edema. Physical findings are usually only present if there is concomitant pulmonary HTN. On physical exam, prominent v waves are seen when examining the jugular venous waveform. Auscultation yields a systolic murmur in the subxiphoid or fourth left intercostal space in the parasternal line **that increases with inspiration** or other activities that increase venous return. TR due to pulmonary HTN is holosystolic and high pitched. TR due to primary valvular dysfunction is lower pitched. The murmur often disappears once atrial and ventricular pressures equalize. Right-sided S_3 or increased P_2 intensity is common. A pulsatile liver, hepatomegaly, lower-extremity edema, ascites, and hepatojugular reflux may be present.

Diagnostic Studies

ECG shows nonspecific findings, including incomplete right bundle-branch block and RV hypertrophy. **Transthoracic echocardiography** illustrates the following important findings: (a) physiologic TR does not occupy >1 cm into the right atrium; (b) the normal TR jet velocity is between 2 and 2.6 m/sec and lasts for <150 msecs in continuous Doppler; and (c) RV overload is exemplified by RV enlargement, septal flattening or paradoxical septal motion, right atrial enlargement, inferior vena cava engorgement, tricuspid valve leaflets that appear thickened and retracted or fixed (carcinoid), and/or tricuspid annulus dilation. In Ebstein's anomaly, the tricuspid valve is displaced downward, and atrialization of the RV occurs.

The severity of TR is assessed in several ways. A TR color jet to right atrial area ratio of <20% is considered mild, 20–40% is moderate, and >40% is severe. Systolic flow reversal of the inferior vena cava is a marker of severe TR. Pulmonary artery systolic pressure is estimated by the simplified **Bernoulli's equation:** pulmonary artery systolic pressure $- (4V^2)$ + right atrial pressure, where **V** is the TR jet velocity. The right atrial pressure is estimated according to inferior vena cava size: 0–5 mm Hg if normal diameter inferior vena cava collapses >50% on inspiration; 5–10 mm Hg if inferior vena cava is mildly dilated and collapses normally; 10–15 mm Hg with mildly dilated inferior vena cava that only partially collapses with inspiration; 15–20 mm Hg with dilated inferior vena cava that does not collapse. Pulmonary artery systolic pressure is considered normal if it is between 18 and 25 mm Hg; a patient is mildly hypertensive if pulmonary artery systolic pressure is 30–40 mm Hg; moderately HTN is associated with 40–70 mm Hg; and severe HTN is associated with pressure >70 mm Hg. Importantly, the severity of TR does not necessarily correlate with the severity of pulmonary HTN. Mild TR can exist with severe pulmonary HTN, and severe TR can exist with no pulmonary HTN or RV outflow tract obstruction. **Right-heart catheterization** is significant for prominent v wave on the RA pressure tracing.

Treatment
Medical therapy is limited to diuretics and afterload reduction to decrease the severity of right-heart failure. Surgical treatment is indicated, depending on the severity of mitral or aortic valve disease. For the tricuspid valve, repair with annuloplasty ring is preferred to replacement. Bioprosthetic valves are preferred to mechanical valves due to the risk of thrombosis (lower pressure on the right side of the heart predisposes to thrombosis of mechanical valves).

Tricuspid Stenosis

Etiology
Tricuspid stenosis is a rare valvular abnormality, generally secondary to

- Rheumatic heart disease
- Carcinoid tumor (± TR)
- Infective endocarditis
- Endocardial fibroelastosis
- SLE
- Fabry's disease
- Methysergide intoxication
- Löeffler's syndrome

History and Physical Exam
Patients complain of easy fatigue and edema correlating to low cardiac output. Palpitations and right upper quadrant pain are also common. A elevated JVP and hepatomegaly are noted. One finds low-pitched diastolic murmur, heard best at the fourth left intercostal space, that increases at postinspiratory apnea. An opening snap is occasionally audible. The liver is often pulsatile and tender. Lower-extremity edema or anasarca are often present.

Diagnosis
Use a high index of suspicion. Right-heart failure without evidence of mitral valve or pulmonary disease suggests the presence of tricuspid stenosis. Due to low pressures, it is difficult to estimate the tricuspid valve gradient by cardiac catheterization, but a suspected diagnosis is confirmed with a mean pull-back diastolic gradient of at least 5 mm Hg from right atrium to RV. On transthoracic echocardiogram, note evidence of right atrial enlargement; the gradient across the tricuspid valve can be calculated by Doppler echocardiography.

Treatment
All valvular abnormalities and their interactions are needed to determine adequate treatment. Diuretics and afterload reducers are used to decrease the severity of right-heart failure. Surgical treatment is indicated, depending on the severity of mitral or aortic valve disease. Tricuspid valvuloplasty or tricuspid valve replacement are indicated for severe tricuspid stenosis. Bioprosthetic valves are preferred to mechanical valves due to the risk of thrombosis.

PULMONARY VALVE

Pulmonary Stenosis

Etiology

- **Congenital:** Most common; seen in 10% of patients with congenital heart disease (e.g., tetralogy of Fallot, Noonan syndrome)
- **Carcinoid heart disease**
- **Rheumatic heart disease:** Most infrequent type of valvular involvement
- **Pseudopulmonary stenosis:** Obstruction of RV outflow tract secondary to aneurysm of the sinus of Valsalva or cardiac tumors, supravalvular stenosis (e.g., Williams syndrome)

History and Physical Exam

Patients exhibit dyspnea on exertion, lower-extremity edema, hepatomegaly, abdominal distention, early satiety, and other signs of right-heart failure. Note systolic ejection murmur at the second intercostal space in the left parasternal line. P_2 may be soft or absent, and the S_2 may be widely split or single. A mid-systolic click of the PV opening may be present as well.

Diagnosis

On the transthoracic echocardiogram, the pulmonary valve may appear thickened or calcified. In severe cases, the RV is hypertrophied in adulthood but may be normal during childhood. Color flow with continuous Doppler quantifies the amount of pulmonary stenosis by gradient: mild disease = 40 mm Hg, moderate = 40–80 mm Hg, severe disease >80 mm Hg gradient across the pulmonary valve.

Treatment

Mild to moderate pulmonary stenosis can be treated medically without major intervention. Pulmonary valvuloplasty is saved for patients with severe disease and decreases the gradient by 75%. Pulmonary valve replacement is reserved for patients with carcinoid syndrome, because they do not respond to valvuloplasty.

Pulmonary Regurgitation

Etiology

- Pulmonary artery HTN (most common by far)
- Congenital valvular disease
- Carcinoid heart disease
- Iatrogenic

History Physical Exam

Symptoms develop slowly. Patients complain of right-heart failure symptoms. The **Graham Steelle's** murmur is classic and is similar to that of AI.

Diagnostic Study

Transthoracic echocardiogram with documentation of the adequate position.

Treatment

Generally depends on the severity of concomitant valvular disease. Valvuloplasty or replacement depend on patient anatomy and physiology.

KEY POINTS TO REMEMBER

- Assessment of valvular heart disease requires careful attention to history and physical exam findings.
- AS is a chronic progressive disease characterized by angina, syncope, and HF, in that order of pathogenesis and prognostic significance (with HF indicating a high mortality).

- Therapy for AS is surgical, with AVR once the patient has become symptomatic in the setting of a high TVG. Patients with severe AS should not be given nitrates.
- Aortic regurgitation (aortic insufficiency) is either an acute or chronic process, the treatment of which depends on patient symptoms and the severity of the process. AVR is usually required. For asymptomatic patients, an LV end-systolic dimension of 55 mm and/or an ejection fraction <55% is classically the threshold to refer for surgery. Medical afterload reduction is appropriate therapy for chronic aortic insufficiency. IABP is contraindicated in moderate to severe aortic insufficiency.
- MR is a common entity with numerous causes that may be acute or chronic. Its therapy is dependent on patient symptoms and the severity of the MR. For asymptomatic severe MR, surgical therapy is warranted if there is pulmonary HTN and/or AF. A dilated LV with an ejection fraction >30% is also a surgical indication if MR is severe. Asymptomatic severe MR due to a flail mitral valve leaflet without these predictors also is usually an indication for surgery. Traditional medical therapy for MR consists of treatment of the underlying cardiac process for secondary MR. For primary severe MR and normal LV function, no form of medical therapy has been shown to slow progression of ventricular dilatation and failure. Beta blockade may be useful; more trials are necessary to assess the role of medical therapy in chronic significant MR.
- MS is usually due to rheumatic fever. Treatment depends on the patient's symptoms and the severity of the obstruction. If there is not significant concomitant MR, percutaneous valvotomy can be performed with good results. If MR accompanies MS, mitral valve replacement is usually required.
- Antibiotic prophylaxis is required for all dental and surgical procedures for significant regurgitant or stenotic lesions.

SUGGESTED READING

Alexander W, Schlant R, Fuster V, ed. *Hurst's the heart,* 9th ed. New York: McGraw-Hill, 1998 (vol. 2).

Carabello B, Crawford F. Valvular heart disease. *N Engl J Med* 1997;337:32–31.

Connolly H, Crary J, McGoon M, et al. Valvular heart disease associated with fenfluramine-phentermine. *N Engl J Med* 1997;337:581–588.

Cooper H, Gersh B. Treatment of chronic mitral regurgitation. *Am Heart J* 1998;135:925–936.

Enriquez-Sarano M, Basmadjian AJ, Rossi A. Progression of mitral regurgitation. A prospective Doppler echocardiographic study. *J Am Coll Cardiol* 1999;34:1137–1144.

Enriquez-Sarano M, Orszulack T, Schaff H, et al. Mitral regurgitation: a new clinical perspective. *Mayo Clin Proc* 1997;72:1034–1043.

Gaasch W, Sundaram M, Meyer T. Managing asymptomatic patients with chronic aortic regurgitation. *Chest* 1997;111:1702–1709.

Giuliani Emilio, ed. *Mayo clinic practice of cardiology,* 3rd ed. St. Louis: Mosby, 1996.

Grigioni F, Enriquez-Sarano M, Ling L, et al. Sudden death in mitral regurgitation due to flail leaflet. *J Am Coll Cardiol* 1999;34:2078–2085.

Grigioni F, Enriquez-Sarano M, Zehr K, et al. Ischemic mitral regurgitation. Long-term outcome and prognostic implications with quantitative Doppler assessment. *Circulation* 2000;103:1759–1764.

Otto CM. Clinical practice. Evaluation and management of chronic mitral regurgitation. *N Engl J Med* 2001;345(10):740–746.

Pellikka P, Nishimura R, Bailey K, et al. The natural history of adults with asymptomatic, hemodynamically significant aortic stenosis. *J Am Coll Cardiol* 1990;15:1012–1017.

Selzer A, Cohn K. Natural history of mitral stenosis: a review. *Circulation* 1972;45:878–889.

Singh J, Evans J, Levy D, et al. Prevalence of clinical determinants of mitral, tricuspid, and aortic regurgitation (The Framingham Heart Study). *Am J Cardiol* 1999;83:897–902.

Tajik AJ. Ischemic mitral regurgitation: role of echo-Doppler in assessment and management. In: *32nd annual New York Cardiovascular Symposium.* New York, December 1999 (vol. 1).

Tornos MP, Olona M, Permanyer-Miralda G. Heart failure after aortic valve replacement for aortic regurgitation: prospective 20 year study. *Am Heart J* 1998;136:681–687.

REFERENCES

1. Wagner S, Selzer A. Patterns of progression of aortic stenosis: a longitudinal hemodynamic study. *Circulation* 1982;65:709–712.
2. ACC/AHA guidelines for the management of patients with valvular heart disease. *J Am Coll Cardiol* 1998;32:1486–1588.
3. Fuster V. The clinical challenge of aortic and mitral regurgitation. In: *32nd annual New York Cardiovascular Symposium*. New York, December 1999 (vol. 2).
4. Bonow RO, Lakatos E, Maron BJ, et al. Serial long-term assessment of the natural history of asymptomatic patients with chronic aortic regurgitation and normal left ventricular systolic function. *Circulation* 1991;84:1625–1635.
5. Scognamiglio R, Rahimtoola S, Fasoli G, et al. Nifedipine in asymptomatic patients with severe aortic regurgitation and normal left ventricular function. *N Engl J Med* 1994;331:689–694.
6. Ling L, Enriquez-Sarrano M, Seward JB, et al. Clinical outcome of mitral regurgitation due to flail leaflet. *N Engl J Med* 1996;335:1417–1423.
7. Gervasio L, Gary M, Greg F, et al. Clinical significance of mitral regurgitation after acute myocardial infarction. *Circulation* 1997;96:827–833.
8. Sharma S. The non-surgical interventional challenge of aortic and mitral stenosis: an update. In: *32nd annual New York Cardiovascular Symposium*. New York, December 1999 (vol. 2).

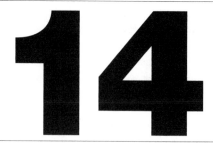

Bradycardia and Permanent Pacemakers

Navinder S. Sawhney and
Peter A. Crawford

INTRODUCTION

When approaching a patient with **bradycardia** [heart rate (HR)] <60 bpm], there are several questions that may affect management:

- Is the patient symptomatic?
- Is there a direct correlation between the symptoms and changes in rhythm?
- Is there a reversible cause?
- Is the bradycardia likely to be transient?
- Could the patient be having an MI?

Bradycardia may result from abnormalities in the **sinus node, AV node,** or **His-Purkinje system.** It may be caused by either intrinsic dysfunction of the **conduction system** or by the response of a heart to extrinsic factors. Table 14-1 lists intrinsic and extrinsic causes of bradycardia.

CONDUCTION SYSTEM

The sinus node is a collection of cells at the junction of the superior vena cava and the right atrium. These cells depolarize spontaneously, and the impulse propagates through the right atrium to the AV node in the low septal right atrium adjacent to the tricuspid annulus. Impulses are conducted through the AV node, during which a delay occurs (this accounts for much of the PR interval). The delay allows time for atrial contraction to effectively contribute to ventricular filling. The impulse then travels to the bundle of His, which courses through the membranous septum and then separates into the right- and left-bundle branches before reaching the ventricular myocardium.

Both the sinoatrial (SA) node and AV node are innervated by the autonomic nervous system, and the relative balance between the parasympathetic and sympathetic nervous systems accounts for the baseline HR. Parasympathetic tone decreases the sinus node automaticity and slows AV conduction, so a strong vagal stimulus can result in marked transient bradycardia or sinus pause. With vagally mediated bradycardia, the ECG shows sinus slowing and prolongation of the PR interval. These bradyarrhythmias are transient and typically require no treatment. If treatment is needed, they should respond to atropine.

CLINICAL PRESENTATION

Cardiac output is equal to stroke volume multiplied by HR. Thus, with decreased HR, if there are compensatory changes in stroke volume, cardiac output may remain the same, and a patient with bradycardia may remain asymptomatic. There is considerable variation in HRs among a normal, asymptomatic population, with the slowest HRs occurring at night. HRs of 30–35 bpm, sinus pauses of ~3 secs, SA block, junctional rhythms, and first-degree and second-degree AV block can all be considered normal variants during sleep.

If the patient is symptomatic, it is important to establish a correlation between symptoms and changes in rhythm. Symptomatic bradycardia may present with syn-

TABLE 14-1. CAUSES OF BRADYCARDIA

Intrinsic
   Congential disease (may present later in life)
   Idiopathic degeneration (aging)
   Infarction or ischemia
   Cardiomyopathy
   Infiltrative disease: sarcoidosis, amyloidosis, hemochromatosis
   Collagen vascular diseases: SLE, rheumatoid arthritis, scleroderma
   Surgical trauma: valve surgery, transplantation
   Infectious disease: endocarditis, Lyme disease, Chagas disease
Extrinsic
   Autonomically mediated
      Neurocardiogenic syncope
      Carotid sinus hypersensitivity
      Increased vagal tone: coughing, vomiting, micturition, defecation, intubation
   Drugs: beta blockers, calcium channel blockers, digoxin, antiarrhythmic agents
   Hypothyroidism
   Hypothermia
   Neurologic disorders: increased ICP
   Electrolyte imbalances: hyperkalemia, hypermagnesemia
   Hypercarbia/obstructive sleep apnea
   Sepsis

cope, presyncope, or confusion; however, the symptoms are often nonspecific (dizziness, fatigue, weakness, heart failure), and establishing a relationship between these nonspecific symptoms and the rhythm disturbance is more difficult.

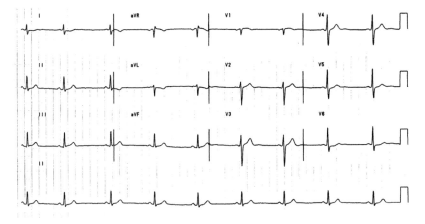

FIG. 14-1. Sinus bradycardia.

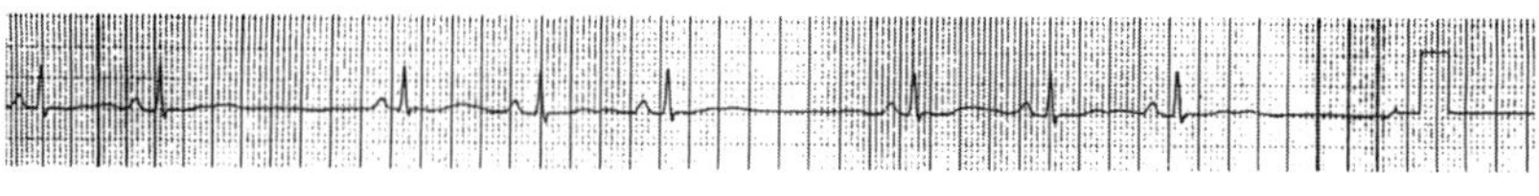

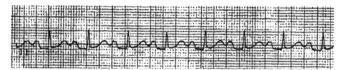

FIG. 14-2. Sinoatrial node exit block. Note that the PP interval in which the pause occurs is exactly twice that of the nonpaused PP interval.

SINUS NODE DYSFUNCTION

Sinus node dysfunction, also referred to as **sick sinus syndrome,** is a common cause of bradycardia. Sinus node dysfunction includes inappropriate sinus bradycardia, sinoatrial exit block, sinoatrial arrest, and tachycardia-bradycardia syndrome. The prevalence is estimated to be as high as 1 in 600 in patients >65, and it accounts for >50% of pacemaker implantations in the United States.

Sinus bradycardia (Fig. 14-1) is defined as an HR <60 bpm and is considered pathologic when the patient is symptomatic or if the HR fails to increase appropriately during activity or exercise. The latter is known as *chronotropic incompetence.* Sinus bradycardia is due to depressed automaticity in the sinus node itself.

Sinus pauses or sinus arrest (Fig. 14-2) may be due to failure of impulse formation or failure of conduction out of the SA node. Pauses >2 secs and <3 secs can be seen in healthy, asymptomatic people. Pauses >3 secs during waking hours are usually due to sinus node dysfunction. SA exit block is similar to sinus arrest; however, it may be distinguished on the ECG by the fact that the duration of the pause is a multiple of the sinus PP interval. They are treated the same, however, so the distinction is not that important. Digoxin toxicity is always a consideration with these rhythms.

Abnormal automaticity and conduction in the atrium predispose patients to AF and atrial flutter, and the **tachycardia-bradycardia syndrome** is a common manifestation of sinus node dysfunction. In the tachycardia-bradycardia syndrome, overdrive suppression of sinus automaticity may result in long pauses and syncope when the tachycardia terminates. Therapy to control the ventricular rate during tachycardia may not be possible due to further depressive effects on the sinus node, and thus, pacemaker implantation may be needed.

AV CONDUCTION DISTURBANCES

AV conduction may be delayed in either the AV node or the bundle of His. Clinically, it is important to distinguish between block within the AV node and the His bundle **(infranodal AV block),** as prognosis and treatment can depend on this distinction. Delays **below** the bifurcation of the bundle of His result in bundle-branch or fascicular blocks, but AV conduction should be maintained unless all three fascicles are simultaneously affected.

Similar to the sinus node, both intrinsic and extrinsic factors can cause disturbances in AV conduction. Unlike the SA node, however, the AV node and bundle of His provide a discrete connection between the atria and the ventricles, so a focal injury (from infarction, infection, or catheter-related trauma) is more likely to cause problems. **Digoxin toxicity is always a consideration with AV block.**

FIG. 14-3. First-degree AV block (prolonged PR interval).

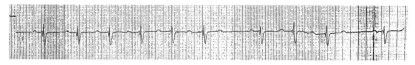

FIG. 14-4. Mobitz type I AV block (Wenckebach). Examples of 6:5 and 4:3 conduction are present on this strip. Variability in ratios within a given patient is not uncommon.

First-Degree AV Block

In **first-degree AV block** (Fig. 14-3), each of the atrial impulses is successfully conducted to the ventricle but with a delay. The delay is usually within the AV node. The PR interval is >0.2 secs with retained 1:1 AV conduction. (The PR interval represents the conduction time from the sinus node through the atrium, AV node, and His-Purkinje system to the onset of ventricular depolarization.) First-degree AV block by itself usually does not cause bradycardia; however, some patients can be symptomatic due to a loss of AV synchrony. These symptoms may resolve with pacing.

Second-Degree AV Block

Second-degree AV block occurs when an organized atrial rhythm fails to conduct to the ventricle in a 1:1 ratio, but some AV relationship is maintained.

Mobitz type I second-degree AV block (Wenckebach) (Fig. 14-4) occurs when there is a stable PP interval and a progressive increase in the PR interval until a P wave fails to conduct. The RR interval progressively shortens, because the **extent** to which the PR prolongs decreases in subsequent cycles. After the blocked P wave, the next PR interval returns to the initial value. The RR interval that contains the nonconducted P wave is by definition shorter than twice the PP interval. Mobitz type I block is usually due to a delay in the AV node **secondary to vagal tone,** but it may be due to a delay in the bundle of His. Mobitz type I block is usually benign.

In **Mobitz type II second-degree AV block** (Fig. 14-5), there is a stable PP interval with no measurable prolongation of the PR interval before an abrupt conduction failure. The RR interval that contains the nonconducted P wave is by definition equal to twice the PP interval. This type of AV block is most often associated with intrinsic disease of the His-Purkinje system (infranodal). **Mobitz type II is frequently confused with premature atrial contractions that are not conducted, the latter being benign.** These can be distinguished by (a) the distinct morphology of the nonconducted P wave, (b) the fact that the blocked P wave comes in earlier than the previous PP intervals, and (c) that the subsequent, conducted P wave follows a compensatory pause that is longer than the prior PP interval. Mobitz II usually requires a pacemaker, because it reflects intrinsic conduction system disease.

In AV block with a 2:1 conduction ratio (Fig. 14-6), designation of type I or type II is not appropriate. Localization of the block to the AV node (vagal tone) vs the His-Purkinje system, **which is, in practical terms, the most important assessment in describing AV block,** can be difficult in this setting. A narrow QRS complex may suggest block within the AV node or His bundle, whereas a wide QRS may suggest the presence of infrahisian block. This analysis can be confounded if the baseline QRS is wide due to baseline Purkinje system disease, and there is superimposed vagal tone

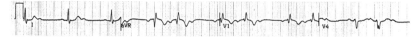

FIG. 14-5. Mobitz type II AV block. Note the normal and fixed PR intervals, with unpredictable failure of P waves to generate QRS complexes.

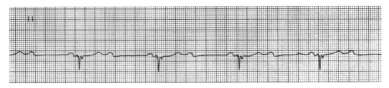

FIG. 14-6. 2:1 AV block.

causing 2:1 AV block. More robust discriminating criteria include improvement of the block with atropine or exercise (treadmill), which suggests a vagal mechanism. Worsening of AV block with these treatments suggests distal conduction system disease.

Third-Degree AV Block

Third-degree AV block (Fig. 14-7) is often referred to as **complete heart block.** Atrial activity and ventricular activity are independent of each other, and there are more P waves than QRS complexes (unless AF is the underlying rhythm). The location of the block is implied by the escape rhythm. A narrow QRS with a rate of 40–60 implies that the block and escape pacemaker are in the AV node, whereas a wide QRS at slower rates implies that the block is located in the His-Purkinje system. The escape rhythm is almost always regular, unless there is intermittent conduction of atrial impulses. **Digitalis toxicity is a common cause of reversible AV block.**

Bi- and Trifascicular Block

Distal conduction system disease can lead to left anterior fascicular block, left posterior fascicular block, left bundle-branch block, or right bundle-branch block. The presence of left anterior fascicular block or left posterior fascicular block **and** right bundle-branch block is commonly referred to as **bifascicular block.** The addition of a prolonged PR interval to this combination is referred to as **trifascicular block.** These conduction patterns increase the likelihood that a patient will require a pacemaker (see Table 14-2).

BRADYARRHYTHMIAS ASSOCIATED WITH ACUTE MI

Bradycardia is present in 4–5% of patients presenting with acute MI. Sinus node dysfunction may manifest as sinus bradycardia, sinus pauses, or sinus arrest and is most common with inferior MI. The bradyarrhythmia may be due to direct effect on the SA node blood supply (the sinus node artery, which originates from the proximal right coronary artery in 65% of patients; the circumflex artery in 25%; and both in 10%), or stimulation of certain receptors in the inferior LV, resulting in increased vagal tone (Bezold-Jarisch reflex).

Prognosis and management depend on the location of the MI, degree of AV block, and hemodynamic stability. During inferior infarction, the site of block is normally the AV node, primarily due to disruption of blood supply to the AV nodal artery, a branch of the right coronary artery, and the Bezold-Jarisch reflex. First-degree, second-degree, and even third-degree AV block in this setting are usually transient and asymptomatic.

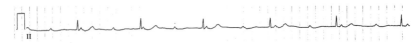

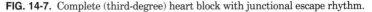

FIG. 14-7. Complete (third-degree) heart block with junctional escape rhythm.

AV block caused by an anterior MI usually involves the His-Purkinje system and results from extensive myocardial damage. This infranodal block is often symptomatic and irreversible, and in this setting, permanent pacing is often indicated.

EVALUATION OF BRADYARRHYTHMIAS

On history and physical exam, look for possible causes of intrinsic or extrinsic sinus node dysfunction or AV block. Clinical attention should focus on identifying and correcting reversible causes (medications, electrolytes, increased vagal tone, thyroid function). Severe nocturnal bradycardia should raise suspicion for obstructive sleep apnea. **Check serum digoxin levels in appropriate patients.**

For patients with intermittent symptoms, correlation of symptoms with bradycardia is important. In patients with frequent symptoms, a 24- to 48-hr continuous monitor may be helpful. A loop recorder may better monitor less frequent symptoms. **For patients with unexplained bradycardia and/or heart block, consider a treadmill exercise test to assess if their block and/or bradycardia improve.** If they do, a pacemaker is unlikely to be necessary, unless the bradycardia causes symptoms. Electrophysiologic testing may be necessary if the mechanism responsible for the bradycardia remains uncertain, because significant His-Purkinje disease is an indication for a permanent pacemaker. However, electrophysiologic testing is not very specific for detection of bradyarrhythmias as a cause for syncope.

MANAGEMENT

Intervention is rarely necessary in patients who are truly asymptomatic from their bradycardia. When bradycardia is present only during sleep, pacing is usually not indicated, unless the HR falls to dangerously low levels or there are very long pauses.

Among symptomatic patients, the correlation between the symptoms and the bradycardia, as well as the potential reversibility of causative factors, is the key to appropriate decision making. Symptoms definitely related to simultaneously confirmed bradycardia caused by intrinsic sinus node dysfunction or AV block should be treated with permanent pacing.

In emergent situations, until pacing can be initiated, atropine is usually used (and is the cornerstone of therapy in ACLS protocol) to increase the activity of the sinus node and improve conduction within the AV node. See Chapter 5, Cardiovascular Emergencies.

- Atropine is not useful and can worsen block if AV conduction abnormalities are due to distal conduction disease.
- If a beta blocker is suspected as a contributor to the bradycardia, **glucagon or milrinone** can be administered to circumvent the antagonized beta-adrenergic receptor and signal downstream.
- If a calcium channel blocker is suspected, **glucagon and calcium** can be administered.
- If digoxin is a suspected culprit, the Fab fragments of digoxin antibodies (Digibind) can be administered in life-threatening situations. Note that this therapy can trigger heart failure or hypokalemia (and associated arrhythmias) and is very expensive. Therefore, its use should be limited to when definitive therapy (i.e., transvenous pacer) is not available or other effects of digoxin toxicity (delirium, hallucinations, vomiting) are problematic.

Temporary pacemakers are available for emergent use to stabilize patients with symptomatic bradycardia, as a bridge to permanent pacing, and for situations in which the dysrhythmia is transient or reversible until the underlying cause can be corrected. See Chap. 24, Procedures in Cardiovascular Critical Care (Intraaortic Balloon Pump, Swan-Ganz Catheterization, Temporary Transvenous Pacemaker), for a description of the procedure. Transvenous pacing is the method of choice for temporary pacing; however, if necessary, transcutaneous pacing can be used as a bridge to transvenous pacing, with variable success in terms of ability to capture the ventricle. This method is also uncomfortable to the patient.

When extrinsic causes of bradycardia are found, make attempts to reverse these causes. With bradycardia due to pharmacologic agents, consider a change in therapy; however, **permanent pacing may be necessary** if no agent with equivalent efficacy is available and that medication is required (commonly seen in patients with CAD and bradycardia who require beta blockers). Pacing is also appropriate in the tachycardia-bradycardia syndrome if the agents required to control the ventricular rate during atrial arrhythmias cause symptomatic bradycardia during sinus rhythm.

PACEMAKERS: CLASSIFICATION, INDICATIONS, AND FUNCTION

Pacemakers are the mainstay of therapy for clinically significant bradyarrhythmias. Their role is to deliver an electronic stimulus to the heart whenever the heart's intrinsic rate falls below a preprogrammed threshold. Therefore, if a patient's heart has a satisfactory intrinsic rate at a given time, there may be no pacing evident on an ECG. This usually indicates completely normal pacemaker function, because the pacemaker is ready on standby. Other times, a given patient may be completely pacer dependent, and pacer spikes may be seen before each QRS complex.

Pacemakers are usually inserted in the left or right pectoral SC tissue, with electronic lead(s) that enter the heart chamber(s) via the central veins. **Complications** of implantation include pneumothorax, cardiac perforation with tamponade, device infection, and bleeding.

In general, the primary indication for pacing is symptomatic bradycardia causing symptoms of CNS hypoperfusion (presyncope, syncope, or confusion) or hemodynamic compromise. Complete indications for permanent pacing are beyond the scope of this chapter, but a brief review is presented. See Table 14-2 for a list of indications for permanent pacemakers.

Acquired AV Block

In acquired AV block, symptomatic bradycardia is still the primary indication for permanent pacing. Occasionally, however, pacing is warranted without symptoms. In symptom-free patients with third-degree AV block with documented periods of asystole >3 secs or an escape rate <40 bpm, pacing is indicated. Also, postop complete heart block that is not expected to resolve is an indication for pacing, as is catheter ablation of the AV junction (pacing is usually preplanned in this situation). Class II indications for pacing include type II second-degree AV block or third-degree heart block with resting awake HR >40 bpm. Asymptomatic infranodal AV block found incidentally during an electrophysiologic study is also a class II indication for pacing.

Chronic Bi- or Trifascicular Block

Advanced heart block (third-degree or type II second-degree) that develops in the setting of chronic bifascicular or trifascicular block is associated with a high mortality rate and a significant incidence of sudden cardiac death and is an indication for pacing. Also, syncope with chronic bifascicular or trifascicular block is associated with an increased risk of sudden cardiac death, so if the cause of syncope cannot be determined with certainty, prophylactic permanent pacing is indicated in this setting. Finally, the PR and HV intervals have been identified as possible predictors of the development of third-degree AV block and sudden death in the presence of underlying bifascicular block; thus, asymptomatic patients with bifascicular block and an HV interval of >100 msecs should be considered for permanent pacing.

Acute MI

The sinus and AV nodes are relatively resistant to permanent injury by infarction, and normal function should be recovered over time; therefore, sinus bradycardia or AV nodal block in these settings rarely requires permanent pacing. The bundle of His

TABLE 14-2. SUMMARY OF COMMON INDICATIONS FOR PERMANENT PACEMAKERS AND RECOMMENDED PACING MODE

Disorder	Class of indication	Recommended pacing mode
Sinus node dysfunction	I Sinus node dysfunction with documented symptomatic bradycardia or chronotropic incompetence	AAI if no evidence of AV node or other conduction system disease
	IIa Sinus node dysfunction with heart rate <40 bpm but no clear association between symptoms and bradycardia Syncope and sinus node dysfunction on EP study	DDD if concomitant AV node disease
	III No symptoms Sinus bradycardia with symptoms due to nonessential drug therapy	
AV block	I Symptomatic bradycardia with complete (third-degree) or advanced second-degree AV block Asymptomatic complete heart block with heart rate <40 bpm or periods of asystole >3 secs Postop complete heart block Neuromuscular disease with complete AV block ± symptoms	DDD if chronotropic competence of the sinus node is preserved VVI if no organized atrial activity DDDR or VVIR if chronotropic response absent
	IIa Asymptomatic second-degree type II block with narrow QRS or complete heart block (especially if LV dysfunction) with heart rate >40 bpm Asymptomatic infranodal block found at EP study First- or second-degree AV block with symptoms attributable to AV dyssynchrony	

(continued)

TABLE 14-2. CONTINUED

Disorder	Class of indication	Recommended pacing mode
	IIb	
	Markedly prolonged PR interval with LV dysfunction and CHF	
	Neuromuscular disease with any degree AV block with or without symptoms	
	III	
	First-degree AV block or asymptomatic type I second-degree AV block, AV block expected to resolve	
Bifascicular or trifascicular block	I	DDD if chronotropic competence of the sinus node is preserved
	Fascicular block with intermittent third-degree AV block or type II second-degree AV block	VVI if no organized atrial activity
		DDDR or VVIR if chronotropic response absent
	Alternating left and right bundle-branch block	
	IIa	
	Syncope not proven to be due to AV block when other likely causes (e.g., VT) have been excluded	
	Incidental finding at EP study of HV interval >100 msecs	
	IIb	
	Neuromuscular disease with any fascicular block with or without symptoms	
	III	
	Asymptomatic fascicular block	
	Fascicular block with prolonged PR interval without symptoms	
Neurocardiogenic syncope	I	DDD or DDI
	Recurrent syncope caused by carotid sinus stimulation	
	Pauses >3 secs induced by minimal carotid sinus pressure	
	IIa	
	Recurrent syncope of unclear origin associated with a hypersensitive carotid response	

(continued)

TABLE 14-2. CONTINUED

Disorder	Class of indication	Recommended pacing mode
	Documented bradycardia during syncope, spontaneously or during tilt-table testing	
	III	
	Syncope in the absence of a cardioinhibitory response	
	Hyperactive cardioinhibitory response to carotid sinus stimulation when no symptoms or vague symptoms, such as nausea, are present	
	Situational vasovagal syncope in which avoidance behavior is effective	

EP, electrophysiologic.
From Gregoratos G, Abrams J, Epstein AE, et al. ACC/AHA/NASPE 2002 Guideline Update for Implantation of Cardiac Pacemakers and Antiarrhythmia Devices. Summary article: a report of the American College of Cardiology/American Heart Association Task Force on Practice Guidelines (ACC/AHA/NASPE Committee to Update the 1998 Pacemaker Guidelines). *Circulation* 2002;106: 2145–2161, with permission.

is subject to permanent damage, however; thus, AV block in the His-Purkinje system due to anterior infarction often justifies the placement of a pacemaker.

Patients with acute MI who develop intraventricular conduction defects (with the exception of an isolated left anterior fascicular block) have an increased risk of sudden cardiac death. The decision to implant a permanent pacemaker for AV or intraventricular conduction block complicating acute MI depends on the type of conduction disturbance, location of the infarction, and the relation of the electrical disturbance to infarct time. Although symptomatic AV block is still the primary indication for pacing, there are times when pacing may be indicated in the absence of symptoms. For example, third-degree AV block within or below the His-Purkinje system after acute MI or advanced (second- or third-degree) infranodal block and associated bundle-branch block are indications for pacing. If the site of the block is uncertain, an electrophysiologic study may be necessary for further evaluation.

Hypersensitive Carotid Sinus Syndrome and Neurally Mediated Syncope

Occasionally, permanent pacing is indicated for hypersensitive carotid sinus syndrome and neurally mediated syncope. In patients who have recurrent syncope caused by carotid sinus stimulation or in whom minimal carotid sinus pressure induces ventricular pauses of >3 secs in the absence of any medication that depresses the sinus node or AV conduction, pacing is indicated. Also, in syncope with significant bradycardia reproduced by tilt-table testing, pacing can be considered. See Chap. 4, Diagnosis and Management of Syncope, for a detailed discussion on the workup and management of syncope.

PACING MODES

Pacemakers are classified according to codes containing 3–5 letters. The first letter denotes the chamber that is **paced: A for atria, V for ventricle, D for dual** (both). The second letter denotes the chamber that is **sensed: A, V, D, O for atrial, ventricle, dual,**

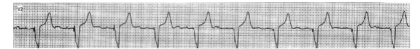

FIG. 14-8. The VVI pacing mode. Note underlying atrial flutter waves.

or none. The third letter indicates the type of **response** the pacemaker makes to a sensed signal: **I for inhibited, T for triggered, or D for dual.** The fourth letter designates the presence of rate-adaptive abilities in which the paced rates vary with metabolic need (denoted with an R). A fifth letter may be used to indicate the presence of antitachycardia pacing capabilities.

CHOICE OF PACING MODE

Once the decision to implant a pacemaker is made, the type of pacing system chosen depends on the primary indication, the accompanying clinical problems, the responsiveness of the sinus node, the presence of any paroxysmal tachyarrhythmias, and the patient's general level of activity.

If the patient has sinus node disease and no evidence of disease in the AV node or His bundle, an AAI pacemaker can be used. However, if the patient has disease in the AV node or His-Purkinje system, a dual-chamber system is more appropriate. The main advantage of a DDD pacemaker is that AV synchrony can be maintained over a wide range of rates; this is associated with reduced incidence of the **pacemaker syndrome** (symptoms from AV dyssynchrony). The main disadvantage of a DDD pacemaker is that it may permit unwanted sensing and tracking of atrial arrhythmias. If a patient has intermittent atrial tachyarrhythmias, then a pacer that can be programmed to the DDI mode should be used. Modern pacemakers can be programmed to **switch modes** from DDD to DDI if the atrial rate is greater than approximately 130 bpm (as seen in atrial flutter, atrial tachycardias, and AF). AV dyssynchrony will

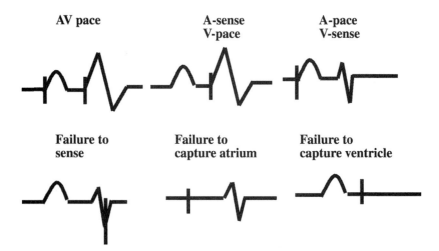

FIG. 14-9. Examples of appropriate and inappropriate dual-chambered pacemaker function. The top row illustrates examples of normal function; the bottom row illustrates common mechanisms of malfunction.

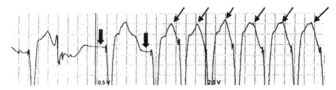

FIG. 14-10. Pacemaker-mediated tachycardia. (From Baim DS, Grossman W, eds., *Grossman's cardiac catheterization, angiography, and intervention,* 6th ed. Philadelphia: Lippincott Williams & Wilkins, 2000, with permission.)

occur, but the ventricular rate will not be rapid. If the patient has chronic AF, a VVI (single-lead) pacemaker should be used. Finally, any patient with chronotropic incompetence should be considered for a rate-adaptive pacemaker **(virtually all modern pacers are rate adaptive).**

PACEMAKER MALFUNCTION

You should assess pacemaker function by obtaining an ECG. Appropriate ventricular pacing only (e.g., VVI mode) produces ventricular spikes followed by ventricular capture, but **only** when there is no intrinsic ventricular activity (Fig. 14-8). VOO pacing is **asynchronous ventricular pacing** (i.e., ventricular pacing independent of intrinsic ventricular activity). These pacing modes are **independent of atrial activity.** Fig. 14-9 illustrates the common cardiac cycles seen with **dual-chamber pacing** (e.g., DDD mode). Below the normal complexes are three examples of abnormal pacer function.

Pacemaker-Mediated Tachycardia

Dual-chambered pacemakers set to the DDD mode are subject to promote a wide-complex tachycardia known as **pacemaker-mediated tachycardia.** This occurs when a PVC conducts retrograde through the AV node to the atrium, which depolarizes the atrium. This activity is sensed by the atrial pacer lead and is interpreted as activity that should trigger a ventricular response. Should retrograde conduction continue through the AV node, an endless cycle will occur that yields a wide-complex tachycardia, with the pacemaker serving as the antegrade limb (Fig. 14-10). The immediate therapy that should be delivered in this setting is the application of a pacemaker magnet over the pacemaker, which will switch the pacer mode to asynchronous DOO. This blocks the antegrade limb, because it prevents the sensing of retrograde P waves. Definitive therapy is to reprogram the postventricular atrial refractory period, so that the retrograde P wave is not sensed by the atrial lead.

KEY POINTS TO REMEMBER

- Bradycardia is caused by a wide variety of pathologies that cause degeneration of the native conduction system or reduce HR secondary to an extrinsic process. Bradycardia due to an extrinsic cause is often reversible.
- It is important to identify the bradycardic rhythm to localize the problem, assess the overall cause, and determine appropriate therapy. Pathology anywhere in the conduction system, from the sinus node through the distal Purkinje fibers, can lead to bradycardia.
- In older patients, think of digoxin toxicity in a patient presenting with a new bradycardia.
- First and foremost, apply BCLS and ACLS protocols for bradycardic patients exhibiting hemodynamic instability.

- Not all bradycardic patients need permanent pacemakers. Guidelines established by the ACC and AHA provide a framework for the decision-making process.
- Understanding the fundamentals of pacemaker function is essential to any internist or cardiologist.

ACKNOWLEDGMENTS

We thank Jane Chen and Morton R. Rinder for providing many of the ECGs presented in this chapter.

REFERENCES AND SUGGESTED READINGS

Gregoratos G, Abrams J, Epstein AE, et al. ACC/AHA/NASPE 2002 Guideline Update for Implantation of Cardiac Pacemakers and Antiarrhythmia Devices. Summary article: a report of the American College of Cardiology/American Heart Association Task Force on Practice Guidelines (ACC/AHA/NASPE Committee to Update the 1998 Pacemaker Guidelines). *Circulation* 2002;106:2145–2161.

Kaushik V, Leon AR, Forester JS, et al. Bradyarrhythmias: temporary and permanent pacing. *Crit Care Med* 2000;28:121–128.

Kusumoto FM, Goldschlager N. Cardiac pacing. *N Engl J Med* 1996;334:89–98.

Mangrum JM, DiMarco JP. The evaluation and management of bradycardia. *N Engl J Med* 2000;342:703–709.

Marso SP, Griffin BP, Topol EJ. *Cardiovascular medicine*. Philadelphia: Lippincott Williams & Wilkins, 2000:281–300.

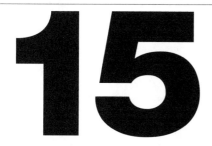

Tachyarrhythmias, Sudden Cardiac Death, and Implantable Cardioverter-Defibrillators

Tuan D. Nguyen and
Peter A. Crawford

INTRODUCTION

When encountering the vast array of tachycardias, even the most astute physician can face difficulties interpreting the correct underlying rhythm and subsequently initiating the appropriate therapeutic measures; however, with the help of an organized, systematic approach and clinical practice, one can become more proficient in this field of cardiac disorders.

Tachycardia is clinically defined as any cardiac rhythm exceeding 100 bpm. Traditionally, the tachyarrhythmias have been categorized as either **narrow-complex** (with a QRS duration <0.12 sec or three small boxes on the standard ECG) or **wide-complex** (with a QRS duration >0.12 sec). As a general rule, narrow-complex tachyarrhythmias are of supraventricular origin (SVT), whereas wide-complex tachycardias (WCT) can arise from supraventricular or ventricular foci (Fig. 15-1). These two general categories of arrhythmias are discussed in Supraventricular Tachycardia and Wide-Complex Tachycardia.

All primary tachycardias, whether supraventricular or ventricular, derive from one of three mechanisms: **abnormal automaticity, reentry,** or **triggered activity** (i.e., early or delayed afterdepolarizations).

SUPRAVENTRICULAR TACHYCARDIA

The initial assessment of narrow-complex tachycardia requires a systematic approach, beginning with the basic ABCs of BCLS. After obtaining vital signs, IV access, and ECG monitoring, assess the patient's clinical status. If unstable (hypotension, active chest pain, dyspnea, or changing mental status), immediate synchronized cardioversion should be performed per ACLS protocol, unless the rhythm is sinus. Alternatively, if there is no hemodynamic compromise, further investigate the nature of the arrhythmia.

Regular Supraventricular Tachycardia

Sinus Tachycardia

Sinus tachycardia is normally a physiologic response to an underlying pathologic insult. The P wave morphology is upright, the rhythm is slow in onset and recovery, and the rate is generally <150 bpm.

Treatment consists of determining and addressing the underlying cause. Etiologies commonly include pain, fever, hypovolemia, hypoxemia (pulmonary embolism), anemia, anxiety, MI, decompensated HF, hyperthyroidism, medications (beta-agonists, caffeine, nicotine), and drug withdrawal (alcohol or illicit drugs).

Other Arrhythmias Mimicking Sinus Tachycardia

INAPPROPRIATE SINUS TACHYCARDIA. Inappropriate sinus tachycardia is an ill-defined clinical entity that generally occurs in young women. The syndrome is characterized by an increased resting heart rate with an exaggerated response to exercise or stress in the setting of a structurally normal heart. At least three of four criteria are required to make the diagnosis of inappropriate sinus tachycardia: (a) resting

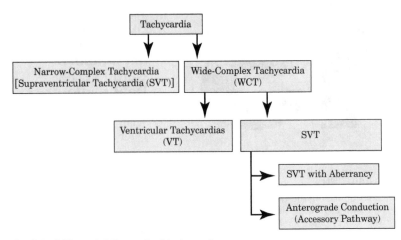

FIG. 15-1. Differential diagnosis of tachycardias.

heart rate >100 bpm, (b) P wave morphology identical to NSR, (c) exclusion of secondary causes of sinus tachycardia, and ± (d) exclusion of sinus node reentry or right atrial tachycardia [via invasive electrophysiologic study (EPS)].

Treatment for this disorder is largely based on clinical judgment, as no firm data currently exist. Initial therapy with beta blockers or verapamil (Calan, Calan SR, Covera-HS, Isoptin, Isoptin SR, Verelan) has been successful in symptomatic patients. For those who fail pharmacologic therapy, invasive interventions, particularly radiofrequency catheter ablation (RFA) of the superior portion of the sinus node, have been pursued with success. Obviously, such options should be instituted only in consultation with appropriate cardiac subspecialists.

SINUS NODE REENTRANT TACHYCARDIA. Sinus node reentrant tachycardia is a rare entity caused by a reentrant circuit within the sinoatrial node and is usually seen in patients with underlying structural heart disease. This arrhythmia can often be mistaken for sinus tachycardia, as the P waves are identical to sinus Ps; however, a history or telemetry strip confirming rapid onset and offset can often identify this tachyarrhythmia. Treatment of sinus node reentrant tachycardia, as well as the remainder of the SVTs, is discussed in greater detail in Acute and Long-Term Medical Therapy.

AV Nodal Reentrant Tachycardia

AV nodal reentrant tachycardia (AVNRT) is the most common regular SVT, with patients usually presenting between 20 and 40 yrs; it commonly affects middle-aged women. The pathologic culprit is a reentrant circuit that resides within the AV node. **For any reentrant circuit to exist, there must be three components: (a) unidirectional conduction block, (b) slow conduction of an impulse, and (c) recovery at the block site.** In AVNRT, EPS delineates two distinct conduction pathways: a slow pathway with sluggish conduction but short refractory period and a fast pathway with rapid conduction but a long refractory period (Fig. 15-2).

"TYPICAL" AV NODAL REENTRANT TACHYCARDIA. Typical AVNRT is often triggered by a premature atrial contraction. The resultant electrical activity travels down (anterogradely) over the slow pathway and is retrogradely conducted back to the atria via the fast pathway. P waves are noticeably absent preceding QRS complexes, and retrograde Ps (P') are either buried in the QRS or cause slurring of the terminal QRS. Hence, the RP' interval is **shorter** than the subsequent P'R interval (RP'<P'R) (Fig. 15-3).

"ATYPICAL" AV NODAL REENTRANT TACHYCARDIA. Atypical AVNRT, in contrast, is often triggered by a PVC and accounts for only 10% of AV nodal tachycardias. The mechanism of this dysrhythmia is the converse of that described for typical AVNRT.

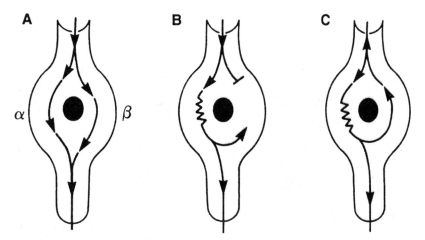

FIG. 15-2. Mechanisms of AV nodal reentrant tachycardia. **A:** Ocassionally, two conduction pathways are present within the AV node. As shown in **(B)**, unidirectional block could occur with a premature upstream impulse (e.g., a premature atrial contraction). Then, as shown in **(C)**, the blocked pathway could recover as the impulse is conducted slowly down the other pathway and conduct retrograde, creating a reentrant loop. (From GJ Klein, EN Prystowsky. *Cardiac arrhythmias.* New York: McGraw-Hill, 1994, with permission.)

Because the retrograde conduction is carried over the slow pathway, the resultant retrograde P (P') can be readily identified on surface 12-lead ECG as a negative deflection generally in the inferior leads (II, III, aVF) (Fig. 15-4). Therefore, the RP' is **longer** than the P'R (RP' >P'R).

AV Reentrant Tachycardia
AV reentrant tachycardia (AVRT), alternatively called "accessory pathway" SVTs, are caused by abnormal bands of conducting tissue located outside the AV node. These

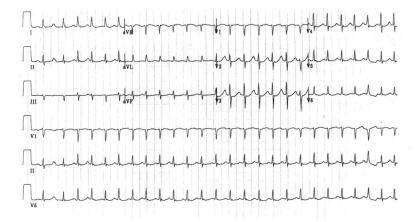

FIG. 15-3. Typical AV nodal reentrant tachycardia. P waves are not readily apparent because they are buried within QRS complexes.

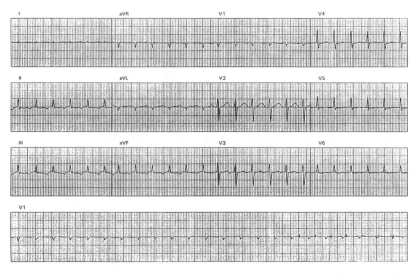

FIG. 15-4. Atypical AV nodal reentrant tachycardia (note retrograde P waves in the inferior leads).

pathways form a circuit that can conduct anterogradely (from atrium to ventricle), retrogradely (from ventricle to atria), or bidirectionally in a given patient.

ANTEROGRADE CONDUCTION AND ANTIDROMIC AV REENTRANT TACHYCARDIA.   While in NSR, anterograde-only and bidirectionally conducting bypass tracts are **manifest** by virtue of a short PR interval and the **delta wave** (or slurred upstroke of the QRS complex). This combination, also referred to as **preexcitation,** is caused by simultaneous activation of the ventricles by the normal conduction system (via the AV node) and the accessory pathway (Fig. 15-5). In patients with these bypass tracts, **antidromic**

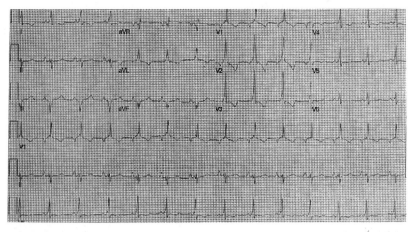

FIG. 15-5. Sinus rhythm in a patient with preexcitation and Wolff-Parkinson-White syndrome. Note the short PR interval and delta wave before the QRS.

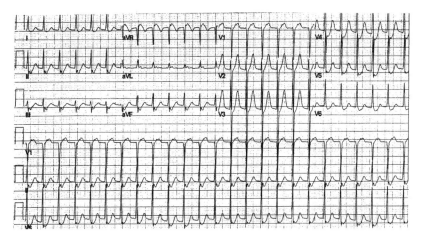

FIG. 15-6. Orthodromic AV reentrant tachycardia. Note retrograde P waves immediately after QRS complexes, especially seen in inferior leads II, III, and aVF.

AVRT can subsequently occur when triggered by a premature atrial contraction or PVC. This rare dysrhythmia involves electrical stimulation traveling anterogradely over the accessory pathway and then reentering the atria via the AV node. The resultant 12-lead ECG displays wide, bizarre QRSs with retrograde Ps noted after each complex (see Fig. 15-7).

RETROGRADE CONDUCTION AND ORTHODROMIC AV REENTRANT TACHYCARDIA. The more typical pattern seen in AVRT is via retrograde conduction through the accessory pathway. In this situation, a premature atrial contraction blocks conduction via the accessory pathway, conducts down the AV node, and then retrograde via the accessory pathway. Electrocardiographically, this arrhythmia is characterized by a normal QRS with retrograde P waves after each complex. A **short RP' tachycardia** results with nondecremental conduction through the bypass tract (Fig. 15-6). The baseline NSR ECG of patients in whom the accessory pathway conducts only retrogradely does not exhibit preexcitation. In this case, the accessory pathway is **concealed.**

Orthodromic AVRT is the most common arrhythmia observed in **Wolff-Parkinson-White (WPW) syndrome.** In WPW, a bypass tract, historically known as the Kent bundle, exists between the atrium and ventricle. While in NSR, WPW is characterized by preexcitation (with the pathognomonic **delta wave**) on ECG, as the abnormal tissue band conducts anterogradely. The baseline delta wave is subsequently lost during the orthodromic reentrant tachycardia, when conduction over the accessory pathway occurs in the opposite direction. Patients with WPW can occasionally develop AF (usually initiated by orthodromic AVRT). In the setting of preexcitation, AF can have serious consequences, because degeneration to VF can occur (discussed in Wide-Complex Tachycardias). To meet the definition of WPW, a patient needs to exhibit preexcitation while in NSR (therefore, the accessory pathway is **manifest**) and exhibit a tachycardia at some point in time.

A distinct form of orthodromic AVRT can occur with a long RP' tachycardia when retrograde bypass tract conduction is **decremental.** This abnormality is sometimes referred to as the permanent form of junctional reciprocating tachycardia (PJRT), which is actually a misnomer, because the tachycardia is not truly junctional in origin.

Fig. 15-7 provides a schematic of the mechanisms of AVRT in the setting of a bypass tract. Remember that a bypass tract can be **concealed** or **manifest,** and it can conduct **nondecrementally** or **decrementally.** As a review, the differential diagnosis of short and long RP' tachycardias can be found in Table 15-1.

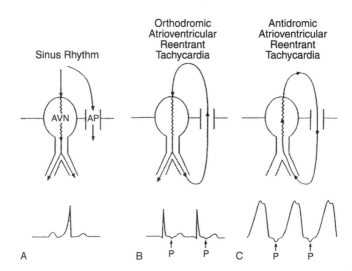

FIG. 15-7. Mechanisms of conduction in the setting of a bypass tract. **A:** Conduction in NSR. **B:** Mechanism of orthodromic reentrant tachycardia. **C:** Mechanism of antidromic reentrant tachycardia, which results in a wide-complex tachycardia. AVN, AV node; AP, accessory pathway. (Adapted from Ganz LI, Friedman PL. Supraventricular tachycardia. *N Engl J Med* 1995;332:162, with permission. © 1995, Massachusetts Medical Society. All rights reserved.)

Nonparoxysmal Junctional Tachycardia
Nonparoxysmal junctional tachycardia, or **junctional ectopic tachycardia,** is caused by increased automaticity within the AV node itself. This is an uncommon arrhythmia that is usually secondary to inflammation near the AV junction (i.e., recent valvular surgery, recent MI), congenital heart disease, or digoxin toxicity. The surface ECG reveals either AV dissociation or a 1:1 ventriculoatrial activation.

Unifocal Atrial Tachycardia
Unifocal atrial tachycardias can result from multiple mechanisms, including ectopic atrial foci or intraatrial reentrant circuits. Typically, the P wave morphology or axis is

TABLE 15-1. DIFFERENTIAL DIAGNOSIS OF NARROW-COMPLEX REGULAR SUPRAVENTRICULAR TACHYCARDIAS[a,b]

Short RP'	Long RP'
Typical AVNRT	Atypical AVNRT
Orthodromic AVRT	Atrial tachycardia
Junctional tachycardia	PJRT (an orthodromic AVRT)
Atrial tachycardia with first-degree AV block	Junctional tachycardia

AVNRT, AV nodal reentrant tachycardia; AVRT, AV reentrant tachycardias; PJRT, permanent junctional reciprocating tachycardia.
[a]These SVT **can occur with a wide complex** if there is aberrant conduction through the His-Purkinje system.
[b]This classification describes SVT with an inverted or abnormal P wave, not upright P waves or flutter waves.

different from that of sinus rhythm, but the QRS complex is identical to those found in NSR.

Intraatrial reentry is generally associated with underlying heart disease or other atrial arrhythmias (i.e., AF) and is usually paroxysmal in nature. In contrast, ectopic atrial tachycardia can occur in structurally normal hearts of younger patients and is more likely to be incessant. Finally, a third variant of atrial tachycardia caused by triggered activity can be seen in digitalis intoxication. In these cases, one frequently sees paroxysms of atrial tachycardia with variable degrees of AV block (**"PAT with block,"** secondary to digoxin's depressive effects on the AV node). Treatment includes correction of electrolytes and phenytoin (Dilantin) administration if the tachyarrhythmia is hemodynamically significant and is associated with digoxin toxicity.

Irregular Supraventricular Tachycardia
Atrial Fibrillation and Atrial Flutter (with Variable AV Block)
Although AF and atrial flutter are obviously supraventricular in origin *(the latter can yield a regular rhythm and should be in considered in the differential in patients with underlying heart disease and a regular tachycardia)*, they are often classified outside of SVTs because of their distinct electrophysiology and acute and long-term management. These arrhythmias are discussed in Chap. 11, Atrial Fibrillation.

Multifocal Atrial Tachycardia
Multifocal atrial tachycardia is generally caused by areas of enhanced automaticity within the atrium, frequently in the setting of concurrent pulmonary disease, such as COPD. The diagnosis is suggested by an ECG showing irregularly irregular ventricular activity and subsequently confirmed by identifying three different P wave morphologies with three different PR-interval lengths. A normal (or flat) isoelectric line between P waves further delineates this rhythm from AF (see Fig. 11-3 for an example).

Treatment of multifocal atrial tachycardia is generally directed at treating or improving the underlying illness. Furthermore, maintenance of electrolytes (particularly potassium and magnesium) can help in suppressing further episodes. Pharmacotherapy, including calcium channel blockers, beta blockers, and amiodarone (Cordarone, Pacerone), has been shown to be efficacious for rate and rhythm control in extreme situations.

ACUTE AND LONG-TERM MEDICAL THERAPY

Acute management of unstable patients in SVT is discussed in Supraventricular Tachycardia. In contrast, when encountering a hemodynamically stable patient, an effort to **diagnose the underlying rhythm** should initially be undertaken. In the case of atrial arrhythmias, such as atrial flutter, AF, atrial tachycardia, or multifocal atrial tachycardia, vagal maneuvers, such as the carotid-sinus massage (do not perform in patients with bruits or a cerebrovascular accident history), **merely slow AV nodal conduction,** reducing ventricular rate and unmasking atrial activity; tachycardia is not terminated in these arrhythmias because they are not dependent on the AV node for their perpetuation (merely for their conduction to the ventricles). However, successful vagal maneuvers **terminate** AVNRT and AVRT. Pharmacologic agents, such as **adenosine (Adenocard)** (6 mg rapid IV push, then 12 mg rapid IV push), transiently block AV conduction and terminate AVNRT or AVRT but only transiently induce AV block with the atrial arrhythmias. Finally, if a patient is unresponsive to vagal maneuvers and adenosine, treatment of choice is a nondihydropyridine calcium channel blocker (diltiazem or verapamil) (see Chap. 11, Atrial Fibrillation, for a list of these medications). These medications have a longer half-life, which enables them to terminate the rhythm or control the ventricular rate over an extended period. Take extreme care in patients with tenuous BPs, as these medications can cause hypotension. Note that beta blockers and digoxin (Lanoxin) can be used as well; digoxin can take hours to take effect, even when given IV.

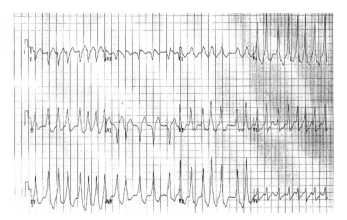

FIG. 15-8. AF with preexcitation (in a patient with Wolff-Parkinson-White syndrome).

Patients experiencing chronic or persistent episodes of SVT not only can develop symptoms of palpitations, but they can also eventually develop a **tachycardia-mediated cardiomyopathy.** Because of this complication, refer these patients (as well as those with recurrent or markedly symptomatic episodes) to cardiologists or electro-physiologists for long-term management.

Current recommendations for long-term treatment depend in part on patient preferences. Long-term pharmacotherapy includes nondihydropyridine calcium channel blockers, beta blockers, or digoxin. If these measures are ineffective or not well tolerated, RFA is often pursued. RFA can also be offered first line. Success rates of up to 95% are possible in AVNRT, 80% in AVRT, and 70–90% in unifocal atrial tachycardia. **Complications** of RFA (~1% rate) include complete heart block requiring a permanent pacemaker and cardiac perforation with pericardial tamponade. The extensive side effects of antiarrhythmic medications (particularly class I and III agents) often limit their use in long-term therapy.

As described in AV Reentrant Tachycardia, special consideration must be taken in the setting of AF in a patient with preexcitation (i.e., AF in a patient with WPW) (Fig. 15-8). **In this situation, AV nodal depressing agents (adenosine, calcium channel blockers, beta blockers, digoxin) are contraindicated.** Blocking AV conduction can provoke selective conduction down the nondecremental accessory pathway, leading to profoundly accelerated ventricular rates and subsequent VF. Ideal treatment would be IV procainamide (Procan SR, Procanbid, Pronestyl, Pronestyl-SR) or amiodarone (which preferentially slow the accessory pathway conduction) or synchronized cardioversion under sedation.

In the case of **asymptomatic** WPW (preexcitation on the ECG while in NSR), there is no indication for medical or ablative therapy, but these patients should be followed, as up to 40% will develop a reentrant tachycardia. Patients with rare episodes of AVRT **may be prescribed AV nodal blocking agents, unless there is a history of (or risk factors for) AF.** AF in patients with WPW is an indication for RFA.

WIDE-COMPLEX TACHYCARDIA

The differential diagnosis of WCTs can be simplistically classified into ventricular tachyarrhythmias and "other" WCTs. The latter group includes any SVT with aberrant conduction through the His-Purkinje system, such as sinus tachycardia, AVNRT, AVRT, or AF/flutter; hyperkalemia; AF with preexcitation; and pacemaker-mediated tachycardia (see Fig. 14-10 for an example of this latter entity). Because of their more grave clinical course, this section focuses on the approach to VTs. As described in the acute management of SVT, the initial approach to WCTs includes the ABCs of ACLS: IV access and continuous ECG monitoring, delivery of O_2, and rapid assessment of vital signs and clinical symptoms. Hemodynamically unstable patients should immediately undergo synchronized cardioversion per ACLS. **Pulseless VT and VF require immediate institution of CPR and rapid defibrillation.** If the patient is stable, however, further investigation into the nature of the arrhythmia is possible.

BRUGADA CRITERIA

Differentiating between VT and SVT with aberrant conduction can often be difficult. Although several criteria have been proposed to help distinguish these two arrhythmias, the stepwise approach introduced by Brugada and Brugada has the greatest sensitivity and specificity (up to 99% and 96%, respectively).

In the Brugada criteria (Fig. 15-9), VT is diagnosed when there is an absence of an RS complex in all of the precordial leads (V_1–V_6). If an RS complex exists, VT can still be diagnosed if the RS interval is >100 msecs in any precordial lead. If this criterion is not met, then findings of AV dissociation (i.e., fusion beats, P and QRS dissociation) can prove VT. Finally, if the previously listed three criteria do not exist, morphologic criteria can be used to rule in or rule out VT (Fig. 15-10).

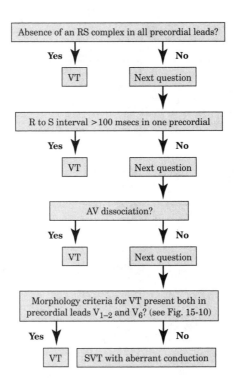

FIG. 15-9. Overview of the Brugada criteria for the differentiation of VT from aberrantly conducted SVT.

Configuration	SVT (n=22)	VT (n=60)	Favors	Sens.	Spec.
Taller left peak 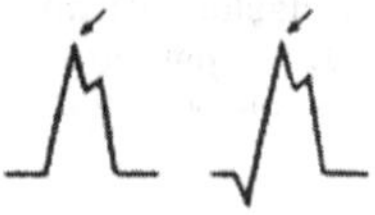	0	14	VT	23%	100%
Biphasic RS or QR 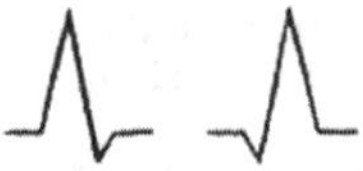	1	11	VT	18%	95%
Triphasic rsR' or rR' 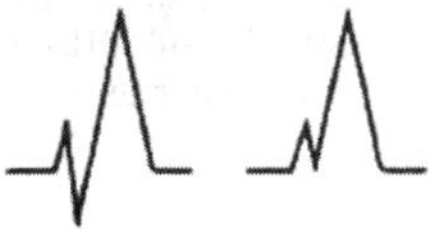	14	8	SVT	64%	87%

A

Configuration	SVT (n=13)	VT (n=38)	Favors	Sens.	Spec.
In V$_1$,V$_2$ any of: (a) r ≥0.04 sec (b) Notched S downstroke (c) Delayed S nadir >0.06 sec 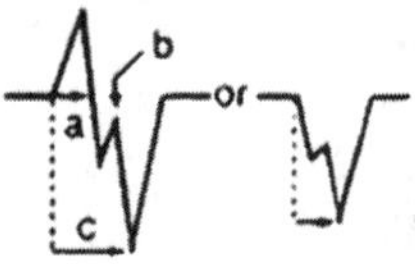	0	33	VT	87%	100%
In V$_1$,V$_2$ absence of: (a) r ≥0.04 sec (b) Notched S downstroke (c) Delayed S nadir >0.06 sec 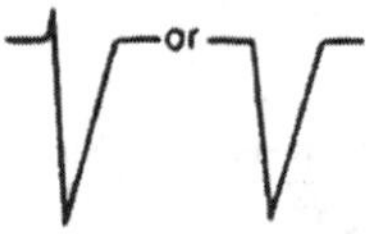	13	4	SVT	100%	89%

B

FIG. 15-10. Brugada morphologic criteria. **A:** Lead V$_1$ criteria in right bundle-branch block (RBBB). R>R' and biphasic RS or QR favor VT, whereas triphasic rSR' or rR' favors SVT. **B:** Lead V$_1$ criteria in left bundle-branch block. r >40 msecs, a notched S, and delayed intrinsicoid deflection (onset of QRS to nadir of S) >60 msecs all favor VT. (*continued*)

Configuration		SVT (n=35)	VT (n=98)	Favors	Sens.	Spec.
Monophasic QS 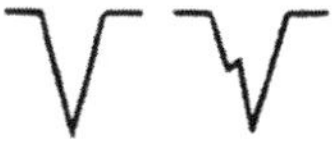		0	29	VT	30%	100%
	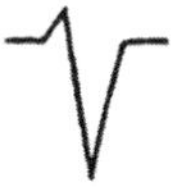 Biphasic rS (RBBB-type)	0	23	VT	38%	100%
	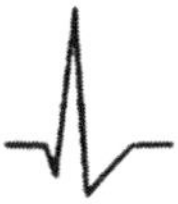 Triphasic qRs (RBBB-type)	8	3	SVT	36%	95%

C

FIG. 15-10. Continued. C: Lead V_6 criteria. Monophasic QS or biphasic rS favors VT. Triphasic qRs favors SVT. (From *Circulation* 1991;83:1649, with permission.)

When faced with an ambiguous or emergent situation, always assume that a WCT is VT until proved otherwise. Furthermore, fairly quick and reliable predictors of VT from a patient's history, such as prior MIs or LV dysfunction, can be obtained. **It is contraindicated to presume or assess a WCT as aberrant SVT by administering adenosine (to determine if it will "break").** In this situation, adenosine administration could precipitate the conversion of infarct-related VT to ischemic VF through alterations in coronary artery hemodynamics. Thus, adenosine administration is only appropriate when one is certain that an arrhythmia is an SVT.

VENTRICULAR TACHYCARDIA AND SUDDEN CARDIAC DEATH

The diagnostic workup and management of VTs is a popular topic that has been extensively studied.

Premature Ventricular Contractions

PVCs are often recognized on ECGs as occasional wide-complex QRSs that lack preceding atrial activity (P waves). PVCs can alternate with normal sinus activity (bigeminy or trigeminy) or occur in pairs or trios (couplets and triplets). Often, these complexes represent a benign event; however, frequent PVCs and nonsustained VT in the setting of LV dysfunction (LV ejection fraction <40%) often identify a group of patients at increased risk for sudden death.

Current treatment strategies regarding PVC suppression are, in large part, defined by the CAST and CAST-II trials. These randomized, controlled trials were designed to test whether suppression of PVCs with class IC antiarrhythmic agents (i.e., flecainide, encainide, and moricizine) could prevent mortality in patients with minimal to no symptoms. **Both trials were prematurely discontinued because of increased mortality (related to proarrhythmias) in patients treated with such agents.**

As a general rule, patients with isolated PVCs, few or no symptoms, and normal cardiac function carry a good long-term prognosis and should not be treated. In those with frequent ectopy or other ventricular dysrhythmias, ensure normalization of potassium and magnesium levels (>4 and >2 mEq/L, respectively). In patients with

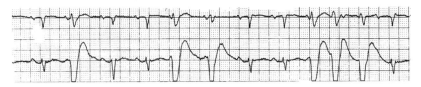

FIG. 15-11. Sinus rhythm with a PVC, couplet, and triplet.

more symptomatic PVCs, beta blockers can be used for control. Finally, in patients with marked symptoms, more aggressive antiarrhythmic therapy beyond the class IC medications (such as amiodarone) may be used to provide relief. Such a regimen would require a cardiology or electrophysiology referral or consult (Fig. 15-11).

Accelerated Idioventricular Rhythm

Accelerated idioventricular rhythm (AIVR) occurs almost exclusively in ischemic heart disease in the periinfarct or postreperfusion settings. The mechanism is believed to be secondary to an ectopic ventricular focus (usually in the reperfusion zone) that accelerates beyond the intrinsic sinus rate. It is usually regular, has a rate of 60–120 bpm, and is of little clinical significance (Fig. 15-12). Treatment for AIVR is rarely necessary. With severe symptoms or hemodynamic compromise, atropine or atrial pacing can be used to stimulate the sinus rhythm to overdrive the ectopic focus.

Nonsustained Ventricular Tachycardia and Sustained Ventricular Tachycardia

Nonsustained VT (NSVT) in the setting of ischemic heart disease has been well described and continues to remain a popular topic for clinical trials. NSVT is defined as three or more QRS complexes of ventricular origin occurring at a rate >100 bpm. Differentiation between NSVT and sustained VT is debated, with some defining NSVT as <30 consecutive beats or <10 secs (Fig. 15-13). As described in High Risk, patients with ischemic disease and a poor LV ejection fraction (<40%) who have NSVT carry an increased risk of sudden cardiac death from ventricular arrhythmia. Indeed, risk stratification plays a crucial role in terms of the management approach for nonsustained VT.

Low Risk

For post-MI **patients with normal LV function** and no or few symptoms during episodes of NSVT, reassurance and appropriate postinfarction pharmacotherapy (beta blocker and ASA) are the treatments of choice.

High Risk

Alternatively, **patients with LV dysfunction and CAD** are stratified into a higher risk group for sudden cardiac death from a sustained ventricular tachyarrhythmia. Man-

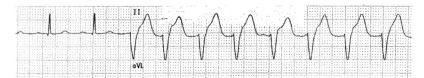

FIG. 15-12. Accelerated idioventricular rhythm.

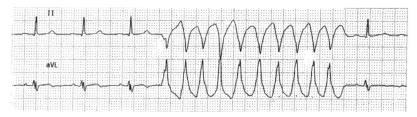

FIG. 15-13. Nonsustained ventricular tachycardia.

agement in this situation has been defined by a myriad of clinical trials that compare standard post-MI/CAD care with antiarrhythmics and implantable cardioverter-defibrillators (ICDs). The EMIAT trial, for example, studied the efficacy of amiodarone vs placebo in reducing mortality in patients with decreased LV ejection fraction in the post-MI setting. Although all-cause mortality and cardiac mortality were not significantly altered, arrhythmic death was reduced with amiodarone. These benefits were potentiated in patients concomitantly treated with beta blockers. Further studies (e.g., CAMIAT) confirm this point.

EPS-directed placement of ICDs in high-risk patients with NSVT, however, currently represents the standard of care for the **primary prevention of sudden cardiac death.** The MADIT study compared ICDs vs "conventional" therapy (mainly amiodarone) in patients with ischemic heart disease and NSVT for the primary prevention of sudden death. In this trial, patients with poor LV ejection fraction (<35–40%), no ischemic events or reperfusion therapy in at least 96 hrs, and NSVT underwent EPS. Those with inducible, nonsuppressible VT (with procainamide) were randomized to amiodarone or ICD. The primary end point of overall survival was significantly improved in the ICD group (a relative risk reduction of 54% in the ICD group). The MUSTT study supported these findings. **Thus, suitable patients with a prior MI, LV ejection fraction <35%, and NSVT are generally referred for EPS to determine if monomorphic VT can be induced, in which case an ICD is often placed.**

A landmark trial, MADIT2 [1], asked whether patients with a **prior MI and depressed LV systolic function (ejection fraction <30%)** benefit from prophylactic ICD implantation, irrespective of the known presence of NSVT (many of these patients do have NSVT, if they are monitored long enough) or an EPS. Investigators found a 19.8% total mortality at approximately 2 yrs in the control group and a 14.2% mortality in the ICD group. This trial provides the theoretical standard by which patients are treated today. **Based on these findings, ICD implantation is an ACC/AHA class IIa indication in patients with these criteria who do not harbor a contraindication.** The **major caveat** with the results of the trial is the health care system's ability to finance such an undertaking, given the extraordinarily large number of patients who, on first glance, meet criteria. The cost of defibrillator implantation is approximately $60,000. At the time of publication, government sources that fund the U.S. Medicare program are in the process of deciding whether MADIT2 criteria will be reimbursed to implanting physicians and facilities. Furthermore, extensive research is under way that is intended to elucidate other features that will risk stratify patients and determine who is at the highest risk for sudden cardiac death due to ventricular arrhythmias.

Secondary prevention of sudden cardiac death from ventricular arrhythmias was studied by the AVID investigators. Patients had LV ejection fraction <40% and were resuscitated from cardiac arrests, presumably due to ventricular arrhythmias, or cardioverted out of sustained VT. Researchers concluded that survivors of VF or sustained VT who had a diminished LV ejection fraction had an increased survival with ICD as compared to class III antiarrhythmics (mainly amiodarone). **Given these convincing findings, ICD placement in this patient population is considered a class I indication.**

In the immediate postinfarction setting (<48 hrs), post-MI monomorphic VT (often derived from a scar) generally does not carry a bad prognosis. Hence, patients with such dysrhythmias should not be subjected to EPS-guided therapy or an ICD as described in High Risk. In contrast, polymorphic VT in the periinfarct setting is a poor prognostic indicator suggestive of recurrent or ongoing cardiac ischemia. In this situation, aim primary efforts at revascularization as opposed to EPS.

Pharmacologic Therapy for Sustained Ventricular Tachycardia

For patients who experience sustained monomorphic VT after ICD implantation, pharmacotherapy with antiarrhythmics is often required to prevent the persistent delivery of ICD shocks. Acutely, IV amiodarone (class III antiarrhythmic) or lidocaine (class Ib antiarrhythmic) are often used. Long-term, amiodarone is commonly chosen first for this purpose, but sotalol (Betapace, Betapace AF) (class III antiarrhythmic) is also effective in patients with or without depressed LV function [3]. Given the population of patients usually requiring pharmacologic VT suppression, however, the widespread use of sotalol is somewhat limited, because it can be dangerous in patients with decompensated HF, is contraindicated in renal failure, and is associated with QTc prolongation and torsades de pointes (see Long QT Syndromes and Torsades de Pointes). Amiodarone is associated with a variety of side effects, including pulmonary fibrosis, transaminitis, hyper- or hypothyroidism, and deposition in the skin and corneas. In situations in which amiodarone and sotalol are ineffective or contraindicated, mexiletine (Mexitil) (class Ib antiarrhythmic) is sometimes used. Remember that treating arrhythmias with antiarrhythmics can lead to proarrhythmia properties. These patients are almost always managed with the assistance of an electrophysiologist. For refractory cases of VT in the setting of ischemic heart disease (in which a scar is the source of the reentrant rhythm that yields VT), EPS and attempted RFA are used, with an approximately 40% success rate.

Dilated and Hypertrophic Cardiomyopathies

Patients with dilated (DCM) and hypertrophic cardiomyopathies (HCM) are at increased risk for sudden death secondary to ventricular tachyarrhythmias.

Dilated Cardiomyopathy

DCM can result from a multitude of disorders and is discussed in greater detail in Chap. 12, Assessment and Management of the Dilated, Restrictive, and Hypertrophic Cardiomyopathies. The clinical data regarding treatment of nonsustained VT in nonischemic DCM are sparse as compared to those for VT in the setting of CAD; however, this topic is currently under intense scrutiny.

Data supporting amiodarone use for prophylaxis against sudden cardiac death in patients with nonischemic cardiomyopathy come from the GESICA and CHF-STAT trials. In the GESICA trial, patients were randomly assigned to standard HF therapy with amiodarone vs standard CHF therapy alone. At an average follow-up of 13 mos, arrhythmia-related mortality was 33.5% in the amiodarone group, as compared to 41.4% in the standard-treatment patients ($p = .02$). In the CHF-STAT trial, no significant difference in total mortality was proven between patients receiving amiodarone vs placebo; however, subgroup analysis of nonischemic HF patients showed a strong trend toward improved survival ($p = .06$).

Currently, there is no role for ICD placement for NSVT in nonischemic cardiomyopathy for the purpose of primary prevention of sudden cardiac death. Limited data from the CASH trial suggest superiority of ICDs over amiodarone and beta blockers in the secondary prevention of sudden death. In this trial, survivors of sudden cardiac death secondary to documented VT and unrelated to MI were randomized to one of four treatment arms: propafenone, metoprolol, amiodarone, or ICD. The propafenone limb was prematurely discontinued because of increased overall mortality as compared to ICD. Although beta blockers and amiodarone produced an equivalent 2-yr reduction in overall mortality, there was an additional 37% relative risk reduction in the ICD group as compared to those treated medically. Only a small portion of the patients included in the study, however, had DCM (the great majority of patients had underlying CAD). Hence, it is difficult to extrapolate clinical guidelines from this limited trial.

As a final note, clinical trials are currently in progress that can further define this patient population. The SCD-HeFT trial, for example, is studying primary prevention of sudden cardiac death in ischemic and nonischemic cardiomyopathy patients with NYHA class II–III HF and an LV ejection fraction of <35%. The three-arm trial compares conventional CHF therapy (beta blockers, ACE inhibitors, and HMG-CoA reductase inhibitors) vs amiodarone vs ICD. Total (overall) mortality, arrhythmic and nonarrhythmic morbidity and mortality, and cost effectiveness are end points under evaluation.

In summary, for nonischemic cardiomyopathy patients experiencing asymptomatic NSVT, current guidelines suggest continued treatment with standard CHF therapy (i.e., ACE inhibitors and beta blockers). **EPS in this subpopulation for NSVT is not currently recommended because of its low sensitivity, specificity, and predictive values.** For symptomatic patients (i.e., severe palpitations), a trial of amiodarone can be used; **however, for a history of syncope concerning for VT/VF or sustained VT, ICD placement is indicated in such patients.**

Hypertrophic Cardiomyopathy

Patients with HCM are at increased risk of sudden death because of VT (see also Chap. 12, Assessment and Management of the Dilated, Restrictive, and Hypertrophic Cardiomyopathies). The ICD plays a critical role in the secondary and primary prevention of sudden cardiac death in this patient population.

In a retrospective, multicenter trial [2] studying the efficacy of implantable defibrillators, ICDs were shown to be highly effective in terminating VT and VF. For survivors of cardiac arrest or sustained VT (secondary prevention), appropriate ICD discharges were reported in 44% at a mean follow-up of 3 yrs. Therefore, an ICD is the treatment of choice for secondary prevention of sudden cardiac death in HCM. For primary prevention of sudden cardiac death, ICD implantation is appropriate in patients considered at high risk for sudden cardiac death, namely those with **sustained VT, family history of sudden death in one or more primary relatives, syncope (especially exertional), frequent NSVT on Holter monitor, and massive LVH of at least 30 mm.** There is virtually no role for EPS in identifying patients at high risk for sudden cardiac death. In general, the role of antiarrhythmics (i.e., amiodarone) is not well defined.

Arrhythmogenic Right Ventricular Dysplasia

Arrhythmogenic RV dysplasia is a rare syndrome characterized by inappropriate myocyte apoptosis and subsequent replacement with adipose and fibrous tissue in the RV. The cardiomyopathy begins in the RV and spreads to eventually include and destroy the LV. The condition is diagnosed by cardiac MRI. Therefore, in the setting of sustained VT that occurs in the absence of LV dysfunction or CAD, MRI is a component of the workup. Monomorphic VT with a left bundle-branch block morphology occurs secondary to reentrant pathways within the diseased RV. A pathognomonic ECG finding (while in NSR) is T wave inversion in the anterior precordial leads with an "epsilon" potential (slurred terminal portion of the QRS complex). Because of VT, patients often present after syncope or sudden death. ICD placement is the only reliable method for primary and secondary prevention against sudden cardiac death. Many of the ventricular arrhythmias in arrhythmogenic RV dysplasia are due to reentrant rhythms that can be ablated.

Ventricular Tachycardia and Ventricular Fibrillation in the Absence of Structural Heart Disease

VT and VF may occur in the absence of any structural heart disease or CAD.

Idiopathic Ventricular Tachycardia

Idiopathic VT is characterized by a normal 12-lead ECG at baseline that converts into a left bundle-branch block or right bundle-branch block pattern on initiation of VT.

RIGHT VENTRICULAR OUTFLOW TRACT. VT originating from the RV outflow tract (RVOT) is often monomorphic and has a left bundle-branch block pattern with an inferior and rightward axis. The dysrhythmia is often triggered by a PVC and, in general, carries a very low risk of sudden death. Patients often present with malaise or lightheadedness. Adenosine has been shown to terminate RVOT VT in the acute setting, and beta blockers and calcium channel blockers have been successfully used for long-term control in symptomatic patients. RFA is also a reliable therapeutic option in refractory cases. An ICD is usually not required.

LEFT VENTRICULAR APEX VENTRICULAR TACHYCARDIA. Monomorphic idiopathic VT can also occur with a nidus in the LV apex. The likely culprit is a reentrant pathway involving the fascicles of the left bundle branch. The arrhythmia has a superior axis and right bundle-branch block pattern and is classically responsive to calcium channel blockers. Possible cure can also be pursued with RFA. An ICD is usually not required.

Brugada Syndrome

The Brugada syndrome *(distinguished from the* **Brugada criteria** *for assessing VT vs aberrant SVT)* is a rare cause of VF and sudden cardiac death due to alterations in sodium-channel function (mutations in the gene encoding the channel SCN5A) in the RVOT region of the myocardium. Patients are typically Asian (with a high prevalence in Thailand), male, and have a positive family history of syncope or sudden death. The baseline ECG is abnormal, showing an incomplete right bundle-branch block pattern with ST elevations noted in the right precordium (V_1–V_2) and early high takeoffs of the ST segment ("J wave") (Fig. 15-14). In addition, patients lack any structural heart disease, as confirmed by echocardiography, MRI, and angiography. Primary prevention of sudden cardiac death in patients with the Brugada-pattern ECG is controversial. Two main groups, led by the Brugada investigators and the Priori investigators, have conducted research in this area. To summarize, the Brugada group concluded that EPS (to induce polymorphic VT) risk stratifies for sudden cardiac death, particularly if class IC (see Chap. 11, Atrial Fibrillation, p. 125) agents are used to enhance the likelihood of inducibility. The Priori group contends that EPS in these patients has poor sensitivity and specificity, and, thus, family history and history of syncope and palpitations are much more reliable indices of the risk of sudden cardiac death. Thus, the decision to implant an ICD in an asymptomatic patient with the Brugada-pattern ECG should be made very carefully, after extensive workup for structural heart disease.

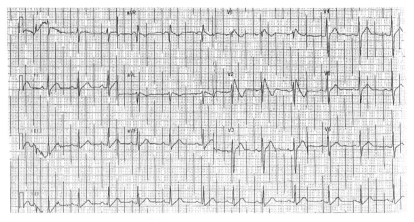

FIG. 15-14. The classic baseline ECG of a patient with Brugada syndrome. Note the coved ST elevations in leads V_1–V_2 and the incomplete right bundle-branch block.

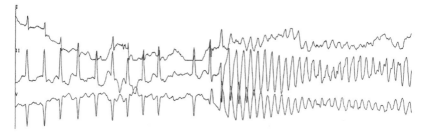

FIG. 15-15. Torsades de pointes.

Long QT Syndromes and Torsades de Pointes

Long QT syndromes (LQTS; QT corrected intervals >450 msecs) can be acquired or inherited diseases. In the case of congenital LQTS, inherited malfunctions in cardiac sodium or potassium channels impair ventricular repolarization, thereby triggering a characteristic polymorphic VT known as **torsades de pointes** (twisting of the points). These mutations can be transmitted as autosomal-recessive (Jervell and Lange-Nielsen syndrome, associated with deafness) or dominant (Romano-Ward syndrome). Acquired LQTS frequently are caused by medications, particularly class I and III anti-arrhythmic drugs **(including quinidine, sotalol, and dofetilide)** and psychotropic medications, such as tricyclic antidepressants and haloperidol (Haldol). Also, combinations of macrolide antibiotics with antifungal "-azoles" or antihistamines have been reported to prolong QT intervals. Finally, metabolic derangements, including hypocalcemia, hypomagnesemia, and hypokalemia, have been implicated in prolonging QT and subsequently inducing torsades de pointes.

Torsades de pointes is a polymorphic VT characterized by wide QRS complexes that vary in amplitude, giving the appearance of twisting around the isoelectric line. The rhythm is often triggered by a PVC and its compensatory pause **("short-long-short" sequence)** (Fig. 15-15).

If torsades de pointes results in hemodynamic compromise, then perform ACLS protocols, including DC cardioversion, promptly. Also, magnesium infusion (2–4 g IV) has been shown to suppress acute recurrences. In the case of acquired LQTS, check and supplement calcium, potassium, and magnesium levels. Remove any offending QT-prolonging medications. Furthermore, because acquired LQTS is often related to bradycardia, overdrive pacing with a transvenous temporary pacer (or rarely, isoproterenol) up to 100 bpm can be performed. Lidocaine has been used to suppress PVCs and further torsades de pointes, but only one-half of cases respond to such therapy. Although many causes of acquired torsades de pointes are discovered and corrected, the precipitating factors surrounding some patients are never definitively determined. In these instances, ICDs play a role in secondary prevention.

The acute treatment of congenital LQTS is similar to that of acquired LQTS. Long-term therapy, however, follows a different approach. Increased sympathetic activity and tachycardia trigger torsades de pointes in some forms of congenital LQTS. Hence, treatments aimed at suppressing adrenergic tone are recommended. Beta blockers are the preferred first-line agents and have been clinically proved to reduce syncope and sudden death. With treatment failure, denervation of the left sympathetic ganglia can be performed. Refractory arrhythmias or those resulting in syncope or sudden cardiac death after conservative pharmacotherapy and left sympathetic ganglia denervation warrant ICD placement.

Inflammatory, Infectious, and Inheritable Diseases

Certainly, ventricular tachyarrhythmias can result from other disorders not mentioned previously in this section. Inflammatory conditions, such as myocarditis and

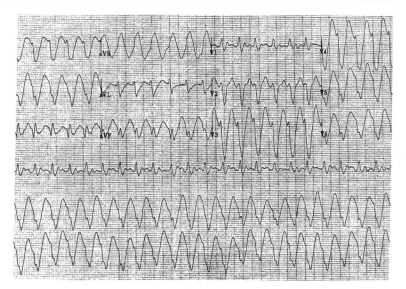

FIG. 15-16. Wide-complex tachycardia induced by hyperkalemia.

sarcoidosis, can create conduction disorders and arrhythmic disease. In sarcoidosis, antiarrhythmics and subsequent ICD placement may be required.

Cardiomyopathies resulting from parasitic infections, such as Chagas' disease, can also present as ventricular tachyarrhythmias, syncope, and sudden death. Again, antiarrhythmic therapy and ICD placement may be indicated in certain situations.

Finally, specific muscular dystrophic disorders can predispose to VT and VF. In Duchenne's muscular dystrophy, for example, there is a predilection for fibrosis of the posterior wall. At baseline, this injured area can often mimic a posterior wall infarct on ECG (large R wave in V_1 and V_2) and creates the nidus for generation of VT. Implantable defibrillators may be indicated in such cases, especially in the setting of syncope.

Digoxin Toxicity

At toxic serum levels, digoxin shifts resting membrane potential to more depolarized levels. This shift enhances automaticity and also yields triggered activity via delayed afterdepolarizations. Occasionally, complex ventricular arrhythmias, such as unifocal or multifocal PVCs, fascicular VTs, and even bidirectional VTs (alternating morphologies and axis in a WCT), occur. As mentioned, digoxin toxicity can also provoke atrial and junctional tachycardias. Calcium loading can **precipitate** these tachyarrhythmias in the setting of digoxin toxicity. Treatment of tachyarrhythmias associated with digoxin toxicity includes correction of electrolytes and use of the Fab fragments of digoxin antibodies (Digibind). Use the latter judiciously, as it can rapidly cause hypokalemia and promote decompensation of HF. It is also expensive. **Phenytoin** is the classic antiarrhythmic used in digoxin-toxic tachyarrhythmias.

Electrolyte Disturbances (Hyperkalemia)

Severe electrolyte imbalances, including hyperkalemia, can cause wide-complex tachyarrhythmias. Typical ECG changes in hyperkalemia (usually >6 mEq/L) include peaked T waves, flattening of the P wave, and prolongation of the PR interval. In general, with further increases in plasma potassium concentration, widening of the QRS complex occurs. Eventual "sine" waves can be seen on surface ECG (Fig. 15-16), looking similar to monomorphic VT, which can subsequently degenerate into VF. In this

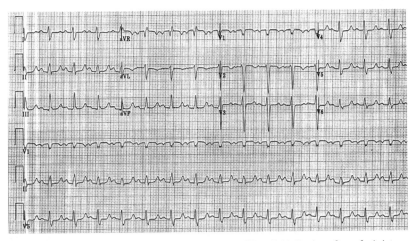

FIG. 15-17. Hyperkalemia in the same patient as in Fig. 15-16, 5 mins after administration of calcium gluconate and sodium bicarbonate.

situation, treat the hyperkalemia and institute ACLS protocols promptly. Calcium and bicarbonate frequently reverse the abnormalities promptly (Fig. 15-17). ICDs have no long-term indication, as this tachyarrhythmia is fully reversible with electrolyte normalization. Similarly, although a hyperkalemic rhythm looks like VT, **it does not respond to cardioversion or antiarrhythmics,** because the underlying rhythm is sinus. The P waves are not visible, most likely because conduction from the sinus node to the AV node occurs over specialized tracts within the atria that do not completely depolarize the atria (sinoventricular rhythm) (Fig. 15-16).

ECG ARTIFACT

It is important to recognize the clinical and financial significance of mistakenly diagnosed ventricular dysrhythmias. One clinical review (see Suggested Reading) showed that ECG artifacts, often caused by patient movement (e.g., Parkinsonian tremors, brushing teeth), can closely simulate VT. 12 patients were described in the synopsis, and misdiagnosis of VT was made by medical house officers, cardiologists, and even an electrophysiologist. In the end, 7 patients were inappropriately treated with lidocaine and 2 were given precordial thumps. Additionally, 3 patients were unnecessarily subjected to cardiac catheterization, one underwent permanent pacemaker placement (for antibradycardic pacing in misdiagnosed torsades de points), and one underwent ICD implantation. See Fig. 15-18 for three examples of ECG artifact.

No formal guidelines currently exist to differentiate artifact from true VT; however, some characteristics of ECG artifact have been described. These findings include

- An unstable isoelectric line preceding or following the questionable event.
- Presence of QRS complexes visible within the event that coincide with the cycle length of the baseline rate.
- Hemodynamic and clinical stability during the event.
- Association of the event with body movement.

IMPLANTABLE CARDIOVERTER-DEFIBRILLATORS

Three major therapeutic options exist for primary and secondary prevention of VT and VF. These include (a) antiarrhythmic agents, (b) surgery or percutaneous catheter–directed ablative techniques, and (c) implantation of ICD. Of course, any combina-

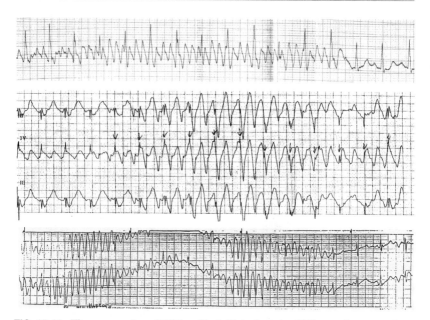

FIG. 15-18. Three examples of ECG artifact. Note that the QRS complexes march at regular intervals throughout the strips.

tion of these measures can also be used. Clinical trials have uniformly documented the benefits of ICD implantation in the secondary prevention of sudden cardiac death. Without devices, recurrence rates of 15–20% per yr are reported. Alternatively, this sudden cardiac death recurrence rate is reduced to 1–2% following ICD implantation. As noted previously in the High Risk section, ICDs play an important role in primary prevention of sudden cardiac death as well.

ICDs usually are programmed to deliver distinct modes of therapy, depending on the rhythm, characteristics, length of time in the rhythm, and outcome of prior attempts at therapy. Most ICDs have the ability to discriminate the morphology of the rhythm in addition to the rate. This characteristic reduces (but does not eliminate) shocks for sinus tachycardia AF or SVT. Furthermore, to minimize the discomfort (which can be substantial) associated with the delivery of shocks, antitachycardia pacing is often delivered first to attempt to pace-terminate VT. VF or failed antitachycardia pacing always leads to the delivery of a shock. **Thus, ICDs do not prevent VT; they treat it after it has occurred, often before hemodynamic instability ensues.** Therefore, ICDs are not a treatment for ongoing incessant VT/VF. Note that most ICDs have back-up pacing capability and thus may serve as a pacemaker as well for bradycardia. The converse is not true of pacemakers, which never have defibrillator capacity. Because a high percentage of patients with an indication for ICD have cardiomyopathy with significant conduction disturbance, the role of biventricular pacemakers with ICD capability is being assessed in the COMPANION trial, whose results will be published in 2003.

The dramatic benefits of ICDs must be weighed against matters of medical and financial practicality, particularly in the setting of primary prevention. Patients who are less likely to benefit from ICDs (i.e., those with transient or reversible disorders or terminal illnesses with life expectancies <6 mos) may be subjected to a procedure in which the associated risk exceeds the potential gain. Additionally, with the high price of ICDs, cost-effectiveness issues must play a role in the decision to implant these devices.

Furthermore, it is critical to be aware of the potential **complications of ICD implantation.** Acutely, pneumothorax, infection, bleeding, and pericardial tamponade are possible. In addition, the ICD must be tested during implantation to confirm that the energy it delivers is sufficient to convert a ventricular arrhythmia (these are called **DFTs,** which determine defibrillator thresholds). To test an ICD, the patient is induced into VF. An extremely small portion of these patients, most of whom have severely diseased hearts, cannot be cardioverted successfully, even externally, leading to death. Later, infection of the system is possible; this frequently necessitates system extraction, a potentially complicated surgery. **Lead fracture** is a problematic complication, because the device interprets the interference generated by the fractured lead ends as VF, leading to the inappropriate delivery of shocks. As mentioned previously in this section, AF and SVTs can also lead to inappropriate shocks, which is a potentially troublesome feature, because dozens of shocks can be delivered for a single episode of AF.

Given these complexities, the ACC/AHA recently published their guidelines for ICD implantation [4,5]:

- **Class I**
  - Cardiac arrest due to VF or VT not due to a transient or reversible cause
  - Spontaneous sustained VT with structural heart disease or in those without structural heart disease who fail pharmacologic or catheter-based therapy
  - NSVT with CAD, prior MI, LV dysfunction, and inducible VF or sustained VT at EPS that is not suppressible with class I antiarrhythmics
  - Syncope of undetermined origin with clinically relevant, hemodynamically significant sustained VT or VF induced at EPS (when pharmacotherapy is ineffective, intolerable, or not preferred)
- **Class IIa:** Patients with CAD, an MI at least 1 mo prior, revascularization at least 3 mos prior, and an ejection fraction <30% (MADIT2 finding)
- **Class IIb**
  - Cardiac arrest presumed to be secondary to VF, with EPS precluded by illness
  - Severe symptoms due to sustained VT for patients awaiting cardiac transplant
  - Inheritable conditions with high risk for VT-associated sudden death (i.e., HCM, LQTs)
  - NSVT with CAD, prior MI, and LV dysfunction and inducible VT/VF
  - Recurrent syncope of unknown etiology in presence of LV dysfunction and inducible VF/VT at EPS
  - Syncope or family history of sudden cardiac death in a patient with a Brugada-pattern ECG at rest
  - Syncope in a patient with advanced structural heart disease in whom no cause can be found
- **Class III (contraindications)**
  - Syncope of unknown etiology without inducible VT/VF and without LV dysfunction
  - Transient or reversible disorder (i.e., acute MI, drugs, trauma) when correction of the problem is thought to dramatically reduce the risk of recurrence
  - Terminal illnesses with life expectancy <6 mos
  - Psychiatric illnesses that may be aggravated by device implantation or may preclude follow-up
  - NYHA class IV drug-refractory CHF in patients who are not candidates for transplantation
  - Incessant VT/VF
  - VF/VT resulting from arrhythmias amenable to ablation (i.e., RVOT)
  - Patients undergoing bypass surgery with LV dysfunction and prolonged QRS in the absence of spontaneous/inducible VT

KEYS POINTS TO REMEMBER

- The most important aspect of the management of acute tachyarrhythmias is to employ BCLS and ACLS protocols.
- Any pulseless tachyarrhythmia must be defibrillated immediately (except sinus tachycardia).
- SVTs usually carry a benign prognosis, unless there is concomitant heart disease present.

- When trying to diagnose a WCT (and discriminate VT from aberrantly conducted SVT), always think about the patient. Does he or she or might he or she have coronary disease and/or a depressed LV ejection fraction? If so, the rhythm is most likely VT. Might he or she have renal failure and hyperkalemia? If so, that may be the cause for the tachyarrhythmia, and antiarrhythmics and cardioversion will be ineffective in that case.
- When your patient exhibits NSVT, always ask first, "Does this patient have CAD and/or an abnormal ejection fraction?" The answers determine the workup and management course.
- In the setting of a prior MI, ejection fraction <35%, and NSVT, an elective evaluation by EPS to assess risk for sudden cardiac death is appropriate. After appropriate discussion, suitable patients will be studied, and if monomorphic VT is induced, an ICD may be placed.
- For patients with only two important historical features—prior MI and an ejection fraction <30%—ICD placement is indicated (class IIa), but at the time of publication, ICD implantation in patients with this indication is not reimbursed for all patients.
- In the setting of nonischemic cardiomyopathy, EPS is very rarely useful to determine the prognosis and need for ICD. In the absence of sustained VT/VF or syncope concerning for VT/VF as etiology, an ICD is not indicated for nonischemic cardiomyopathy at this time; however, in the presence of these features, ICD is always indicated in suitable patients.

ACKNOWLEDGMENT

The authors acknowledge Jane Chen for contributing several of the ECGs presented in this chapter.

SUGGESTED READING

Alings M, Wilde A. Brugada syndrome: clinical data and suggested pathophysiological mechanism. *Circulation* 1999;99:666–673.

American College of Cardiology/American Heart Association Task Force on Practice Guidelines. ACC/AHA guidelines for implantation of cardiac pacemakers and antiarrhythmia devices: executive summary. *Circulation* 1998;97:1325–1335.

Antiarrhythmics Versus Implantable Defibrillators Investigators. Comparison of antiarrhythmic drug therapy with implantable defibrillators in patients resuscitated from near-fatal ventricular arrhythmias: AVID. *N Engl J Med* 1997;337:1576–1583.

Brugada P, Brugada J, Mont L, et al. A new approach to the differential diagnosis of a regular tachycardia with a wide QRS complex. *Circulation* 1991;83:1649–1659.

Buxton AE, Lee KL, Fisher JD, et al., for the Multicenter Unsustained Tachycardia Trial Investigators. Randomized study of the prevention of sudden death in patients with coronary artery disease: MUST. *N Engl J Med* 1999;341:1882–1890.

Cairns J, Connolly SJ, Roberts R, et al., for the Canadian Amiodarone Myocardial Infarction Arrhythmia Trial Investigators. Randomized trial of outcome after myocardial infarction in patients with frequent or repetitive premature depolarizations: CAMIAT. *Lancet* 1997;349:675–682.

Camm A, Julian D, Janse G, et al., for the European Myocardial Infarct Amiodarone Trial Investigators. Randomized trial of effect of amiodarone on mortality in patients with left ventricular dysfunction after recent myocardial infarction: EMIAT. *Lancet* 1997;349:667–674.

Cannon DS, Prystowsky EN. Management of ventricular arrhythmias: detection, drugs, and devices. *JAMA* 1999;281:172–179.

Cardiac Arrhythmia Suppression Trial II Investigators. Effect of the antiarrhythmic agent moricizine on survival after myocardial infarction. *N Engl J Med* 1992;327:227–233.

Cardiac Arrhythmia Suppression Trial Investigators. Preliminary report: effect of encainide and flecainide on mortality in a randomized trial of arrhythmia suppression after myocardial infarction. *N Engl J Med* 1989;321:406–412.

Domanski MJ, Douglas ZP, Schron E. Treatment of sudden cardiac death: current understandings from randomized trials and future research directions. *Circulation* 1997;95:1694–2699.

Doval HC, Nul DL, Grancelli HO, et al. Randomized trial of low-dose amiodarone in severe congestive heart failure: CHF-STAT. *Lancet* 1994;344:493–498.

Dresing T. Tachyarrhythmias. In: Marso SP, Griffin BP, Topol EJ. *Manual of cardiovascular medicine*. Philadelphia: Lippincott Williams & Wilkins, 2000.

Ganz LI, Friedman PL. Supraventricular tachycardia. *N Engl J Med* 1995;332:162–173.

Grubb NR, Newby DE. Acute Arrhythmias. *Churchill's pocketbook of cardiology*. London: Harcourt, 2000.

Knight B, Pelosi F, Michaud G, et al. Clinical consequences of electrocardiographic artifact mimicking ventricular tachycardia. *N Engl J Med* 1999;341:1270–1275.

Krahn AD, Yee R, Klein GJ, et al. Inappropriate sinus tachycardia: evaluation and therapy. *J Cardiovasc Electrophysiol* 1995;6:1124–1128.

Maron MS, Olivotto I, Betocchi S, et al. Effect of left ventricular outflow tract obstruction on clinical outcome in hypertrophic cardiomyopathy. *N Engl J Med* 2003;348:295–303.

Maron BJ, Shen WK, Link MS, et al. Efficacy of implantable cardioverter-defibrillators for the prevention of sudden death in patients with hypertrophic cardiomyopathy. *N Engl J Med* 2000;342:365–373.

Moss AJ, Hall WJ, Cannom DS, et al., for the Multicenter Automatic Defibrillator Implantation Trial Investigators. Improved survival with an implanted defibrillator in patients with coronary disease at high risk for ventricular arrhythmia: MADIT. *N Engl J Med* 1996;335:1933–1939.

Siebels J, Cappato R, Ruppel R, et al., and the CASH Investigators. Implantable cardioverter defibrillator compared with antiarrhythmic drug treatment in cardiac arrest survivors: CASH. *Am Heart J* 1994;127:1139–1144.

Viskin S. Long QT syndromes and torsade de pointes. *Lancet* 1999;354:1625–1633.

REFERENCES

1. Moss AJ, Zareba W, Hall WJ, et al. Prophylactic implantation of a defibrillator in patients with myocardial infarction and reduced ejection fraction. *N Engl J Med* 2002;346:877–883.

2. Maron BJ, Shen WK, Link MS, et al. Efficacy of implantable cardioverter-defibrillators for the prevention of sudden death in patients with hypertrophic cardiomyopathy. *N Engl J Med* 2000;342:365.

3. Pacifico A, Hohnloser SH, Williams JH, et al. Prevention of implantable-defibrillator shocks by treatment with sotalol. d,l-Sotalol Implantable Cardioverter-Defibrillator Study Group. *N Engl J Med* 1999;340:1855–1862.

4. Gregoratos G, Abrams J, Epstein AE, et al. ACC/AHA/NASPE 2002 Guideline Update for Implantation of Cardiac Pacemakers and Antiarrhythmia Devices—summary article: a report of the American College of Cardiology/American Heart Association Task Force on Practice Guidelines (ACC/AHA/NASPE Committee to Update the 1998 Pacemaker Guidelines). *J Am Coll Cardiol* 2002;40:1703–1719.

5. Gregoratos G, Abrams J, Epstein AE, et al. ACC/AHA/NASPE 2002 guideline update for implantation of cardiac pacemakers and antiarrhythmia devices: summary article: a report of the American College of Cardiology/American Heart Association Task Force on Practice Guidelines (ACC/AHA/NASPE Committee to Update the 1998 Pacemaker Guidelines). *Circulation* 2002;106:2145–2161.

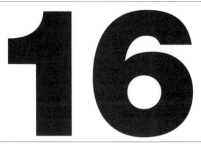

Diseases of the Pericardium

Adam B. Stein and
Peter A. Crawford

INTRODUCTION

The term **pericardium** refers to the visceral pericardium and the parietal pericardium. The two are separated by a total of approximately 30–50 cc of lubricating fluid. The role of the pericardium is to prevent motion of the heart within the chest cavity, but it is not required for normal function of the heart under most conditions.

ACUTE PERICARDITIS

Acute pericarditis is diagnosed in 1 in 1000 hospital admissions. The hallmarks of acute pericarditis are chest pain, a friction rub, and characteristic ECG findings. Pericarditis is often classified by etiology (Table 16-1). Most cases are idiopathic and are thought to be virally mediated.

Specific Pericarditis Etiologies

Postcardiac Injury Syndrome
Postcardiac injury syndrome is pericarditis that occurs after injury to the myocardium from either surgery, trauma, or MI. Generally, patients present with chest pain 1–4 wks postcardiac injury. The disease is usually controlled with NSAIDs, but prednisone may be used in more refractory cases. Prednisone is generally avoided in the postinfarct setting, due to risk of myocardial rupture. **Dressler's syndrome** refers to pericarditis that occurs weeks to months post-MI with an incidence of 1%.

Uremic Pericarditis
Uremic pericarditis usually occurs in one-third of patients with chronic uremia, most of whom are on hemodialysis. It is often associated with a pericardial effusion. Adequate treatment usually consists of NSAIDs and adequate hemodialysis.

Collagen Vascular Diseases
Collagen vascular diseases, such as SLE, may be complicated by pericarditis.

Tuberculous Pericarditis
Tuberculous pericarditis should be suspected in high-risk patients (immunocompromised). Often, patients present with pericardial effusion, CHF, and fever. Initiate therapy when tuberculous pericarditis is suspected and not when finally diagnosed.

History and Physical Exam

Many patients with acute pericarditis complain of **chest pain.** Pain can range from severe, which is often the case with infectious causes, to absent. Pain is often sharp, retrosternal, and radiating to the back, neck, and shoulders. It may be pleuritic in nature. Classically, pain is worse when the patient is supine and improved when the patient leans forward. Patients may also complain of fever accompanying their pain.

Physical exam of patients with acute pericarditis classically reveals a **pathognomonic pericardial rub** caused by friction between the inflamed, juxtaposed visceral

TABLE 16-1. ETIOLOGIES OF ACUTE PERICARDITIS

Infections

    Viral (coxsackie A and B, echovirus, HIV, adenovirus, Epstein-Barr, hepatitis B)

    Bacterial

    TB

    Fungal

Uremia

Neoplastic (lung, breast, lymphoma, leukemia)

Radiation

Autoimmune disease and inflammatory disorders (acute rheumatic fever, lupus, rheumatoid arthritis, scleroderma, polyarteritis nodosa, Wegener's granulomatosis, sarcoidosis, inflammatory bowel disease, Whipple's disease)

Drugs (hydralazine, procainamide, phenytoin, isoniazid, doxorubicin, penicillin)

Postinfarction (acute)

Postinfarction (late), Dressler's syndrome

Postcardiotomy (postcardiac surgery)

Aortic dissection

Trauma

Idiopathic

From Braunwald E, ed. Pericardial disease. In: *Heart disease: a textbook of cardiovascular medicine,* 4th ed. Philadelphia: WB Saunders, 1992:1469, with permission.

and parietal pericardia. The rub is described as high pitched, grating, and scratching. Classically, the rub has three components per cardiac cycle; these three components correspond to atrial systole, ventricular systole, and rapid ventricular filling.

The ventricular systole portion is the most often heard component present in nearly all cases. Rubs are best heard with the diaphragm of the stethoscope at the left lower sternal border with the patient leaning forward during respiratory expiration. Rubs can often be exacerbated with exercise.

Lab Data and Studies

Serial ECGs must be done in patients suspected of having acute pericarditis. ECG changes are present in 90% of cases. ECGs reveal characteristic changes that evolve through four stages. *Stage 1* changes are the characteristic changes associated with acute pericarditis; there is diffuse ST-segment elevation with upright T waves and depressed PR intervals in all leads except aVR and, occasionally V_1, in which the PR segment is elevated and the ST is depressed. One must differentiate acute STEMI patterns from the changes of acute MI and early repolarization (Fig. 16-1). In *stage 2*, the ST segments normalize, and the T wave amplitude drops. In *stage 3*, the T waves invert. Finally, in *stage 4*, the ECG becomes normalized again. **The important distinction from the injury pattern of STEMI is that chronologically, the ST segments normalize before T wave inversion in pericarditis, whereas the T waves invert before ST normalization in MI.** Low voltage and electrical alternans on an ECG suggest that the patient has developed an effusion.

    Chest x-ray is not helpful in the diagnosis of acute pericarditis. Obtain a chest x-ray to see if the patient has an enlarged water bottle–shaped cardiac silhouette suggestive of an effusion. Chest film may also reveal the cause of the effusion.

    Lab tests may reveal nonspecific markers of inflammation, such as ESR, CRP, and leukocytosis. More specific tests, such as ANA, rheumatoid factor, thyroid function, TB tests (PPD), and blood cultures, should be sent based on the clinical scenario.

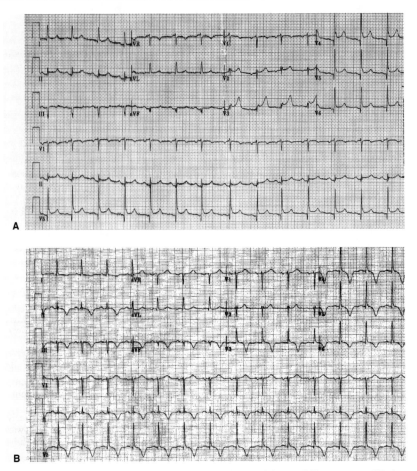

FIG. 16-1. ECG in pericarditis. **A:** Stage 1 pericarditis, exhibiting diffuse concave ST elevations and PR depression except in aVR, where the abnormalities are reversed. **B:** Stage 3 pericarditis, 1 day later in the same patient, showing diffuse T wave inversion after ST segments had normalized.

Echocardiogram does not aid in the diagnosis of pericarditis but is important to evaluate the size of the pericardial effusion, which is usually small or barely visible.

Treatment

Almost all patients should be admitted to the hospital to assess for effusive pericarditis and tamponade (15%) and to assess for MI. Direct therapy at the underlying disease. Treat uncomplicated pericarditis with high-dose NSAIDs, such as ibuprofen, 800 mg PO tid for 3 wks. If symptoms are not relieved with NSAIDs, a prednisone taper can be started at 60 PO mg daily until pain is controlled and then tapered slowly over the course of 3 wks. Continue bed rest until pain and fever resolve. Discontinue PO anticoagulants. If anticoagulation is absolutely necessary, IV heparin has been recommended over Coumadin due to its reversibility.

Complications
- Recurrent pericarditis occurs in approximately 25% of patients. It can usually be controlled with high-dose NSAIDs and/or steroids. If the steroids cannot be tapered because of pain relapses, consider chronic colchicine.
- Development of a large effusion with consequent pericardial tamponade occurs in 15% of patients.
- Constrictive pericarditis.

PERICARDIAL EFFUSION

Fluid in the pericardial sac can present variably. It can be an asymptomatic fluid collection incidentally noticed on diagnostic testing, or it can present as life-threatening cardiac tamponade, in which the intrapericardial pressure compresses the heart. The diverse clinical presentations depend on the **rate** of accumulation of fluid in the pericardial sac, the total **amount** of fluid, and underlying **characteristics** of the pericardium. Patients with a normal pericardium can accommodate 80–200 mL of fluid fairly quickly without causing tamponade physiology. >200 mL may cause increased intrapericardial pressure and tamponade. If fluid accumulates slowly, the pericardial sac can stretch and accommodate up to 1 L without tamponade. A stiff pericardial sac can obviously not accommodate as much fluid as a normal pericardium. Table 16-2 lists the etiologies of pericardial effusion.

TABLE 16-2. ETIOLOGIES OF PERICARDIAL EFFUSION

Idiopathic	Infectious mononucleosis
Acute MI	Influenza
Delayed postmyocardial-pericardial injury syndromes	Lymphogranuloma venereum
	Varicella
Post-MI (Dressler's) syndrome	HIV
Postpericardiotomy syndrome	Fungal infections
Pulmonary HTN (chronic)	Histoplasmosis
Metabolic	Aspergillosis
Uremia	Blastomycosis
Myxedema (hypothyroidism)	Coccidioidomycosis
Hypoalbuminemia	Fungal endocarditis
Radiation	Other infections
Dissecting thoracic aneurysm	Amebiasis
Trauma	*Echinococcus*
Pericardiotomy	Lyme disease
Indirect trauma to the chest	*Mycoplasma pneumoniaeRickettsia*
Percutaneous cardiac interventions	Tumors
Perforation of the heart by indwelling catheters	Primary
Viral infections	Mesothelioma
Coxsackie A, B5, B6	Teratoma
Echovirus	Fibroma
Adenovirus	Leiomyofibroma and sarcoma
Mumps virus	Leukemia
Hepatitis B	Lipoma angioma

(continued)

TABLE 16-2. CONTINUED

Metastatic	Phenylbutazone
Breast carcinoma	Cromolyn sodium
Bronchogenic carcinoma	Dantrolene
Lymphoma	Methysergide
Melanoma	Doxorubicin
Others	Penicillin
Bacterial infections	Minoxidil
Staphylococcus	Colony-stimulating factor
Streptococcus	Interleukin-2
Pneumococcus	Immunologic/inflammatory disorders
Haemophilus influenzae	Rheumatic fever
Neisseria gonorrhoeae	SLE
Neisseria meningitidis	Ankylosing spondylitis
Legionella hemophilia	Rheumatoid arthritis
TB	Vasculitis
Salmonella	Wegener's granulomatosis
Psittacosis	Polyarteritis nodosa
Tularemia	Scleroderma
Bacterial endocarditis	Dermatomyositis
Familial Mediterranean fever	Sarcoidosis
Drugs	Inflammatory bowel disease
Procainamide	Whipple's disease
Hydralazine	Behçet's syndrome
Heparin	Reiter's syndrome
Warfarin	Temporal arteritis
Phenytoin	Amyloidosis

Adapted from Marso SP, Griffin BP, Topol EJ, eds. *Manual of cardiovascular medicine.* Philadelphia: Lippincott Williams & Wilkins, 2000.

History and Physical Exam

Patients with slowly accumulating fluid often are asymptomatic. Occasionally, patients may complain of a dull ache or pressure in their chests. Large effusions may compress extrinsic structures and lead to complaints of dysphagia, hiccups, dyspnea, hoarseness (due to recurrent laryngeal nerve impingement), or cough.

Physical exam often yields no unique findings unless tamponade is present. In large effusions, one may notice muffled heart sounds, dullness to percussion below the angle of the left scapula due to compression of the left lung (**Ewart's sign**), or rales from compression of lung parenchyma.

Diagnostic Studies

- **ECG** may reveal low voltage of the QRS complex with flattening of the T waves. **Electrical alternans** suggests large effusion and possibly tamponade.
- **Chest x-ray** may reveal enlargement of the cardiac silhouette if >250 mL of fluid has accumulated. The classic globular or water bottle–shaped heart may occasionally be

seen. Normally, the parietal pericardial and epicardial fat layers are separated by 1–2 mm. More marked separation may be seen in 25% of patients with effusion.

- **Transthoracic echocardiography** is the study of choice for diagnosing and following pericardial effusions due to its rapidity and accuracy. Fluid is seen as an echo-free space between the posterior LV wall and posterior parietal pericardium and between the anterior RV wall and surrounding pericardium. M-mode echocardiography can detect as little as 20 mL of fluid. Quantification of fluid is generally done by location of the fluid and the time in the cycle during which it is seen. Very small effusions are often seen as a posterior echo-free space during systole. Small to moderate effusions are also seen posteriorly but often throughout the cardiac cycle. Moderate effusions of approximately 300 mL can be seen anteriorly and posteriorly. Moderate to large effusions may be associated with a swinging motion of the heart in the pericardial sac. Transthoracic echocardiography can often detect if the pericardial fluid is likely blood based on the acoustic density of the fluid; it is also effective at detecting loculated pericardial effusion.
- **MRI** detects pericardial effusions with great sensitivity. It is very effective at detecting loculated effusions and pericardial thickening.
- **CT** is also effective at detecting effusions. It can provide fairly detailed information about the quality of fluid in the pericardial sac. CT also relays information about any underlying thoracic pathology that may yield an effusion (e.g., malignancy). Therefore, this modality is an important tool in the assessment of idiopathic effusions, particularly ones that are large.
- **Pericardiocentesis** is indicated if there is tamponade physiology or to establish diagnosis. Diagnostic pericardiocentesis should be pursued if the cause is suspected to be infectious (TB, bacterial or fungal infection) or malignant, although the diagnostic yield is in the range of only 5–10%. Often, the likely diagnosis can be made with history, physical exam, and noninvasive diagnostic tests (e.g., PPD or serologic assays). Pericardiocentesis may be indicated for large effusions without clear etiology.

Therapy

Therapy for pericardial effusion depends on the presence or absence of tamponade, underlying etiology, and fluid volume. Pericardiocentesis should be done if malignancy or bacterial, mycobacterial, or fungal infection is suspected. Pericardiocentesis is appropriate for any effusion that is hemodynamically significant (see Chap. 5, Cardiovascular Emergencies, as well as Management and Cardiac Tamponade). Avoid anticoagulation until the effusion resolves.

CARDIAC TAMPONADE

Tamponade is a result of increased intrapericardial pressure from pericardial fluid accumulation characterized by elevated intracardiac pressures, progressive limitation of ventricular diastolic filling, and a decrease in cardiac output.

Pathophysiology

Fluid in the pericardial sac causes an increase in intrapericardial pressure. As this pressure increases, a decrease in transmural distending pressure results. As the intrapericardial pressure approaches atrial and ventricular diastolic pressure, the transmural distending pressure approaches zero, and cardiac output drops. In most cases, as intrapericardial pressure increases, adrenergic surge allows some hemodynamic compensation by inducing tachycardia and increased vascular tone. If tamponade progresses, the compensatory mechanisms eventually fail, resulting in a cycle of severely decreased cardiac output and coronary hypoperfusion, leading to further decreased cardiac output.

Etiology

The causes of tamponade are essentially the same as causes of acute pericarditis. The most common causes are malignant disease, idiopathic disease, uremia, cardiac rupture, iatrogenic disease, bacterial infection, TB, radiation, myxedema, dissecting aortic aneurysm, postcardiotomy, and lupus.

Clinical Features

Patients with a slowly developing pericardial effusion often present only with dyspnea, and their BP is normal, as the pericardium can stretch with time. Patients with an effusion developing more rapidly or chronic effusions that reach a critical volume yield more significant signs and symptoms. These would include decreased mental status, decreased urine output, dyspnea, chest pain, fatigue, weakness, and agitation. On physical exam, seek the classic findings of tachycardia, JVD, hypotension, and distant heart sounds. **The most sensitive sign is JVD.** The neck veins should be examined for a **prominent *x* descent and lack of *y* descent,** characteristic of tamponade. The only situation in which tamponade can occur without JVD is isolated left atrial tamponade post–cardiac surgery. **Pulsus paradoxus,** an exaggerated drop in systolic pressure on inspiration, should be assessed. It occurs because inspiration increases RV filling. This increase in RV filling shifts the intraventricular septum to the left and thus compromises LV filling, along with decreased pulmonary venous filling. Pulsus paradoxus can be checked by inflating the BP cuff above the systolic pressure and deflating until Korotkoff sounds are heard only during expiration. Further deflate the cuff until Korotkoff sounds are heard with both inspiration and expiration. The pulsus paradoxus is the difference between these pressures. A drop in pressure by >10 mm Hg is significant. Other disorders with pulsus paradoxus include obstructive pulmonary disease, constrictive pericarditis, and RV failure from infarction and pulmonary embolism. However, tamponade in the presence of ASD, aortic insufficiency, LV dysfunction, or a loculated effusion may not yield a pulsus paradoxus.

Diagnostic Studies

- **ECG** may show features of pericarditis or pericardial effusion. **Electrical alternans** is a more specific finding of tamponade and is caused by the heart swinging within the pericardium during systole and diastole.
- Perform **transthoracic echocardiography** in any patient with signs and symptoms suggestive of tamponade. Note that tamponade is a clinical diagnosis, and echocardiography studies should be used to further substantiate the diagnosis. The lack of effusion practically excludes the diagnosis of tamponade, except in post–cardiac surgery patients who may have compression from a loculated effusion or thrombus. The echocardiographic findings of tamponade are pericardial effusion, right atrial diastolic collapse, RV early diastolic collapse, left atrial collapse, abnormal inspiratory increase in tricuspid valve flow velocity (>40%) and >15% inspiratory decrease of LV dimension, inspiratory decrease (>25%) of mitral valve diastolic inflow velocity, inferior vena cava plethora, and a swinging heart (late finding). Pulmonary HTN will delay the onset of RV collapse, because the pressure within the chamber overcomes intrapericardial pressure. The size of the pericardial effusion has been shown to be the best predictor of outcome.
- **Right-heart catheterization** can detect hemodynamic changes associated with tamponade, including elevated right atrial pressure with preserved *x* descent and absent *y* descent (Fig. 16-2). One can also show that (a) RV mid-diastolic pressure, (b) right atrial pressure, (c) PCWP, (d) pulmonary artery diastolic pressure, and (e) LV diastolic pressure **are all elevated and equal** (within 4 mm Hg) to intrapericardial pressure. PCWP can be shown to be slightly greater than intrapericardial pressure during expiration and slightly lower than intrapericardial pressure during inspiration.

Management

Patients with clinical tamponade need to be drained expediently. If possible, experienced physicians should perform drainage. Options for drainage include percutaneous needle

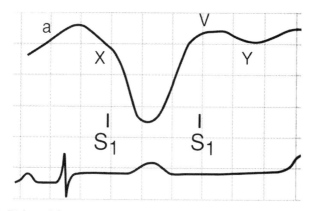

FIG. 16-2. Right atrial pressure tracing in pericardial tamponade. Note the prominent *x* descent and absent *y* descent. (From Murphy JG. *Mayo Clinic cardiology review,* 2nd ed. Philadelphia: Lippincott Williams & Wilkins, 2000:854.)

pericardiocentesis and pericardiotomy (pericardial window). Different drainage procedures should be selected on an individual basis determined by the clinical situation (degree of exigency, location of effusion, likelihood for recurrence). Before drainage, **resuscitate patients with volume-expanding agents** to delay RV diastolic collapse. Add norepinephrine (Levophed) for BP support if absolutely necessary.

Percutaneous needle pericardiocentesis is a rapid method for draining pericardial fluid. It requires relatively little preparation. Complications include damage to the lungs, heart, and coronary arteries. An experienced cardiologist should perform pericardiocentesis. Hemodynamic and/or echocardiographic monitoring concomitantly with pericardiocentesis is recommended. See Chap. 5, Cardiovascular Emergencies, for a detailed description of the procedure. Percutaneous pericardiocentesis will likely be unsuccessful in acute traumatic hemopericardium, a small or loculated pericardial effusion, lack of anterior effusion, and clot or fibrin causing compression. After needle access to the effusion has been acquired, a pericardial drain is usually left in place for 24–48 hrs. Occasionally, sclerosing agents, such as thiotepa, bleomycin, or doxycycline, can be instilled after the drain output rate has decreased to <100 cc/day.

Percutaneous balloon pericardiotomy can be performed by obtaining access via needle pericardiocentesis and then inserting and inflating a balloon to cause a rent in the pericardium. This technique is effective for tamponade and large pericardial effusions, especially malignant effusions, as it allows for a pericardial window through which fluid can drain.

Surgical pericardial drainage is generally more invasive than percutaneous drainage and requires a longer recovery period; however, it allows for more complete drainage and examination of the pericardium grossly and via biopsy. A limited pericardiectomy or pleuropericardial window allows for drainage of pericardial fluid into the left pleural space and requires a left thoracotomy. Subtotal and total pericardiectomy involves resection of all or nearly all the pericardium. In general, surgical pericardial drainage is preferred in patients with loculated effusions (immediately postop from cardiac surgery), effusoconstrictive pericarditis, and in effusions likely to recur (e.g., malignancy). See Chap. 5, Cardiovascular Emergencies, for additional information regarding pericardiocentesis.

CONSTRICTIVE PERICARDITIS

Constrictive pericarditis occurs when there is a thickened and noncompliant pericardium that restricts diastolic filling. Usually, the two pericardial layers fuse and form a noncompliant symmetric sac surrounding the heart.

Pathophysiology

Constrictive pericarditis results in restricted diastolic filling in all four chambers of the heart. As a result, all four chambers have elevated and equal filling pressures. The elevated filling pressures cause a rapid and accentuated filling during early diastole that is abruptly halted as the maximal volume allowed by the constricting pericardium is attained. This abnormal pattern of filling accounts for the classic **dip-and-plateau** waveform seen in the ventricles. The dip corresponds to the early rapid diastolic filling, and the plateau represents end diastole when the constricting pericardium slows filling. The venous wave forms show an M or W configuration from a prominent and **deep y descent during diastole** and a present x descent during systole. In normal physiology, venous blood flows into the atria maximally during ventricular systole. In constrictive pericarditis, venous flow into the atria is maximal during early diastole and occurs with the prominent y descent.

Etiology

All etiologies of constrictive pericarditis result in chronic inflammation and fibrosing and thickening of the pericardium.

- Idiopathic constrictive pericarditis represents the most common cause of constriction. It is thought to be from previous unrecognized viral pericarditis.
- Radiation therapy can cause constrictive pericarditis that generally occurs many years after radiation therapy.
- A late complication of cardiac procedures involving the pericardium, usually associated with extensive valve repairs and CABG surgeries.
- Infectious disease, including viral, fungal, bacterial, parasitic, and tuberculous infections. TB and bacterial etiologies are more common in developing nations, where antibiotics and antitubercular medicines are not readily available.
- Inflammatory and immunologic diseases, including rheumatoid arthritis, SLE, sarcoid, and scleroderma.
- Neoplastic diseases, commonly lung cancer, breast cancer, Hodgkin's disease, and lymphoma.
- End-stage renal disease treated with hemodialysis.

Clinical Findings

The signs and symptoms of constrictive pericarditis are a result of elevated filling pressures and symptoms synonymous with left- and right-sided HF. In early stages, patients may complain of fatigue, weakness, and decreased exercise tolerance. As filling pressures continue to rise, patients complain of left-sided symptoms, such as dyspnea on exertion, orthopnea, paroxysmal nocturnal dyspnea, and cough, and right-sided symptoms, such as lower-extremity edema, increased abdominal girth, and ascites. The physical exam is critically important in constrictive pericarditis.

Jugular Venous Distention
JVD is the most important aspect of the physical exam. Almost all patients with constrictive physiology have elevated neck veins from the elevated filling pressures. Both x and y descent can be appreciated. Close exam of the veins should reveal the rapid y descent seen as a rapid collapse that results from the rapid early diastolic filling of the ventricles. Look for **Kussmaul's sign,** an inspiratory increase in systemic venous pressure that occurs because blood cannot fill the RA/RV to a further extent and, therefore, fills the jugular veins. This sign is also seen in RV infarct and in pulmonary embolism.

Cardiac Exam
Perform a cardiac exam with careful attention for a diastolic **pericardial knock** (difficult to appreciate). A knock is the result of sudden impedance to diastolic ventricular filling by constriction. It corresponds to the nadir of the diastolic y descent. It is best heard at the left lower sternal border during early diastole. It generally occurs before S_3 and is a higher-pitched sound than an S_3 gallop.

Pulmonary Exam

Perform a pulmonary exam to assess for a pleural effusion or rales suggestive of HF, **although pulmonary edema is rare with constrictive pericarditis.**

Abdominal Exam

On abdominal exam, pay careful attention for signs of right-sided HF. **Hepatomegaly** is often present, and **pulsation in the liver** may be appreciated that corresponds to central venous pressures. Splenomegaly is another possible finding.

Extremities Exam

Examine extremities for evidence of edema, which can be severe.

Diagnostic Studies and Testing

No study alone provides definitive evidence of constrictive pericarditis; it is often necessary to obtain several different studies to support clinical suspicion.

* **Chest x-ray** could reveal a calcified pericardium, which suggests the possibility of a calcified and constricted pericardium. Pericardial calcification is generally over the right heart chambers and in the AV groove. Calcification over the LV apex or posteriorly suggests LV aneurysm. **Findings of pulmonary edema are uncommon,** but pleural effusions are common.
* **ECG** findings commonly include low QRS voltage, generalized T wave inversion or flattening, and left atrial enlargement. AF is fairly common and is seen in <50% of cases.
* Three types of **echocardiography** studies—M-mode, two-dimensional, and Doppler—provide evidence of constrictive physiology.
  * **M-mode findings**
    * Thick pericardium: one thick line or multiple lines in parallel (train-tracking)
    * Abrupt posterior motion of the interventricular septum during early diastole and anterior motion of the septum during atrial systole (late ventricular diastole)
    * Constant total volume between LV and RV, with alternation of septal position with respiration to accommodate filling of each ventricle
    * Decreased amplitude of the LV posterior wall motion
    * Early opening of the pulmonic valve due to increased RV end-diastolic pressure (RVEDP) that exceeds pulmonary artery pressure
  * **Two-dimensional findings**
    * Immobile and dense pericardium
    * **Septal bounce:** abrupt displacement of interventricular septum during early diastolic filling
    * Inferior vena cava plethora
    * Decreased angle between LV and left atrium
  * **Doppler findings**
    * In constrictive physiology, the heart chambers are isolated from changes in intrathoracic pressure. As a result, during inspiration, the interventricular septum shifts to the left (or right-sided volume increases) and the driving gradient from pulmonary capillaries to left atrium is decreased. Thus, during inspiration, one sees decreased mitral valve flow velocities and decreased pulmonary venous flow velocities, repectively. This results in decreased LV filling. Leftward shift of the septum allows augmented RV volumes and a resultant **increase** in tricuspid and hepatic vein flow rates with inspiration, and decreased forward velocities with expiration (expiratory **reversal** of hepatic vein flow is seen). These variations in flow through the valves and in the hepatic and pulmonary venous system are useful in **distinguishing constrictive pericarditis from restrictive cardiomyopathy.**

Right- and left-heart **catheterizations** are done simultaneously to document elevated and equal diastolic pressures, assess cardiac output and myocardial function, and help differentiate constrictive from restrictive physiology. Hemodynamic measurements reveal elevated and **equal pressure in all four chambers** in diastole before the a

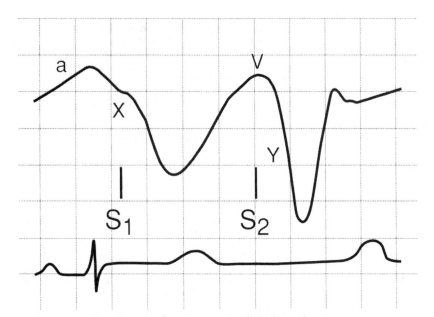

FIG. 16-3. Right atrial pressure tracing in constrictive pericarditis. Note the prominent *y* descent. (From Murphy JG. *Mayo Clinic cardiology review,* 2nd ed. Philadelphia: Lippincott Williams & Wilkins, 2000.)

wave. Right atrial measurements reveal an M or W waveform. There is a **preserved *x* descent and a steep *y* descent** from the increased flow during early diastole (Fig. 16-3). Ventricular hemodynamic measurements reveal **the dip-and-plateau (square root sign) during diastole** (Fig. 16-4). This is a result of rapid early diastolic filling, which is abruptly halted once the constricted volume is reached. Also, end-diastolic pressures of both ventricles are equal. A **Kussmaul's sign** is apparent by the increase in right atrial pressure on the pressure tracing during inspiration.

CT and MRI are useful for detecting pericardial thickening, dilated hepatic veins, dilated right atrium, and other findings that support constrictive pericarditis. These studies are not diagnostic and should only be used to support a diagnosis of pericardial constriction.

Hemodynamic Differentiation of Constrictive Pericarditis from Restrictive Cardiomyopathy

Although the steep *y* descent, square root sign, and equalization of pressures are classic, they do not distinguish constrictive pericarditis from restrictive cardiomyopathy (see Chap. 12, Assessment and Management of the Dilated, Restrictive, and Hypertrophic Cardiomyopathies). This is a common diagnostic branch point in the workup of a patient with edema, elevated neck veins, dyspnea, and malaise. Specificity features that suggest the diagnosis of constrictive pericarditis over restrictive cardiomyopathy include the following:

- **Dissociation of intrathoracic and intracardiac pressures,** which yields a decreased diastolic filling gradient in the left atrium during inspiration, because the PCWP decreases while the LV diastolic pressure remains the same. Thus, during inspiration, LV filling is impaired. This is due to the physical encasement of the heart by the pericardium.

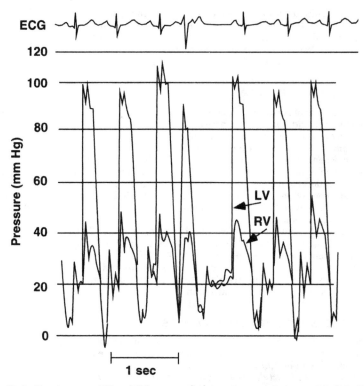

FIG. 16-4. Simultaneous RV and LV pressure tracings in constrictive pericarditis. Note the prominent dip and plateau (square root sign), particularly post-PVC. (Adapted from Marso SP, Griffin BP, Topol EJ, eds. *Manual of cardiovascular medicine.* Philadelphia: Lippincott Williams & Wilkins, 2000.)

- **Ventricular interdependence,** which means that the RV and LV peak systolic pressures vary inversely with inspiration with constriction. Inspiration increases the RV peak systolic pressure.
- **The absence of pulmonary HTN** (pulmonary artery systolic pressure <55 mm Hg), in the setting of the above findings, suggests constrictive pericarditis, whereas restrictive cardiomyopathy is often associated with pulmonary HTN.
- LVEDP = RVEDP suggests constriction, whereas LVEDP > RVEDP by approximately 5 mm Hg suggests restriction.
- **RVEDP > one-third of RV systolic pressure** suggests constriction.

The first two features are considered more specific and highlight that in the setting of equalized pressures and a square root sign, it is respiratory variation of ventricular filling that truly distinguishes constrictive pericarditis from restrictive cardiomyopathy.

Management

Constrictive pericarditis is a difficult disease to manage medically. Treat the underlying cause if possible. Diuretics and a low-salt diet form the cornerstone of therapy but often meet with limited success. **Surgical pericardiectomy** (stripping) is the definitive therapy of choice in surgical candidates; however, the operative mortality rate can be as high as 15%. 90% of patients report symptomatic improvement. Treat patients with comorbid conditions that limit life expectancy medically with diuretics and a low-sodium diet. Perform surgery early, as constrictive pericarditis is a progressive disease, and patients with poor functional class are at higher risk of periop death.

KEY POINTS TO REMEMBER

- The spectrum of pericardial disease includes acute pericarditis, pericardial effusion, tamponade, and constrictive pericarditis. A variety of etiologies underlie each pathology, with at least partial overlap among them.
- The history and physical exam are cornerstones of assessment and management.
- Management of acute pericarditis and pericardial effusion (without tamponade) is focused on treating the underlying cause, antiinflammatory medication, and monitoring for development of a hemodynamically significant effusion.
- Management of pericardial effusion with tamponade is focused on fluid resuscitation, draining fluid before hemodynamic collapse, assessing etiology, and delivering long-term preventative therapy.
- Diagnosis of constrictive pericarditis is one of the most elegant in medicine. A patient presenting with edema, elevated neck veins, and the absence of pulmonary edema should trigger the possibility. It is associated hemodynamically with the square root or dip-and-plateau sign (as is restrictive cardiomyopathy), but it is the respiratory variation of ventricular filling that truly distinguishes constrictive pericarditis from restrictive cardiomyopathy.

REFERENCES AND SUGGESTED READINGS

Appleton PA, Hatle LK, Popp RL. Cardiac tamponade and pericardial effusion: respiratory variation and transvalvular flow velocities studied by Doppler echocardiography. *J Am Coll Cardiol* 1988;11:1020.

Braunwald E, ed. *Heart disease: a textbook of cardiovascular medicine,* 5th ed. Philadelphia: WB Saunders, 1997:1481–1533.

Fuster V, Alexander RW, O'Rourke RA, eds. *Hurst's the heart,* 10th ed. New York: McGraw-Hill, 2000:2064.

Guberman BA, Fowler NO, Engel PJ, et al. Cardiac tamponade in medical patients. *Circulation* 1981;64:633.

Hatle LK, Appleton CP, Popp RL, et al. Differentiation of constrictive pericarditis and restrictive cardiomyopathy by Doppler echocardiography. *Circulation* 1989;79:357–370.

Marso SP, Griffin BP, Topol EJ, eds. *Manual of cardiovascular medicine.* Philadelphia: Lippincott Williams & Wilkins, 2000:354–383.

Oh J, Hatle LK, Seward JB, et al. Diagnostic role of Doppler echocardiography in constrictive pericarditis. *J Am Coll Cardiol* 1994;23:154–162.

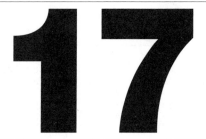

Infective Endocarditis and Acute Rheumatic Fever

Adam B. Stein and
Peter A. Crawford

INTRODUCTION

Definition and Terms

Infective endocarditis (IE) is infection involving the cardiac endothelium. IE has been divided into many different descriptive categories.

- **Acute bacterial endocarditis (ABE)** has a clinical course that rapidly develops over 1–2 days. Generally, the infecting organism is highly pathogenic (e.g., *Staphylococcus aureus*).
- **Subacute bacterial endocarditis (SBE)** has a more indolent clinical course with symptoms that evolve for weeks to months. Often, the infecting organism is less virulent [e.g., *Streptococcus viridans, Streptococcus bovis* (associated with colonic polyps and cancer), HACEK group organisms (*Haemophilus aphrophilus, Actinobacillus actinomycetemcomitans, Cardiobacterium hominis, Eikenella corrodens,* and *Kingella kingae*) (gram-negative bacilli)].
- **Native valve endocarditis** is infection of a native, although usually not normal, valve.
- **Prosthetic valve endocarditis (PVE)** is infection of a prosthetic valve. Defined as **early** if it occurs within first 2 mos after valve surgery and **late** if it occurs thereafter.

The annual incidence of endocarditis is 10– 20 per million, with a mortality of 16–27%.

CAUSES

Epidemiology and Etiology

Different patient populations have different infecting organisms and different courses of disease (Table 17-1).

Native valve endocarditis in adults ages 15–60 yrs, excluding IV drug users and nosocomial infections, most commonly occurs with MVP and an associated murmur (7–30% of the time). In decades past, rheumatic heart disease was the most common predisposing condition. Congenital heart disease accounts for 6–24% of cases. The most common infectious organism is *Streptococcus* (most commonly *viridans*); *Staphylococcus* is the second most common organism isolated. Species in the HACEK group are responsible for approximately 5% of SBE and often portend a poor prognosis. These organisms are a normal part of the mouth flora and can be translocated with a dental procedure.

Age has been found to be a risk factor for endocarditis. 25% of cases are in patients >60 yrs. The annual risk increases fivefold in patients >80 yrs. Older patients most commonly have underlying degenerative and calcific valve disease.

IV drug users have a high risk for IE. They have a high proportion of right-sided endocarditis from nonsterile injection methods and contamination with skin flora. The tricuspid valve is most commonly involved. *S. aureus* accounts for >60% of cases. Patients generally have an acute but less severe course. *Pseudomonas* is also a common organism in the setting of IV drug use, and its course is usually severe.

Early PVE occurring within the first 2 mos after surgery is most commonly caused by coagulase-negative staphylococci. These patients are thought to be inoculated at the time of surgery. The risk of PVE peaks at 3–9 wks postop.

TABLE 17-1. FREQUENCY OF VARIOUS ORGANISMS CAUSING INFECTIVE ENDOCARDITIS[a]

Organism	NVE (%)	IV drug abusers (%)	Early PVE (%)	Late PVE (%)
Streptococci	60	15–25	5	35
Viridans, alpha-hemolytic	35	5–10	<5	25
Streptococcus bovis	10	<5	<5	<5
Enterococcus faecalis	10	10	<5	<5
Other streptococci	<5	<5	<5	<5
Staphylococci	25	50	50	30
Coagulase positive	23	50	20	10
Coagulase negative	<5	<5	30	20
Gram-negative aerobic bacilli	<5	5	20	10
Fungi	<5	<5	10	5
Miscellaneous bacteria	<5	5	5	5
Diphtheroids, propionibacteria	<1	<5	5	<5
Other anaerobes	<1	<1	<1	<1
Rickettsiae	<1	<1	<1	<1
Chlamydiae	<1	<1	<1	<1
Polymicrobial infection	<1	1–5	5	5
Culture-negative endocarditis	5–10	<5	<5	<5

NVE, native valve endocarditis; PVE, prosthetic valve endocarditis.
[a]Variations are to be expected.
From O'Rourke RA, Fuster V, Alexander RW, eds. *Hurst's the heart,* 10th ed. New York: McGraw-Hill, 2000:596, with permission.

Late PVE is most commonly caused by *S. viridans* and is thought to be related to incidental bacteremias and not associated with surgery.

Nosocomial endocarditis is probably more common than suspected. Patients often have infections and multiple portals of entry (e.g., catheters), which can serve as sources of bacteremia. Statistically, the most common offending organisms are staphylococci, enterococci, *Candida* spp., and gram-negative bacilli.

Culture-negative endocarditis has an incidence of 5–10%. It usually results from prior antibiotic use but may occur from fastidious or slow-growing organisms (HACEK), *Coxiella, Brucella,* and *Legionella.*

Fungal endocarditis generally occurs in patients with prosthetic valves, indwelling catheters, immunosuppression, or IV drug use. *Candida* and *Aspergillus* are common.

Pathophysiology

The first step in development of IE involves formation of a sterile, platelet–fibrin complex termed **nonbacterial thrombotic endocarditis (NBTE).** Endothelial injury and hypercoagulable states predispose to NBTE formation. Endothelial injury may be caused by a high-velocity jet, flow from a high-pressure to a low-pressure system, or flow across a narrow orifice (creating **turbulence**). Primary valvular abnormalities (stenosis, regurgitation), as well as secondary abnormalities (Libman-Sacks lesions in lupus, marantic lesions in neoplasia, and nodules in antiphospholipid syndrome) are all predisposing factors. Thus, most patients with infective endocarditis have an underlying cardiac abnormality. NBTE generally develops on the ventricular surface of the aortic and pulmonic valves and on the atrial side of the tricuspid and mitral valves. The next step in IE development is the presence of bacteremia with organisms that have the propensity to adhere and multiply within the NBTE. The infected vegetation then becomes a nidus for more platelet–thrombin deposition and a source of recurrent bacteremia, possible embolization, and valvular dysfunction.

PRESENTATION

Clinical Findings

A detailed history and physical exam are the keys to diagnosing IE. The clinical spectrum varies widely between ABE presenting rapidly with catastrophic symptoms and SBE with a more insidious course. **Fever and a new murmur are the most common manifestations.** Prolonged malaise is common in SBE. Clinical manifestations in IE can be attributed to systemic infection, intravascular infection, or immunologic response to infection.

A plethora of physical exam findings can be found with IE.

- **Neurologic:** Significant neurologic findings are present in 30–50% of patients. These findings include confusional states, focal neurologic findings from emboli, hemorrhages from **mycotic aneurysms,** and cerebritis symptoms.
- **Cardiac:** Examine the heart for evidence of new or changing murmurs. Also seek evidence of **CHF** on exam, as it occurs in up to 55% of patients. **Heart block** can occur with aortic valve endocarditis with aortic root abscess. **Angina and positive troponins** can occur due to embolization to the coronary arteries.
- **Abdominal:** Exam should include signs of emboli resulting in bowel ischemia or splenic infarcts. Splenomegaly is common and is found in 15–55% of patients, in whom splenic abscesses have formed.
- **Skin and extremities:** Check the extremities for peripheral pulses and other evidence of emboli. Seek signs of IV drug use. In addition, some of the more interesting manifestations include
  - **Petechiae:** Thought to be a result of microembolization, it is most often found in the conjunctiva, palate of the mouth, behind the ears, and on the chest.
  - **Osler's nodes:** Thought to be a result of septic emboli and **immunologic** reaction, they are **painful** erythematous nodules usually found on hands. They may have pale central areas without necrosis.
  - **Janeway lesions: Painless,** macular red spots found on the palms and soles of some patients. They blanch with pressure and are a **vascular** phenomenon.
  - **Splinter hemorrhages:** Seen within the nail bed; due to emboli.
- **Ophthalmologic:** In addition to conjunctival petechiae, a funduscopic exam should be done to look for retinal hemorrhages, **Roth's spots,** and evidence of ophthalmitis. Roth's spots are immunologic lesions with a pale center surrounded by a red halo.

MANAGEMENT

Lab Tests and Diagnostic Studies

Lab Tests

- **Blood cultures** are of utmost importance. Draw a total of at least three sets (anaerobic and aerobic) from three different sites over the course of 24 hrs.
- **CBC** may reveal evidence of a leukocytosis. **Platelet count** may be elevated or depressed. Patients often develop a hypoproliferative normocytic normochromic anemia with SBE.
- Check **creatinine** and **BUN** to see if there is evidence of immune complex glomerulonephritis.
- **ESR, rheumatoid factor,** and **CRP** are elevated in most cases.

- **UA** can reveal a microscopic hematuria and proteinuria. Immune-complex glomeru-lonephritis is associated with red-cell casts, gross proteinuria, and decreased total complement levels. Renal infarction from embolic disease may manifest as gross hematuria.

Diagnostic Studies

- Obtain **chest x-ray** to confirm clinical findings of HF and assess for septic emboli in IV drug use with suspected right-sided endocarditis.
- Obtain **ECG** for evidence of embolic disease to coronary arteries (yielding ischemic changes) and to assess for conduction delays (AV block) suggestive of abscess formation. Patients with ABE should be followed on telemetry while inpatients.
- **Echocardiogram** is important in patients suspected of having IE and is helpful in diagnosis and management. When IE is suspected, patients should initially undergo **transthoracic echocardiography,** which has a sensitivity of 60–75%. If patients have negative or nondiagnostic transthoracic echocardiography and the diagnostic suspicion is high, they should undergo **TEE,** which has a sensitivity of up to approximately 95%. If the TEE is positive, a transesophageal echocardiography is **sometimes** still warranted to carefully evaluate the anatomy of the affected valve and vegetation, particularly if the integrity of the valve is compromised to an extent that may require surgery.
- **Cardiac catheterization** is not routinely necessary. Cardiac catheterization is generally done to further evaluate patients needing surgery.

Diagnosis

In 1994, Durack et al. published the criteria by which IE is currently diagnosed, known as the **Duke criteria.** These criteria were updated from the previous von Reyn criteria, which did not take into account the role of new technologies and the higher incidence of IV drug use. Table 17-2 presents the criteria.

Complications

The development of **CHF** has the greatest impact on prognosis. It occurs more frequently with AV endocarditis than that of the mitral valve. It is due to perivalvular extension, leading to abscess formation and severe aortic insufficiency. A ruptured chorda on the mitral valve apparatus can yield CHF via a flail leaflet and acute severe mitral regurgitation.

    Embolization occurs more frequently with mitral valve endocarditis, particularly with vegetations >1 cm on the anterior leaflet. The consequences of embolization can be disastrous (see Clinical Findings).

    Perivalvular extension (abscess formation in the aortic root) occurs more commonly with AV endocarditis than mitral valve endocarditis. AV block can result from this extension, as can CHF.

Medical Treatment

In general, obtain an infectious diseases consult in patients being treated for endocarditis. Use bactericidal antibiotics whenever possible.

    Institute empiric therapy while the etiologic organism and antibiotic sensitivities are being determined. Initiate empiric therapy based on whether the patient has SBE or ABE. For SBE, streptococci must be covered, and the initial choice is ampicillin, 2 g IV q4h, plus gentamicin, 1.5 mg/kg IV q8h. **For ABE, therapy must cover for S. aureus, streptococci (and Enterococcus spp.) and gram-negative bacilli.** Initial coverage includes nafcillin, 2 g IV q4h, plus ampicillin, 2 g IV q4h, plus gentamicin, 1.5 mg/kg IV q8h. If methicillin-resistant *S. aureus* is likely, substitute vancomycin, 1 g IV q12h, for nafcillin. *Pseudomonas* usually requires a combined medical and surgical approach to therapy, as infections are usually invasive. Fungal IE generally

TABLE 17-2. DUKE CRITERIA FOR THE DIAGNOSIS OF INFECTIVE ENDOCARDITIS

Pathologic criteria

Microorganisms demonstrated by culture or histology in a vegetation, embolus, or intracardiac abscess

Pathologic lesions; vegetation or intracardiac abscess present, confirmed by histology

Clinical criteria (two major criteria, or one major and three minor, or five minor criteria)

Possible infective endocarditis (falls short of definition but does not meet rejected criteria)

Rejected infective endocarditis (firm alternative diagnosis, resolution of manifestations with therapy of ≤ 4 days, or no pathologic evidence at surgery or autopsy)

Major criteria

Positive blood culture for endocarditis

Typical organism (*viridans* streptococci, *S. bovis*, HACEK group, community-acquired *S. aureus* or enterococci in the absence of a primary focus from two separate cultures)

Persistence of positive blood culture (blood cultures drawn >12 hrs apart, or all of three or a majority of four separate cultures drawn at least 1 hr apart)

Evidence of endocardial involvement

Positive echocardiogram (oscillating intracardiac mass on valve or supporting structures, abscess, partial dehiscence of a prosthetic valve, new valvular regurgitation)

Minor criteria

Predisposition (heart condition or IV drug use)

Fever >38°C

Vascular phenomena (major arterial emboli, septic pulmonary infarcts, mycotic aneurysm, intracranial hemorrhage, conjunctival hemorrhages, Janeway lesions)

Immunologic phenomena (glomerulonephritis, Osler's nodes, Roth's spots, rheumatoid factor)

Microbiologic evidence (positive blood cultures not meeting major criteria or nonculture evidence of endocarditis-causing organism)

Echocardiogram consistent with endocarditis but not meeting major criterion

From Durack DT, Lukes AS, Bright DK. New criteria for diagnosis of infective endocarditis: utilization of specific echocardiographic findings. Duke Endocarditis Service. *Am J Med* 1994;96:200, with permission.

requires medical and surgical therapy. Medical therapy includes amphotericin B (Amphocin, Fungizone), 0.5 mg/kg daily ± flucytosine (Ancobon).

Once the organism and antibiotic sensitivities have been determined, tailor the antibiotic regimen accordingly. **Duration** depends on multiple factors, including the organism, severity of infection, and underlying patient characteristics. Usually 4–6 wks of IV antibiotics are required.

Anticoagulation has not been shown to be beneficial in the treatment of IE. On the contrary, the combination of heparin and penicillin has been shown to increase the risk of intracerebral hemorrhage. In general, avoid heparin unless there is an urgent indication. Also avoid warfarin unless there is necessary indication, such as a mechanical prosthetic valve.

Monitor response to therapy with surveillance blood cultures, fever, and WBC count. Treatment failure may indicate a need for a change in medical therapy or addition of surgical therapy.

Surgical Treatment

Surgery is ultimately required in approximately one-third of patients. The major indications for surgery are

- Moderate to severe HF (due to valve dysfunction) not responding to medical therapy
- PVE (very rarely responds to medical therapy)
- Valvular obstruction, periannular or myocardial abscess, uncontrollable infection despite antibiotics
- Perivalvular extension, causing obstruction; periannular or root abscess; fistula; heart block
- ≥ 2 major embolic events, assuming patient remains an operative candidate after the event (e.g., mental status that is stable and/or likely to improve if impaired)
- Fungal infections
- Vegetations that enlarge despite treatment
- Recurrent endocarditis

Often with IE, it is difficult to determine (a) which patients should receive surgical therapy and (b) when they should receive it. Surgery done prematurely subjects patients to unnecessary risks from the surgery itself, combined with risks of an inadequately controlled infection. Surgery postponed too long could result in patients deteriorating rapidly to the point that surgery is too high risk. As a result, patients with IE in whom surgery might be indicated must be evaluated closely, both clinically and with serial echocardiograms.

The type of valve depends on a multitude of factors, including the ability to anticoagulate the patient postop. A mycotic brain aneurysm, for example, precludes anticoagulation.

Prophylaxis

Prophylaxis is recommended for patients with cardiac conditions that place them at risk for endocarditis when undergoing procedures that could cause bacteremia. Clinicians must assess the risk posed by the underlying cardiac lesion and the risk posed by the procedure when deciding on prophylaxis.

Endocarditis prophylaxis is recommended for high- and moderate-risk patients. **High-risk patients** include those with prosthetic heart valves, prior endocarditis, VSD, patent ductus arteriousus, cyanotic congenital heart disease, and surgically constructed systemic-pulmonary shunts or conduits. **moderate-risk patients** are those with most uncorrected congenital heart diseases, rheumatic and other acquired valvular disease, HCM, and MVP with regurgitation. **Low-risk patients** are those with isolated MVP and no regurgitation; isolated secundum atrial septal defect; surgically repaired atrial septal defect, VSD, or patent ductus arteriosus; prior CABG; prior rheumatic heart disease without valve dysfunction; pacemaker and implantable cardioverter-defibrillators; and flow murmurs.

Dental procedures; procedures in the respiratory, GI, or genitourinary tracts; and cardiac procedures require prophylaxis in high- and moderate-risk patients, depending on the procedure.

Prophylactic regimens for dental, respiratory, or esophageal procedures include amoxicillin (Amoxil), 2 g PO or IV, and clindamycin (Cleocin), 300 mg PO, if the patient is penicillin allergic within 1 hr before the procedure. For genitourinary or GI procedures, ampicillin, 2 g IV, plus gentamicin, 1.5 mg/kg IV, within 30 mins of the procedure is appropriate (vancomycin, 1 g IV, if penicillin allergic). For complete guidelines of antibiotic prophylaxis, see References and Suggested Readings.

For further information on the assessment and treatment of IE, review *The Washington Manual*™ *Infectious Diseases Subspecialty Consult,* Chap. 5, Cardiovascular Hardware Infections.

Acute Rheumatic Fever

Acute rheumatic fever is usually an immunologic response to group A streptococci. The risk is related to untreated streptococcal pharyngitis, of which 3% of untreated infections result in the disease. Host and organism susceptibility and virulence factors, respectively, also play important roles. The incidence in the United States is low, approximately 2 in 100,000, whereas it is 100 in 100,000 in Asia, Africa, and South America.

Rheumatic fever is a pancarditis, involving the endocardium, myocardium, and pericardium. It also affects the skin and connective tissues. The **Jones criteria** were established to solidify the diagnosis. Major criteria are carditis, polyarthritis, Sydenham's chorea, erythema marginatum, and subcutaneous nodules; minor criteria are fever, arthralgia, elevated ESR, elevated CRP, and a prolonged PR interval. Two major criteria or one major criteria and two minor criterion are required to make the diagnosis. The most common manifestation of carditis is mitral valvulitis, resulting in MR. Sinus tachycardia, HF, and ventricular arrhythmias are present in severe cases. The pathognomic, pathologic feature of rheumatic carditis is the **Aschoff body.**

Treatment includes support for HF and valvular abnormalities, penicillin or erythromycin, and high-dose ASA (75 mg/kg PO qd). Prednisone (1 mg/kg PO qd) may be used for severe carditis. Secondary prophylaxis is used in patients for durations that depend on the severity of carditis. Prophylaxis with penicillin (daily PO or q3wks IM) until age 40 is employed for patients with persistent valvular heart disease. The chronic sequela of rheumatic heart disease, chronic valvular dysfunction, are discussed in Chap. 13, Valvular Heart Disease.

KEY POINTS TO REMEMBER

- Infective endocarditis should be high in the differential diagnosis for any patient presenting with fever of unclear etiology, especially if there is a new murmur.
- Blood cultures are the essential first test in the diagnostic workup. Transthoracic echocardiography with Doppler is usually the correct test to order next.
- The most common complication of mitral valve endocarditis is embolization; the most common complication of aortic valve endocarditis is HF. Heart block can also result from aortic valve endocarditis.
- Acute rheumatic fever is uncommon in industrialized nations but should be considered for any patient (particularly those visiting from countries with poor access to health care) presenting with acute valvular disease and/or cardiomyopathy. The Jones criteria are clinical characteristics that help pinpoint the diagnosis.

REFERENCES AND SUGGESTED READINGS

Bayer AS, Bolger AF, Taubert KA, et al. Diagnosis and management of infective endocarditis and its complications. *Circulation* 1998;98:2936–2948.

Braunwald E, ed. *Heart disease: a textbook of cardiovascular medicine,* 5th ed. Philadelphia: WB Saunders, 1997:1077–1104.

Dajani, et al. Guidelines for the diagnosis of rheumatic fever: Jones criteria. *Circulation* 1993;87(1):302.

Dajani AS, Taubert KA, Wilson W, et al. Prevention of bacterial endocarditis. Recommendations by the American Heart Association. *JAMA* 1997;277:1794–1801.

Dajani AS, Taubert KA, Wilson W, et al. Prevention of bacterial endocarditis. Recommendations by the American Heart Association. *Circulation* 1997;96:358–366.

Durack DT, Lukes AS, Bright DK. New criteria for diagnosis of infective endocarditis: utilization of specific endocardiographic findings. *Am J Med* 1994;96:200–209.

Durack DT. Prevention of infective endocarditis. *N Engl J Med* 1995;332:38–44.

Marso SP, Griffin BP, Topol EJ, eds. *Manual of cardiovascular medicine.* Philadelphia: Lippincott Williams & Wilkins, 2000:629–643.

O'Rourke RA, Fuster V, Alexander RW, eds. *Hurst's the heart,* 10th ed. New York: McGraw-Hill, 2000:2087–2125.

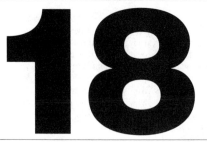

18

Pulmonary Hypertension, Right-Heart Failure, and Pulmonary Embolism

Alan Zajarias and
Peter A. Crawford

INTRODUCTION

Anatomy

The RV is formed by an inferior, anterior, posterolateral wall and shares the interventricular septum with the LV. With the exception of the conus arteriosus, the RV surfaces are irregular and generated by the trabecular muscles. The RV walls are formed by the superficial, deep sinospiral muscles and subendocardial fibers, which originate from the free walls of both ventricles and form the interventricular septum. The fibers shared by both ventricles allow them to work in relative dependence. The branches of the right coronary artery and posterior descending artery perfuse its walls.

The RV pumps deoxygenated blood to the pulmonary circulation, a circuit of low resistance and low pressure. Under normal circumstances, the RV does not experience pressures >20 mm Hg and, thus, has thin walls (0.9 cm in thickness during systole). The pulmonary circulation is thought to be able to maintain low pressure due to the continuous recruitment of capillaries in the lung fields, not by vascular distention.

The sudden increase in pulmonary vascular resistance causes right-heart strain or overload and leads to **acute cor pulmonale. Chronic cor pulmonale** refers to the hypertrophy and dilatation of the RV secondary to disease of the pulmonary parenchyma, pulmonary artery, or veins.

Etiologies of Right-Heart Failure and Pulmonary Hypertension

Right-heart failure (RHF) and pulmonary HTN can be envisioned as a Venn diagram in which the two often overlap, as pulmonary HTN often causes RHF. RHF can occur independently of pulmonary HTN, however, and pulmonary HTN can exist without RHF [although if severe and left untreated, it usually leads to RHF **(cor pulmonale)**]. In fact, the prognosis of isolated pulmonary HTN depends most significantly on the function of the right side of the heart.

Thus, independent differential diagnoses for these processes should be appreciated. In these patients, it is important to recognize whether a single process is responsible or both processes are ongoing.

CAUSES

Differential Diagnosis of Right-Heart Failure

1. Left-heart failure (LHF)
   a. Systolic dysfunction
   b. Diastolic dysfunction
   c. Valvular disease
   d. Left-sided cardiac tumors
2. Chronic volume overload
   a. Valvular abnormalities (pulmonary and tricuspid regurgitation)
   b. Congenital abnormalities
      i. Atrial septal defects (ASDs) [septum primum, secundum (most common), sinus venosus]
      ii. VSD (usually leads to left-sided failure first)

iii. Anomalous connection of the pulmonary veins to the right atrium
iv. Ebstein's anomaly
c. Portosystemic shunting [e.g., transjugular intrahepatic portosystemic shunt (TIPS)]
3. Acute pressure overload as seen in pulmonary embolism
4. Chronic pressure overload
   a. Valvular abnormalities (pulmonary stenosis)
   b. Congenital heart disease (tetralogy of Fallot)
   c. Pulmonary HTN
      i. Pulmonary parenchymal abnormalities (COPD, interstitial fibrosis)
      ii. Pulmonary vascular processes (primary or secondary pulmonary HTN)
5. RV infarction
6. Arrhythmogenic RV dysplasia
7. Uhl's anomaly/parchment heart

Differential Diagnosis of Pulmonary Hypertension, Anatomic Scheme

1. Precapillary (pulmonary arterial or arteriolar disease)
   a. Vascular obliteration or obstruction
      i. Parenchymal lung disease (e.g., pneumonias, pneumonitides, neoplasms, COPD, infiltrative lung disease, idiopathic pulmonary fibrosis, sickle cell disease, sarcoid, alveolar proteinosis)
      ii. Pulmonary vasculitis (Wegener's, Churg-Strauss, polyarteritis nodosa, Behçet's syndrome, Henoch-Shönlein purpura)
      iii. Collagen-vascular disease (e.g., scleroderma)
      iv. Thromboembolic disease, acute and/or chronic
      v. Contaminants (certain preparations of L-tryptophan and rapeseed oil have been associated); talc granulomata (IV drug users)
      vi. Schistosomiasis
      vii. Medications (e.g., phentermine/fenfluramine, aminorex)
      viii. HIV
      ix. Idiopathic (primary pulmonary HTN)
      x. Pulmonary emboli
   b. Vasoconstriction (hypoxia): COPD, sleep apnea, parenchymal lung disease, hypoventilation syndromes (obesity-hypoventilation, neuromuscular diseases)
   c. High-flow/pressure left-to-right shunt, ASD/VSD, portopulmonary shunting (i.e., hepatopulmonary syndrome)
   d. Peripheral pulmonic stenosis
2. Postcapillary (pulmonary venous or cardiac disease)
   a. Elevated left atrial pressure (LHF)
      i. Systolic dysfunction
      ii. Diastolic dysfunction
      iii. Valvular heart disease
      iv. Left atrial/LV tumors
   b. Venoocclusive disease
   c. Fibrosing mediastinitis

Pathophysiology of Right-Heart Failure

Volume Overload

The pulmonary circulation is normally a low-resistance circuit. It has the capacity to recruit more blood vessels in the lung parenchyma, thereby increasing the capillary surface area. This quality permits it to accommodate up to 5 × the blood volume before pulmonary HTN develops.

In ASD/VSD, in which left-to-right intracardiac shunt exists, blood flow within the cardiac cavities is unidirectional. As the pressures in the left and right cavities equalize over time, blood tends to follow the path of least resistance, initially moving through the RV. The flow depends on the magnitude and direction of the shunt. The magnitude of the shunt depends on the size and relative flow resistance or compliance of the ventricle. The increase in pulmonary flow causes pulmonary venous congestion and, eventually, pulmonary HTN if not corrected. Pulmonary HTN is seen in 5% of patients <20 with ASD and may increase to 50% in patients >40. Right-to-left shunting is only seen in 6% of patients with ASDs. Reversal of the shunt, seen in untreated VSDs and other congenital disease, is known as **Eisenmenger syndrome** (see Chap. 19, Congenital Heart Diseases in the Adult) and is associated with a high mortality. The only definitive treatment is heart–lung transplant. Chronic volume overload eventually causes right atrial enlargement that develops AF in 25–45% of patients by age 45.

Pressure Overload

- **Hypoxic vasoconstriction:** Hypoxia causes capillary closure in lung areas of low oxygenation to improve effective oxygenation. Persistent vasoconstriction becomes irreversible after the arteries develop medial hypertrophy and increase musculature.
- **Vascular obstruction:** Two-thirds of the vascular bed needs to be destroyed to cause pulmonary HTN. PA obstruction causes an increase in the pulmonary vascular resistance, which increases the PA pressure, causing an increase in the RV work and eventually causing RV dilation.

In previously healthy patients, acute pressure overload causes the RV to dilate and will not be accompanied by pulmonary pressures >40 mm Hg, because the normal RV cannot generate higher pressures. Therefore, a large acute pulmonary embolus is associated with RV enlargement and dysfunction but not markedly increased PA systolic pressure, unless underlying pulmonary HTN has already conditioned the RV. Chronic pulmonary HTN causes RV dilation to ensure adequate contraction by Frank-Starling mechanisms and results in hypertrophy to decrease wall stress.

RV Failure Due to Intrinsic Processes

RV infarct and conditions such as arrhythmogenic RV cardiomyopathy (or dysplasia) are associated with normal volumes and normal to slightly elevated right-sided BPs. Nevertheless, the RV fails and can yield clinical signs of RHF.

PRESENTATION

History and Physical Exam

Patients with RHF and/or pulmonary HTN generally complain of fatigue, lower-extremity edema, early satiety, anorexia, weight gain, dyspnea, and palpitation. Take a careful social and medication history, as well as a family history for primary pulmonary HTN.

On exam, jugular venous distention (JVD) is apparent if RHF is present. A large v wave may be present if there is pulmonary HTN and associated tricuspid regurgitation. Other signs of RHF include pulsatile hepatomegaly, ascites, and lower-extremity edema. Jaundice may be obvious secondary to chronic passive congestion of the liver. Specific signs of pulmonary HTN may be evident on exam by an RV heave, pulmonary artery tap (second intercostal space parasternal line), a loud P_2, and a widely split S_2.

DIAGNOSIS

Lab Tests

Expect elevation of AST, ALT, alkaline phosphatase, bilirubin, and PT secondary to liver congestion. In a new pulmonary HTN workup, evaluate HIV, ANA, rheumatoid factor, TSH, hemoglobin electrophoresis, Scl-70 (for scleroderma), and antiphospholipid panel (for hypercoagulable state) as appropriate.

ECG

ECG may evidence right-axis deviation, right bundle-branch block, or RV hypertrophy. AV blocks may accompany sinus venosus ASDs. RV infarctions are seen as an extension of inferior wall infarct (ST elevations in II, III, aVF) and are evidenced by

ST-segment elevation in V_3R and V_4R (and occasionally in V_1). The $S_1Q_3L_3$ pattern is seen in patients with RV strain or horizontalized hearts, and is the classic "pimp" sign for pulmonary embolism (despite its lack of sensitivity or specificity). The most reliable finding suggestive of acute PE is sinus tachycardia alone, possibly with right axis deviation and/or incomplete right bundle-branch block.

Chest X-Ray

Chest x-ray is critical for the assessment of the heart, pulmonary arteries, and lung parenchyma. RV enlargement and increased pulmonary arteries are identifiable findings on chest x-ray.

Echocardiography

In the absence of RV outflow tract obstruction or pulmonic stenosis, pulmonary HTN may be assessed by the degree of tricuspid regurgitation by the modified Bernoulli equation [see Chap. 13, Valvular Heart Disease, and Chap. 22, Imaging and Diagnostic Testing Modalities (Nuclear Imaging, Echocardiography, and Cardiac Catheterization)]. The right atrial pressure is estimated according to inferior vena cava (IVC) size: 0–5 mm Hg if normal diameter IVC collapses >50% on inspiration; 5–10 mm Hg if IVC is mildly dilated and collapses normally; 10–15 mm Hg if mildly dilated IVC that only partially collapses with inspiration; 15–20 mm Hg if dilated IVC does not collapse. Thus, for a velocity of 3.5 m/sec in the setting of a normal IVC, the pulmonary artery systolic pressure is 54 mm Hg. End-systolic flattening of the interventricular septum is specific for RV pressure overload. Complete evaluation with Doppler interrogation of the valves and saline contrast **(bubble study)** to evidence right-to-left shunting. Several additional features on M mode and Doppler are also indicative of pulmonary HTN. If the integrity of the atrial or ventricular septum is in question, a TEE may be obtained.

Pulmonary Function Testing

Administer if pulmonary HTN is present, including spirometry, diffusion capacity, and ambulatory oximetry.

Cardiac Catheterization

Right-heart catheterization with determination of O_2 saturations may be used for the diagnosis of ASD, VSD, or congenital anomalous pulmonary venous drainage. This is performed by serially measuring the O_2 saturation of blood at various anatomic points in the circuit from the systemic veins to the pulmonary arteries. Should a "step-up" in the oxygenation occur, a left-to-right shunt is suggested. A shunt fraction can be calculated [see Chap. 24, Procedures in Cardiovascular Critical Care (Intraaortic Balloon Pump, Swan-Ganz Catheterization, and Temporary Transvenous Pacemaker)]. Determination of the pulmonary vasculature resistance and its response to vasodilators (adenosine, calcium channel blockers, sodium nitroprusside) is crucial for the treatment option of pulmonary HTN.

Ventilation/Perfusion Scan

A $\dot{V}/\dot{Q}$ scan is obtained in patients with suspected acute or chronic pulmonary embolic disease. A **pulmonary angiogram** is useful in selected cases.

CT Scan

CT scan with pulmonary embolus protocol (helical or spiral CT) is obtained to document acute or chronic obstruction of the pulmonary arteries and their major branches. Obtain a **high-resolution CT scan** if lung parenchymal disease is suspected.

Polysomnogram (Sleep Study)

Obtain in patients in whom a cause for pulmonary HTN is not otherwise determined.

6-Minute Graded Walk

A paraclinical test to objectively quantify a patient's level of activity to document improvement or failure of therapeutic regimens.

Radionuclide Ventriculogram

Nuclear medicine techniques can be used to determine the ejection fraction of the RV by first-pass or equilibrium ventriculography.

TREATMENT

Pulmonary Embolism

Anticoagulation with IV heparin to obtain a PTT twice the upper limit of normal is the goal. Administer a bolus of 60 U/kg of weight, followed by an infusion of 14 U/kg/hr. Continue heparin for at least 5 days and until the INR is >2 for 2 consecutive days. SC low-molecular-weight heparin may be substituted for unfractionated heparin. Continue PO anticoagulation with warfarin (Coumadin) for a minimum of 4 mos depending on the origin of the embolus. Treat patients with modifiable risk factors and idiopathic pulmonary emboli for 4–6 mos. Patients with hypercoagulable states (pregnancy, antiphospholipid syndrome, malignancy, activated protein C resistance–factor V Leiden) should be kept on PO anticoagulants until the hypercoagulable state is reversed (if possible). The use of warfarin in early pregnancy of course is problematic, due to teratogenicity. Chronic pulmonary embolism and associated pulmonary HTN may be treated with pulmonary thromboendarterectomy.

COPD

Treat RHF due to COPD symptomatically. **The only treatment known to reduce mortality and increase functional activity is supplemental O_2.** Supplemental O_2 decreases hypoxic vasoconstriction and decreases pulmonary pressures. Treat with bronchodilators and steroids when appropriate. The resection of bullous lung parenchyma (lung volume reduction surgery) improves FEV_1, reduces dyspnea on exertion, increases exercise tolerance, and decreases O_2 requirements in appropriately selected patients.

Congenital Heart Disease

A multidisciplinary approach involving appropriate surgical intervention, medical management, optimal pulmonary rehabilitation, and physical therapy is required for adequate development for these patients. Surgical correction before the pulmonary vasculature develops fixed resistances is crucial for further development (see Chap. 19, Congenital Disease in the Adult).

Pulmonary Hypertension

- **Treatment of the underlying cause** is the most successful; e.g., treatment of underlying heart disease is appropriate if this is the underlying etiology (see Chap. 10, Management of Acute and Chronic Heart Failure). Patients with RV failure usually do not benefit from digoxin unless the LV is involved.
- **Supplemental O_2** is required if O_2 saturation <89%.
- **Pulmonary vasculature reactivity,** as evidence by a decrease in the pulmonary vascular resistances and increase or maintenance of the cardiac output, is essential for treatment. If responsive (to adenosine while a pulmonary catheter is present), initiate nifedipine or diltiazem. If unresponsive, continuous infusion epoprostenol, a prostacyclin analog that induces pulmonary vasodilation, inhibits platelet aggregation, and attenuates vascular cell migration and proliferation, is often used. Its use has been widespread in primary pulmonary HTN, in which it shows a mortality benefit, and in scleroderma-mediated pulmonary HTN. It is contraindicated in the setting of LHF, as unloading the right heart leaves the left heart unprotected from the displaced volume

that was previously pooled in the right-sided circulation. Furthermore, treatment of the pulmonary circulation in this manner does not treat the underlying cause of pulmonary HTN due to LHF. Bosentan (Tracleer), PO endothelin-receptor antagonist, has also gained acceptance for indications similar to those of epoprostenol. Other forms of therapy, including SC prostacyclin analogs, endothelin antagonists, and even medicines such as sildenafil (Viagra), are being investigated. Inhaled **nitric oxide (NO)** (10–40 ppm) can be used in the acute setting to reduce pulmonary pressures.

* **Anticoagulation** with Coumadin is appropriate (INR, 2–3) for many patients with severe pulmonary HTN to prevent recurrent thromboembolic events, as well as thrombosis *in situ*. It is contraindicated, however, in Eisenmenger syndrome due to the risk of pulmonary hemorrhage.
* **Atrial septostomy,** or creation of an ASD, is used for salvage in some patients with refractory RHF and volume overload. Hypoxemia due to right-to-left shunt is a complication of the procedure.
* **Lung or heart–lung transplantation** is an option for some patients who are refractory to pharmacologic treatment. Heart transplant is rarely necessary if the source of RHF is exclusively pulmonary HTN, as it will recover. Pulmonary HTN due to systemic disease is usually a contraindication for lung transplant.

OUTCOMES

The course of patients with RHF and/or pulmonary HTN depends on the cause. Patients suffering RV infarcts usually recover; the course of arrhythmogenic RV cardiomyopathy/dysplasia is usually more dependent on rhythm issues than RV failure (see Chap. 15, Tachyarrhythmias, Sudden Cardiac Death, and Implantable Cardioverter-Defibrillators). Patients with isolated pulmonary HTN without RV failure fare better than those with evidence of RV failure. If the source for pulmonary HTN is LV failure, then the outcome depends on (a) the severity of the LV dysfunction and (b) reversibility of the pulmonary HTN. Poor reversibility with nitroprusside, adenosine, or calcium channel antagonists portends a poor prognosis. For appropriate candidates, epoprostenol improves morbidity and mortality, but the disease often progresses to the development of cor pulmonale. In this setting, lung transplantation is the only option, but this form of therapy is severely limited by availability of donor organs.

KEY POINTS TO REMEMBER

* RHF (cor pulmonale) and pulmonary HTN have partially overlapping causes, because pulmonary HTN often causes RHF. However, these entities may also be distinct: There are other important causes of RHF, and in chronically progressive pulmonary HTN, the right heart does not fail initially.
* The physical exam is very telling in both conditions.
* Diagnostic testing and treatment of the condition(s) depend in part on the etiology but share some common threads. The transthoracic echocardiogram with Doppler is a good initial test.

REFERENCES AND SUGGESTED READINGS

Hankins SR, Horn EM. Current management of patients with pulmonary hypertension and right ventricular insufficiency. *Curr Cardiol Rep* 2000;2:244–251.

Klings ES, Farber HW. Current management of primary pulmonary hypertension. *Drugs* 2001;61:1945–1956.

Lee F. Hemodynamics of the right ventricle in normal and disease states. *Cardiol Clin* 1992;10:59–67.

McIntyre K, Sasahara A. Determinants of right ventricular function and hemodynamics after pulmonary embolism. *Chest* 1974;65:534–543.

Nocturnal Oxygen Therapy Trial Group. Continuous or nocturnal oxygen therapy in hypoxemic chronic obstructive lung disease. *Ann Intern Med* 1980;93:391–398.

Schulman DS, Matthay R. The right ventricle in pulmonary disease. *Cardiol Clin* 1992;10:111–136.

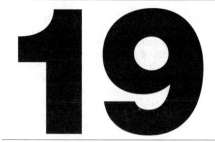

Congenital Disease in the Adult

Richard G. Garmany

INTRODUCTION

As more patients with congenital disease survive into adulthood, the number of patients with corrected and uncorrected congenital abnormalities is increasing. It is estimated that there are 1 million adult patients in the United States with congenital cardiac abnormalities. In the past, surgeries were palliative, and most patients with severe abnormalities did not survive past childhood. Through the 1980s and 1990s, palliative techniques improved, and corrective surgeries advanced significantly. Many patients can be expected to have near-normal life expectancies.

Doppler echocardiography is the single most important diagnostic tool, and along with newer techniques in CT and MRI, the frequency of cardiac catheterization is reduced in a given patient.

MINOR CONGENITAL LESION

Bicuspid aortic valve is among the most common congenital abnormalities, usually causing no hemodynamic significance until the sixth decade. Aortic stenosis and regurgitation usually result over time, requiring aortic valve replacement. The main complication of this condition is infective endocarditis, and for that reason, patients should receive antibiotic prophylaxis before procedures. This lesion is occasionally associated with aortic coarctation as well as thoracic aortic aneurysm.

ACYANOTIC DISORDERS

Atrial Septal Defect

Atrial septal defect **(ASD)** is the most common significant heart defect seen in adults, accounting for approximately one-third of the cases of congenital disease diagnosed in adults. ASD is different from patent foramen ovale (PFO), which occurs in 25–30% of the general population and usually does not allow a left-to-right shunt.

Etiology

The etiology of ASD depends on the anatomic defect. There are three primary abnormalities:

- **Ostium secundum defects** are the most common (75% of cases) and occur in the fossa ovalis. These occur much more frequently among women and are occasionally associated with MVP.
- **Ostium primum defects** (15% of cases) affect the lower aspect of the interatrial septum. Given their location, they are commonly associated with endocardial cushion defects and cleft mitral valve abnormalities causing mitral regurgitation (MR). This is frequently in the setting of trisomy 21 (Down syndrome).
- **Sinus venosus defects** (10% of ASDs) occur in the superior interatrial septum and are frequently complicated by partial anomalous venous return to the right atrium.

Complications

Complications of ASD depend on the size of the defect. Defects <0.5 cm are associated with small shunts and rarely cause serious consequences. Larger ASDs, particularly those >2 cm, allow blood to flow from the left atrium to the right, a shunt favored by the normal lower pressure in the right heart. This leads to increased pulmonary arterial flow, and pulmonary HTN develops over time. The result is dilatation of the right atrium and ventricle and decreased right-heart function. This leads eventually to right-sided pressures that equal or exceed those of the left heart, and the shunt decreases or even reverses, becoming a right-to-left shunt **(Eisenmenger syndrome)**.

Clinical Presentation

The clinical presentation of ASD is frequently very subtle, with nonspecific signs and symptoms. Patients are generally asymptomatic early in the course of the disease and develop fatigue and dyspnea in the later stages. Clinical complications include those of right-sided HF, supraventricular arrhythmias, and paradoxical embolism (venous thrombosis that liberates an arterial embolus via the ASD or PFO, commonly producing a stroke). On **physical exam,** patients may have a palpable RV impulse. The S_1 is normal, with **a widely split and fixed S_2.** S_2 is fixed because of the minimization of the normal effect of inspiration due to increased flow across the ASD on inspiration. A soft systolic-flow murmur may be present at the second left intercostal space due to increased pulmonary blood flow (not due to flow across ASD).

ECG findings are also usually nonspecific. Classic findings in **secundum** defects include **right** axis deviation, RV hypertrophy (RVH), right atrial enlargement, and first-degree AV block. In defects in the **primum,** typical findings are **left** axis deviation, biventricular hypertrophy, and AV block. The classic ECG pattern of septal defects includes an incomplete right bundle-branch block or an rSR' pattern. AF is common in patients with significant ASD after the third decade.

Chest x-ray may show cardiomegaly and increased pulmonary vascular markings.

Diagnosis

The diagnosis of ASD can usually be made based on echocardiographic findings. Transthoracic echocardiography can be used to visualize ostium primum and secundum defects. Assessment of color flow across the interatrial septum in the subcostal long axis is the most helpful window. TEE is frequently needed to characterize the exact location of the defect. The sensitivity of echocardiography in the diagnosis of ASD can be improved by injecting IV contrast of agitated saline ("saline contrast") during imaging **(bubble study).** The microbubbles are visualized moving across the ASD, **but only if there is any component of right-to-left shunt** (the Valsalva maneuver increases the sensitivity of the test by decreasing LV filling). The role of cardiac catheterization in ASD is limited to measuring the direction of the shunt by oximetry and pulmonary pressures as part of an evaluation before correction of the defect. Angiography is sometimes performed before surgery to evaluate for coronary disease.

Management

Management of ASD depends on the ratio of pulmonary to systemic blood flow (Qp/Qs). If this ratio is <1.5, the ASD usually causes no significant hemodynamic complications, and intervention to close the defect is not indicated. Most adults diagnosed with ASD have more severe defects and should be considered for closure. If the Qp/Qs ratio is >1.5, the RA/RV is enlarged, or there is pulmonary HTN, the patient should be considered for closure of the defect. Irreversible pulmonary HTN is a contraindication to closure and may prevent correction in adults diagnosed with ASD. Recurrent thromboembolic events, usually in the setting of Coumadin failure, are another indication for closure of PFO or ASD. Both surgical and percutaneous techniques (with Amplatzer or CardioSEAL closure devices) are available for ASD closure.

Antibiotic prophylaxis is not indicated in ASD unless valvular abnormalities are present. Of note, prophylaxis should be given to patients with corrected ASD in the 6 mos after repair.

Ventricular Septal Defect

VSD is the most common congenital cardiac condition in children. Because 25–40% close spontaneously by age 2 and 90% close by age 10, they are usually not corrected unless hemodynamic abnormalities are present. VSDs also occur as a complication of acute MI (see Chap. 5, Cardiovascular Emergencies, and Chap. 8, Acute ST-Segment Elevation Myocardial Infarction).

Etiology
Etiology of congenital VSDs is as follows:

- 70% of congenital VSDs occur in the membranous portion of the interventricular septum **(perimembranous VSD)**; such VSDs have the highest rate of spontaneous closure.
- 20% of VSDs occur in the muscular portion of the septum; many of these close as well.
- 5% of these lesions occur inferior and adjacent to the aortic valve (subaortic or supracristal VSD).
- 5% are defects of the AV canal; these rarely close and are frequently associated with abnormalities of the AV valves.

Complications
Complications of VSD include LV volume overload and left-sided CHF due to increased pulmonary venous return. Because of the chronically increased right-sided volumes, equalization of ventricular pressures can occur if the defect is large. Given the lower compliance of the RV, this leads to a right-to-left shunt and increased pulmonary vascular flow. Pulmonary vascular hypertrophy and fibrosis can consequently develop with time. This leads to pulmonary HTN and RV dilatation and failure, and ultimately, Eisenmenger syndrome, a cyanotic condition.

Clinical Presentation
Patients are usually asymptomatic until late in the disease, when dyspnea with exertion is the most common symptom. **Physical exam** findings include a laterally displaced left point of maximal impulse. The pulmonary component of the second heart sound may be loud if pulmonary HTN is advanced. The murmur of VSD is typically holosystolic at the left lower sternal boarder and frequently associated with a palpable thrill. An additional middiastolic murmur due to increased mitral flow may be present. The murmur diminishes late in the disease, and patients may develop signs of systemic cyanosis, including digital clubbing.

ECG findings in VSD include left atrial enlargement and LVH early in the course, with the QRS axis shifting right as pulmonary HTN develops.

Chest x-ray findings vary from normal to increased pulmonary vascular markings with cardiomegaly.

Diagnosis
The diagnosis and surgical evaluation of VSD can usually be done with echocardiogram. **Transthoracic echocardiography** is the initial diagnostic study, although **TEE** is often required in adults. Catheterization is usually not required unless there is uncertainty about the echocardiography findings.

Management
Management of VSD in adults is similar to ASD. Most adults with a small VSD do not develop symptoms and do not require intervention. These patients do **require endocarditis antibiotic prophylaxis** (see p. 218). Large VSDs or those associated with increased pulmonary pressures should be considered for closure. In general, if Qp/Qs is >1.5, the LV is enlarged, or pulmonary HTN exists, the VSD should be closed. In the absence of these manifestations, a VSD is termed **restrictive.** For significant VSDs, surgical closure is usually performed, although percutaneous techniques are under investigation. Patients with more irreversible pulmonary HTN and pulmonary-to-systemic vascular resistance >0.7 should not undergo closure. Medical management in these patients includes managing HF with diuretics, digoxin, and afterload reduction.

Patent Ductus Arteriosus

The ligamentum arteriosus is the normal remnant of the ductus arteriosus, the embryonic vessel connecting the left pulmonary artery with the descending aorta. In the fetus, it allows shunting of blood oxygenated in the placenta around the pulmonary circulation. The ductus normally closes within 1–2 days after birth, when the aortic pressure rises and the pulmonary pressure falls. If it fails to close, then flow is directed from the aorta to the pulmonary artery.

Clinical Presentation

Physical exam of patent ductus arteriosus (PDA) may include a hyperdynamic LV impulse and wide-pulse pressures. The S_1 is normal. The classic murmur of PDA is continuous and loudest over the second left intercostal space, frequently obscuring the S_2. The murmur is often described as a **washing machine murmur.** Of note, PDA is the most common cause of a continuous murmur, although other conditions may produce this finding. Additionally, the murmur may be replaced by a murmur of pulmonary regurgitation as pulmonary HTN worsens.

ECG findings are nonspecific and include LVH and left atrial enlargement.

Chest x-ray findings include pulmonary vascular congestion later in the disease. The ascending aorta is prominent, and PDA may be visualized at area of the aortic knob.

Echocardiogram with Doppler study is usually sufficient to measure flow across PDA. Catheterization is usually reserved for therapeutic purposes.

Management

PDAs rarely close spontaneously after infancy. A small PDA poses only the risk of infective endocarditis. Larger PDAs cause fatigue by early adulthood due to increased pulmonary pressures. Eventually, patients develop LV failure due to volume overload. Additional complications, regardless of the size of the PDA, are aneurysm and rupture. One-third of patients with uncorrected PDA die by age 40 and two-thirds die by age 60. For these reasons, all PDAs should be ligated or closed. Percutaneous closure devices are the standard of care in most centers. Surgical ligation is also possible, frequently with minimally invasive surgery. As with ASD and VSD, irreversible pulmonary HTN precludes closure of PDA.

Aortic Stenosis

Aortic stenosis is a common complication of **congenital bicuspid aortic valve** (see Chap. 13, Valvular Heart Disease). This occurs much more commonly in men. Symptoms include angina, syncope, and those resulting from CHF; mean survival of patients with these symptoms is 5, 3, and 2 yrs, respectively.

Clinical Presentation

On physical exam, classic findings include delayed carotid upstrokes, a decreased aortic component of the S_2, and presence of an S_4. The murmur is typically a harsh, systolic, crescendo–decrescendo murmur over the aortic area. The murmur peaks later in systole with more advanced disease.

Management

Adults with asymptomatic aortic stenosis have a normal life expectancy and should be followed for development of symptoms and receive antibiotic prophylaxis. For the management of severe or symptomatic aortic stenosis, see Chap. 13, Valvular Heart Disease.

Subvalvular Aortic Stenosis

Subvalvular aortic stenosis (subaortic membrane) is a congenital condition that produces an obstruction to blood flow from the LV outflow tract to the ascending aorta. Over time, it yields **aortic insufficiency** due to the diversion of a discrete jet against the aortic valve leaflets. In this case, resection of the membrane and aortic valve replacement are both required.

Pulmonary Stenosis

Pulmonary stenosis accounts for approximately 10% of cases of adult congenital disease (see Chap. 13, Valvular Heart Disease). 90% of the cases are valvular, and 10% are supra- or infravalvular. The normal pulmonary valve area is 2 cm with no gradient across the valve.

- **Mild:** area >1 cm/m body surface area and transvalvular gradient <50 mm Hg
- **Moderate:** area 0.5–1.0 cm and transvalvular gradient 50–80 and RV systolic pressure 75–100
- **Severe:** valve area <0.5 cm and transvalvular gradient >80 or RV systolic pressure >100

Clinical Presentation
Clinical signs include symptoms of dyspnea and fatigue. If pulmonary HTN develops, a right-to-left shunt may occur across a PFO, causing cyanosis and clubbing. Physical exam findings include a prominent RV impulse and a possible thrill at the left second intercostal space. Patients have a normal S_1 and a wide, split S_2 with normal respiratory variations. There is a harsh systolic crescendo–decrescendo murmur. P_2 component may be absent. A mid-systolic click may be present. Signs of right-heart failure may be evident on exam if pulmonary stenosis is severe and prolonged. Typical ECG findings are right-axis deviation and RVH. Echocardiography demonstrates RVH and paradoxical septal motion.

Management
Management of asymptomatic adults involves antibiotic prophylaxis and surveillance for signs or symptoms. For moderate pulmonary stenosis, percutaneous balloon valvuloplasty is indicated. Valve replacement is reserved for severe regurgitation occurring after valvuloplasty.

Aortic Coarctation

Coarctation of the aorta is most commonly due to a ridge of tissue in the aortic lumen, creating a "shelf" distal to the left subclavian artery at the site of the ligamentum arteriosus. In some cases, the coarctation is proximal to the left subclavian artery. HTN develops proximal to the coarctation, including the upper extremities and cranial circulation. In addition, **extensive collaterals** develop via the internal thoracic, intercostal, and subclavian arteries. Of note, aortic coarctation is occasionally associated with bicuspid aortic valve.

Complications
Complications of coarctation include HTN, LV failure, aortic aneurysm, dissection, and cerebral embolic disease. Infective endocarditis occurs with increased frequency. Due to these complications, 75% of patients with uncorrected coarctation die by age 50.

Clinical Presentation
Patients may present with **symptoms** of lower-extremity hypotension or CHF, although most are asymptomatic. The **physical exam** of aortic coarctation is significant for widened pulse pressures proximal to the defect. Given the fall in pressure across the lesion, it is important to document BP in all four extremities, considering coarctation as a diagnosis. Additional findings include a thrill appreciated over the suprasternal notch. The S_2 is loud, with a harsh systolic murmur at the left sternal boarder radiating to the back.

ECG may be normal or show LVH. **Chest x-ray** classically shows **rib notching** of the third through eighth ribs due to collateral vessels. In addition, the coarctation may be visualized at the aortic knob, giving rise to the **"3 sign."**

Echocardiogram is the primary diagnostic study, with MRI reserved for patients with nondiagnostic echocardiograms.

Management
Management is surgical excision if the transcoarctation pressure gradient is >30 mm Hg. Early repair is felt to improve survival, and many are repaired in childhood. Late

complications of surgery include aneurysms and recurrence of the coarctation. Although surgery is the first-line treatment, balloon angioplasty and stenting can be performed safely in many patients, particularly those with recurrence of the coarctation. The position of the coarct precludes percutaneous intervention in some patients.

CYANOTIC CONDITIONS

Cyanotic conditions are the result of venous blood being shunted into the arterial circulation. These conditions remain more common in children than in adults, because without correction, very few survive to adulthood. Adult patients with a history of corrected cyanotic congenital heart disease are becoming increasingly common as survival of these conditions improves. The two most common cyanotic conditions in adults are **tetralogy of Fallot (TOF)** and **Eisenmenger syndrome.**

Tetralogy of Fallot

TOF is the most common cyanotic condition occurring after infancy. The four associated findings occur with varying severity and include

- VSD, typically large
- An aorta that overrides the LV and RV
- Some degree of RV outflow tract obstruction, which may be subvalvular, valvular, supravalvular, or occurring in the pulmonary circulation
- RVH
- Other associated findings include ASD (occurring in 10% of cases; so-called pentalogy of Fallot), right-sided aortic arch (occurs in 25%), and coronary arterial anomalies (occur in 10%)

Complications
The complications of TOF are due to equalization of ventricular pressures across the VSD and shunting of blood from the RV to the LV due to obstruction of the RV outflow tract. As systemic vascular resistance falls to allow adequate cardiac output, this right-to-left shunt worsens. Without surgical correction, survival is 40% at age 3, 11% at age 20, and 3% at age 40.

Clinical Features
The child with uncorrected TOF has cyanosis and sudden episodes of hypoxia ("tet spells") characterized by tachypnea, increased cyanosis, squatting, then loss of consciousness and even sudden death. Adults with TOF typically have dyspnea and frequently show complications of erythrocytosis, cerebroembolic disease, and endocarditis. **Physical exam** is significant for cyanosis and digital clubbing. Pulses are normal, and an RV heave may be present. The S_1 is normal; however, the S_2 lacks a pulmonic component. A systolic ejection murmur at the lower sternal boarder, often accompanied by a thrill, is due to flow across an obstructed RV outflow tract. The **ECG** findings are right-axis deviation and RVH. On **chest x-ray,** the classic finding is of a "boot-shaped" heart. The diagnosis and characterization of the defects is made by echocardiogram.

Management
Current management of TOF is surgical corrective repair of the defect, closure of the VSD, and repair of the RV outflow tract obstruction. This procedure is usually performed as one step in early childhood, with a very low operative mortality. All patients with a history of TOF **require antibiotic prophylaxis** (see p. 218) before procedures. Late complications after repair of TOF include arrhythmias, and Holter monitoring should be considered in any patient with repaired TOF and symptoms of arrhythmia. In particular, AF and atrial flutter occur with high frequency and are tolerated poorly. Pulmonary regurgitation, as well as recurrent obstruction of the RV outflow tract, are other late complications.

Before corrective surgery, patients with TOF were managed with one of three palliative repairs of TOF. The goal of this series of procedures was to increase pulmonary blood flow.

A Waterson procedure, consisting of a side-to-side anastomosis of the ascending aorta to the right pulmonary artery, was performed first. The Potts procedure, or side-to-side anastomosis of the descending aorta to the left pulmonary artery, was also effective. Finally, a Blalock-Taussig procedure was performed by anastomosing the end of the subclavian artery to the side of the left pulmonary artery. This series helped relieve symptoms; however, it is complicated by eventual pulmonary HTN, distortion of the pulmonary vasculature, and HF. Almost all adults with repaired TOF at this time had one of these three procedures before more definitive correction.

Eisenmenger Syndrome

The **pathogenesis** of Eisenmenger syndrome is initiated by a left-to-right shunt (due to uncorrected VSD, ASD, PDA, or other condition creating single-ventricle physiology) that causes pulmonary vascular overload and pulmonary HTN due to pulmonary vascular fibrosis. As the pulmonary HTN worsens, the compliance of the RV increases, and the shunt decreases and eventually reverses, causing blood to flow from right to left and systemic cyanosis. The condition is irreversible if pulmonary HTN becomes severe.

Clinical Features
The typical clinical picture is that of a patient with a childhood murmur that resolved as the shunt decreased. Cyanosis is one of the early findings, followed by symptoms of dyspnea. Complications include atrial arrhythmias, heart failure, and sudden death. Erythrocytosis occurs, leading to fatigue, headache, and neurologic defects due to hyperviscosity. In addition, paradoxical emboli arise and may lead to CNS symptoms. **Hemoptysis occurs due to pulmonary infarction.**

   Physical exam reveals cyanosis and digital clubbing. Jugular venous v waves are prominent as tricuspid regurgitation develops. A right parasternal heave is often present. The pulmonic component of the S_2 is loud, and a right-sided S_4 is present. **Chest x-ray** typically reveals proximal pulmonary artery enlargement with "pruning" of the pulmonary vessels. **Saline-contrast echocardiogram** can be used to visualize most right-to-left shunts. **Left- and right-heart catheterization** is useful to assess severity of pulmonary vascular disease and determine reversibility of pulmonary HTN.

Management
Management of established Eisenmenger syndrome involves avoiding intravascular volume depletion as well as exertion, high altitude, vasodilators, surgical procedures, and pregnancy. Phlebotomy with crystalloid replacement is used for hyperviscosity syndromes due to secondary erythrocytosis. Iron is given for microcytosis, which can occur due to relative iron deficiency, resulting in reduced deformability of erythrocytes. Epoprostenol (Flolan) has been used to decrease the pulmonary HTN. PALL filters should be used with IV catheters to prevent air embolism. Heart–lung transplant is an option for a few of these patients. The 10-yr survival after diagnosis is 80%, with most patients dying from arrhythmias or massive hemoptysis. **Coumadin is relatively contraindicated.** Antibiotic prophylaxis is of course required (see p. 218).

Ebstein's Anomaly

Ebstein's anomaly is a tricuspid valve abnormality in which the septal and posterior leaflets are displaced into the ventricle. Abnormalities of the anterior leaflet are common. Portions of the RV are superior to the tricuspid valve ("atrialization of the RV"), resulting in a small RV. The valve is generally regurgitant and may be stenotic. The cyanotic component of this condition is due to the 80% incidence of ASD or PFO, allowing right-to-left shunting. **Maternal lithium** use during pregnancy is a risk factor for Ebstein's anomaly.

Clinical Features
Physical exam reveals hepatic congestion due to tricuspid regurgitation. The S_1 is widely split, and a systolic tricuspid regurgitation murmur may be present. S_3/S_4 are

common. **ECG** findings include tall P waves, right bundle-branch block, and first-degree AV block. In addition, 20% of patients with Ebstein's abnormality have an accessory pathway, so delta waves (Wolff-Parkinson-White) are common.

Diagnosis

Echocardiogram is the principal diagnostic tool, allowing characterization of the leaflets and shunt. Cardiac catheterization is of limited use; angiography is useful to exclude CAD before valve surgery in adults at risk.

Management

Management of Ebstein's abnormality includes **antibiotic prophylaxis** (see p. 218). CHF is managed with diuretics and digoxin. If an accessory pathway is present, patients should be considered for ablation. Valve repair with closure of the septal defect is the definitive treatment, with valve replacement reserved for cases in which repair is impossible. If the condition is severe in childhood, patients are managed with a palliative surgical series for single-ventricular physiology (see Conditions of Single-Ventricle Physiology).

Transposition of the Great Arteries

Transposition occurs when the aorta arises from the RV and the pulmonary artery from the LV. In **D-transposition** with situs solitus (normal positioning of the atria), two parallel circulations exist, resulting in the inability for oxygenated blood to reach systemic organs. In the absence of a septal defect or PDA, this is not compatible with survival after birth. Survival at birth is dependent on mixing of blood from the two circulations via a PFO or PDA. If the infant does not have a large ASD or VSD, prostaglandin E is given to keep the ductus arteriosus patent, and then a Rashkind procedure (atrial septostomy) may be performed shortly after birth. This creates or enlarges an ASD.

Historically, this condition was palliated in early childhood with an atrial-switch procedure (Mustard or Senning), resulting in creation of a baffle system in the atria. This allowed systemic venous blood to be directed across the mitral valve into the LV and then the pulmonary circulation, while pulmonary venous blood was directed across the tricuspid valve and into the aortic circulation. The RV still must function as the systemic ventricle, which with decades becomes problematic. Adults who received these surgeries often exhibit atrial flutter, sick sinus syndrome, and varying degrees of baffle leak. Now, the definitive arterial switch (Jatene) procedure is favored, in which the pulmonary artery and aorta are transected superior to the semilunar valves and reanastomosed in their correct anatomic positions. The coronary arteries are reimplanted so that they receive oxygenated blood.

In **L-transposition** ("congenitally corrected" transposition, an acyanotic defect), the aorta still arises from the RV, and the pulmonary trunk still arises from the LV; however, there is AV discordance, in which the position of the ventricles is reversed. Consequently, the systemic veins drain into the right atrium, to the LV, and then to the pulmonary artery, and the pulmonary veins drain into the left atrium, the RV, and then the aorta. Thus, the circuits are appropriate, and the condition is compatible with life *ex utero*. Most patients do well until the RV begins to fail because of chronic exposure to systemic BPs, usually in the fourth or fifth decade.

Conditions of Single-Ventricle Physiology

Single-ventricular physiology includes several rare conditions. Adults with these conditions may have undergone the palliative procedures described. The most common single-ventricular states include **hypoplastic left heart, tricuspid atresia, pulmonary atresia,** and **complete AV canal.** These conditions are managed with a series of palliative surgeries during childhood. The end result is the elimination of the right heart and pulmonary perfusion by systemic venous pressure. The Norwood procedure creates a single functioning aorta from elements of both aorta and pulmonary artery arising from a single ventricle. Pulmonary circulation is provided by anastomosing the subclavian artery to the left pulmonary artery (the Blalock-Taussig). This is followed by the Glenn procedure (and repair of the subclavian to pulmonary artery shunt), which is anastomosis of the superior vena cava to the pulmonary artery. Finally, a Fontan procedure is performed, and the inferior vena cava and hepatic veins are anastomosed to the pulmonary artery. The latter is often complicated later by protein-losing enteropathy and pulmonary AV malformations later in life.

KEY POINTS TO REMEMBER

- When thinking about congenital heart disease, attempt to classify the abnormality by the following parameters:
  - Is the condition cyanotic?
  - Is the pulmonary artery flow low or high?
  - Is the left- or right-sided circulation the origin of malformation?
  - What is the dominant ventricle?
  - Is there pulmonary HTN?
- Surgical repairs have become more corrective, rather than palliative. Consequently, many patients have much longer life expectancies.
- The consequences of a palliative surgery, which are necessary for compatibility with life, currently create many of the management dilemmas of adult patients with congenital heart disease.

REFERENCES AND SUGGESTED READINGS

Brickner ME, Hillis LD, Lange RA. Congenital heart disease in adults. First of two parts. *N Engl J Med* 2000;342:256–263.
Brickner ME, Hillis LD, Lange RA. Congenital heart disease in adults. Second of two parts. *N Engl J Med* 2000;342:334–342.

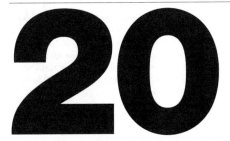

Diseases of
the Aorta

Richard G. Garmany

ANATOMY

The aorta is comprised of the ascending aorta, which is the site of the left, right, and non-coronary sinuses of Valsalva, and the origins of the coronary arteries. It continues as the aortic arch, the site of the great vessels of the head and upper extremities, followed by the descending thoracic aorta and abdominal aorta, which terminates at the bifurcation of the iliac arteries. **Histologically,** the aorta is comprised of a thin, physiologically important intima. This is surrounded by a thick media providing much of the aortic tensile strength. Finally, the adventitia surrounds the outside surface and is responsible for supplying blood flow to the outer layers of the media through vaso vasorum.

ABDOMINAL AORTIC ANEURYSM

Abdominal aortic aneurysm (AAA) is defined as a pathologic dilatation of all layers of the aorta >1.5× the normal diameter (~3 cm). They may be classified as fusiform (symmetric) or saccular (asymmetric outpouching). "True" aneurysms involve all three layers of the aorta. Pseudoaneurysms result from damage to the intima, allowing blood to dissect into the media and resulting in dilation of the media and adventitial layers. 75% of all aortic aneurysms occur in the abdominal aorta; the majority of these are infrarenal.

Etiology

The etiology of AAAs is usually multifactorial. In >90%, atherosclerosis is a major contributing feature; other causes include inflammatory arteritis and infectious causes.

Risk Factors

Risk factors include HTN, hyperlipidemia, tobacco use, diabetes, male sex, and age (>55 yrs in men, >70 yrs in women). Family history is a risk factor as well.

Clinical Presentation

On presentation, most patients are asymptomatic, and aneurysms are discovered incidentally on exam (pulsatile abdominal aorta >4 cm). Severe back or flank pain is the most common symptom of a rapidly enlarging or ruptured AAA. **Pulsatile abdominal mass, hypotension, and abdominal pain merit an immediate vascular surgery consult.**

Physical Exam

Exam frequently shows asymptomatic pulsatile mass.

Rupture Risk

The main factor in determining risk of rupture is aneurysm size. AAAs typically enlarge by 0.4 cm/yr. Larger aneurysms enlarge more rapidly, according to the law of

Laplace (tension = pressure × radius). At 5–6 cm, a 6% annual risk of rupture exists; at >7 cm, this increases to 20%. Before the availability of surgery, the survival rates at 3 and 5 yrs were 49% and 19%, respectively. The most frequent site of rupture is the left retroperitoneal space, which may increase the chances of tamponade and temporary hemodynamic instability. AAAs may also rupture into the GI tract and present with a small herald bleed or by massive GI hemorrhage. Always consider this in a patient with a history of AAA presenting with any GI bleed.

Diagnostic Imaging

Diagnostic imaging is used for diagnosis, surveillance of stable aneurysms, and operative planning. U/S has the advantage of being rapid and readily available; it can give a rough estimate of aneurysm size. Contrast CT has the advantages of yielding more accurate size estimates and allowing some assessment of branch vessels. CT is, in most cases, the test of choice for diagnosis and ongoing surveillance. Inability to determine patency of renal and mesenteric vessels limits the value of CT in preop evaluation; furthermore, it requires IV contrast, which can be problematic in patients with renal insufficiency. Aortography was the classic study performed preop due to its ability to visualize renal and iliac vessels and their potential involvement by the AAA. Given the invasive nature and dye load required for this test, in addition to improvements in CT and availability of MRI/magnetic resonance angiography (MRA), many surgeons no longer request aortography in all AAA patients preop. MRI/MRA allows precise definition of anatomy and is useful in planning elective repair. Limitations include expense and availability. Suspected ruptured AAA should ideally be diagnosed in the OR, and no imaging is indicated before consultation with an experienced vascular surgeon, but impending rupture may be diagnosed by CT scan.

Screening

Screening asymptomatic patients without known AAA is controversial. There are no official recommendations based on large studies. Some physicians advocate screening men >60 yrs with at least one additional risk factor.

Treatment

Treatment of stable AAA involves risk factor reduction, with control of HTN and smoking cessation while monitoring AAA size to determine appropriate time of elective surgical repair. Most physicians would recommend screening with CT or U/S q3–6mos, depending on size and other risks. Guidelines recommend elective repair of an AAA >4 cm or expanding at a rate >0.5 cm/yr in a patient of reasonable surgical risk. Consider repair of an AAA >6 cm regardless of surgical risk. Two recent studies [1,2] demonstrated no mortality benefit to operating on an AAA <5.5 cm.

Treatment of acutely enlarging or suspected ruptured AAA is limited to lowering aortic pressure with IV agents (Table 20-1) while awaiting surgical repair. Establish IV access and send blood for type and cross in addition to standard labs.

Preop Evaluation

Preop evaluation should include cardiac risk assessment in all AAA patients. The **prevalence of CAD is extremely high among patients with aortic aneurysms,** and MI is the most common surgical complication of AAA repair. Assessment is best achieved with a pharmacologic stress nuclear perfusion study or echocardiogram, as most patients with AAA have poor exercise tolerance due to comorbidities.

THORACIC AORTIC ANEURYSM

Thoracic aortic aneurysms (TAAs) are less common than AAAs and have more varied etiologies. They are classified by the anatomic segment involved.

TABLE 20-1. IV ANTIHYPERTENSIVES FOR ACUTE MEDICAL MANAGEMENT OF AORTIC DISEASE

Agent	Dosage
Propranolol	Starting: 1 mg IV q3–5 mins to goal HR of 60 (max. 6.15 mg/kg)
	Maintenance: 2–6 mg IV q4–6h as needed to maintain MAP and HR
Labetalol	Starting: 20 mg IV over 2 mins, followed by 40–80 mg q10–15mins to goal HR and BP (max. 300 mg)
	Maintenance: 2 mg/min IV gtt, titrated to effect (max. 5–10 mg/min)
Esmolol	Starting: 500 μg/kg IV bolus
	Maintenance: 50 μg/kg/min IV infusion, titrate to max. 200 μg/kg/min
Metoprolol	Starting: 5 mg IV q5mins
	Maintenance: 10 mg IV q4–6h to goal MAP and HR
Sodium nitro-prusside	Starting: 20 μg/min IV infusion
	Maintenance: Titrate up to max. 800 μg/min
Enalaprilat	Starting: 0.625 mg IV
	Maintenance: 0.625 mg IV q4–6h, titrate to max. 5 mg IV q6h
Diltiazem	Starting: 0.25 mg/kg IV over 2 mins
	Maintenance: 5 mg/hr IV infusion, titrate to max. 15 mg/hr
Verapamil	Starting: 5–10 mg IV over 2 mins, with 10-mg dose repeated after 15 mins if no effect
	Maintenance: 5 mg/hr IV infusion, titrate to max. 15 mg/hr

HR, heart rate; MAP, mean arterial pressure.
Adapted from Marso SP, Griffin BP, Topol EJ. *Manual of cardiovascular medicine.* Philadelphia: Lippincott Williams & Wilkins, 2000.

Etiology

Etiologies include Marfan syndrome, Ehlers-Danlos syndrome, cystic medial degeneration (a nonspecific pathologic descriptor comprised of many entities), atherosclerotic disease, trauma (including postprocedural), inflammatory states (Takayasu's and giant cell arteritis), infections (syphilis), and, occasionally, bicuspid aortic valve.

Clinical Presentation

Presentation varies with location of the aneurysm. 40% of all TAAs are asymptomatic and discovered incidentally. Vascular complications include aortic insufficiency; myocardial ischemia; thromboembolic disease; and rupture of aneurysm into the right atrium, causing a left-to-right shunt. The mass effect of the TAA may cause compression of other structures in the thorax, presenting as superior vena cava syndrome, dysphagia, hoarseness, wheezing, dyspnea, chest pain, and postobstructive pneumonia.

Imaging

Imaging studies are similar to those used to assess AAAs. Contrast CT is the typical method of diagnosis and surveillance imaging, whereas MRI/MRA is reserved for operative planning. CT screening q6–12mos for asymptomatic patients with TAAs <5 cm and q3–6mos for those >5 cm is a reasonable strategy.

Management

Management of TAAs is similar to AAAs, with the goal of avoiding the catastrophic complication of rupture. **Activity restriction** is designed to prevent acute dissection or rupture caused by a high-output state. **Beta blockade** is often appropriate, especially if the patient is chronically hypertensive. Timing of surgery is less well defined than for abdominal aneurysms. 1-, 3-, and 5-yr survival without surgery is 65%, 36%, and 20%, respectively, for TAAs >6 cm. Surgery is currently recommended when an ascending aortic aneurysm is >5.5–6 cm and when a descending aneurysm is >6 cm. **Most authorities recommend surgery earlier in patients with Marfan syndrome due to their high risk of rupture. TAA of 5 cm would be an indication for repair in such patients and earlier if it is enlarging rapidly.**

AORTIC DISSECTION

Aortic dissection, in most cases, begins with damage to the aortic intima, allowing blood to extravasate into a diseased and partially weakened aortic media. Under the ongoing pulse pressure, blood moves longitudinally between the aortic layers for some distance, creating a **false aortic lumen.** This is separated from the true lumen by an **intimal flap,** which may develop further tears and communication between the true and false lumens. The risk of death from aortic dissection is due to involvement of branch arteries (such as coronaries and carotids), external rupture, and pericardial tamponade. Mortality for unrecognized acute aortic dissection is 1% per hr during the first 48 hrs after symptom onset.

Etiology

The etiology of dissection includes several conditions, including Marfan and Ehlers-Danlos syndromes, and other causes of cystic medial necrosis predisposed to dissection through the mechanism of aortic medial degeneration. It is clear that this process is involved in dissection in a number of individuals without known predisposing connective tissue disorders. Other predisposing factors include **aging; HTN; coarctation with or without bicuspid aortic valve; and trauma, including placement of an intraaortic balloon pump and other intraaortic devices.** Pregnancy in combination with another risk factor further predisposes to aortic dissection.

Classification Schemes

The two predominant classification schemes for aortic dissections are based on anatomy, time course, and management. 65% of dissections arise in the ascending aorta, whereas 20% arise in the descending aorta. In general, dissections are classified as **acute** (more common), in which symptoms have been present for <2 wks, and **chronic** or **symptomatic,** featuring symptoms present for >2 wks. This has prognostic significance, as most patients who survive 2 wks are found to have stable dissections, and the high mortality curve levels off at this point. The two schemes based on anatomy are the Stanford (types A and B) and DeBakey (types I–III) (Fig. 20-1). **Type A** or **proximal dissections** involve the ascending aorta and, in general, are almost always managed with urgent or emergent surgery. **Type B** or **distal dissections** do not involve the ascending aorta and are initially managed medically (aggressive control of heart rate and HTN). Surgery does not offer benefit to these patients unless there are complications, such as end-organ or limb ischemia.

Clinical Presentation

Clinical presentation is with severe chest or back pain in 75–90% of patients. The pain is typically **sudden and maximal at onset,** as compared with more gradual onset of

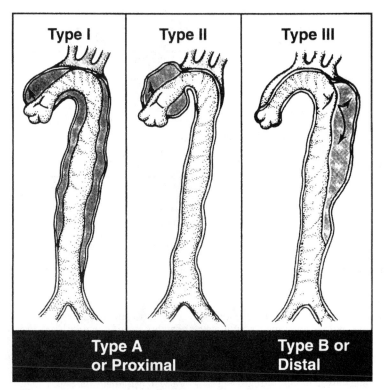

FIG. 20-1. The two classification schemes based on anatomy are the Stanford (types A and B) and DeBakey (types I–III). (From Marso SP, Griffin BP, Topol EJ. *Manual of cardiovascular medicine*. Philadelphia: Lippincott Williams & Wilkins, 2000, with permission.)

pain in acute MI. The quality of the pain is classically described as **tearing, ripping, or stabbing.** Presentation may be clinically indistinguishable from an acute MI, which frequently complicates proximal dissections with coronary ostial involvement (usually right coronary artery). Because of the position of the flap and the direction of blood flow, dissections **usually** extend distally from the initiation point of the flap. **Diagnosis requires a high index of suspicion, as it can be commonly overlooked.**

Marfan syndrome should be strongly considered in patients with pectus carinatum or excavatum, long arms, arachnodactyly, hyperextendable joints, scoliosis, highly arched palate, ectopia lentis (dislocated lenses), MVP, stretch marks, and/or a family history of Marfan. Because of the pleomorphic nature of the disease, patients with Marfan syndrome do not always present with the classic lanky appearance.

Physical Exam

Findings typical of proximal and distal dissections are shown in Table 20-2. Of note, none of these findings should be considered specific of either class of dissection.

Diagnostic Considerations

Diagnostic considerations in acute dissection include MI, acute aortic regurgitation, nondissecting TAA or AAA, pericarditis, mediastinal tumors, and musculoskeletal pain.

TABLE 20-2. PHYSICAL EXAM FINDINGS IN AORTIC DISSECTION

Proximal (type A) dissections	Distal (type B) dissections
Hypotension	HTN
Unilateral pulse defects in upper extremities and neck (take BP in each arm)	Pulse defects in lower extremities
Murmur of aortic insufficiency, frequently with signs of CHF, given acute nature of aortic insufficiency	Rare paraparesis due to anterior spinal artery involvement
CNS and cranial nerve neurologic defects due to involvement of carotids	
Cardiac tamponade is a late complication	

Nonspecific Studies

Nonspecific studies include chest x-ray, which frequently shows a wide aortic silhouette and evidence of displacement of a calcified intima from the aortic wall (calcium sign). The most common ECG finding is LVH, although evidence of acute MI will be present if there is coronary involvement. The most frequent coronary artery involved is the RCA; thus, an inferior infarction pattern is compatible with concomitant dissection.

Diagnostic Studies

Diagnostic studies are similar to those used for aortic aneurysms and have similar advantages and limitations. Institutional availability should guide decisions regarding which study to obtain.

- **MRI/MRA** with a sensitivity and specificity of 98% is the current reference standard for diagnosis and surveillance of aortic dissection. It remains expensive, of limited availability in urgent settings, and slow for use in potentially unstable patients.
- **Echocardiography** is rapid and readily available. **Transthoracic echocardiography** is of limited utility in diagnosis given its low sensitivity (59–85%). **TEE**, however, has a sensitivity of 98% and is extremely useful in the acute setting, allowing safe patient triage. The ability to identify aortic insufficiency and pericardial effusion extends the utility of TEE. If available, TEE is probably the optimal study in the acute setting.
- **Contrast CT**, with a sensitivity of 83–94%, is the most useful study in the acute setting if TEE is not readily available.
- **Aortography** has a sensitivity of 88%; however, the time and personnel required to perform it limit its usefulness in the acute setting. Furthermore, it requires an invasive procedure and dye load. For these reasons, reserve aortography for cases in which results of other studies are inconclusive.

Management

Management of dissections depends on anatomic location and complications. In general, **proximal (type A) dissections require immediate operative repair.** The management of all dissections requires diligent and immediate antihypertensive control. Studies comparing surgery with medical therapy for distal (type B) dissections show no survival advantage to surgical strategy. Therefore, type B dissections and chronic dissections of all types are generally managed medically. Indications for surgery in these patients are listed in Table 20-3. General therapeutic considerations in **any** patient with aortic dissection include

- Admit to ICU
- Decrease aortic pressure and the force of ventricular ejection with IV medications to a goal systolic BP of 100–120 mm HG or a mean arterial pressure of 60–75 (Table 20-1).

TABLE 20-3. INDICATIONS FOR SURGERY IN ANY AORTIC DISSECTION

End-organ dysfunction

Suspected aortic rupture

Acute aortic insufficiency

Dissection in a patient with known or suspected Marfan syndrome

Retrograde extension of the dissection into the aortic arch

Development of hemodynamic instability

Intractable pain

Beta blockers are first-line agents with target heart rate of 60 bpm. Esmolol (Brevibloc) is a particularly short-acting beta blocker that is useful if there is concern about how these agents will be tolerated. The calcium channel blockers diltiazem or verapamil are second-line agents used in patients intolerant of beta blockers. Sodium nitroprusside (Nipride) is started if needed for additional BP control **after** adequate beta blockade. Enalaprilat is an IV ACE inhibitor that is useful in cases of refractory HTN in addition to beta blockers.

- Place an arterial line for accurate pressure recording, avoiding the femoral arteries if possible, given the potential need for these sites as graft material.
- Obtain IV access, generally with a central line allowing central venous pressure monitoring and large-volume infusions.
- If pressors are required for hypotension, norepinephrine (Levophed) or phenylephrine (Neo-Synephrine) are preferred over epinephrine or dopamine, as they are less likely to increase the force of LV ejection (dP/dT).
- **Thrombolytics are absolutely contraindicated, even in the presence of acute MI, if aortic dissection is suspected.** Thrombolysis has been shown to increase the risk of catastrophic hemorrhage.
- Control pain with IV morphine.
- Routine cardiac catheterization and coronary angiography before surgery are controversial. In small studies, the surgical delay due to angiography resulted in higher overall mortality. The presence of coronary ostial occlusion or severe chronic CAD is significant before surgery, as repair of an aortic dissection at the same time as CABG is possible with acceptable mortality. Therefore, in stable patients with strongly suspected CAD, angiography is sometimes performed preop.

Long-Term Management
Long-term management of dissection involves aggressive BP control with PO beta blockers or calcium channel blockers (see Chap. 6, Stable Angina). Additional agents will frequently be necessary. It is important to start direct vasodilators, such as minoxidil (Loniten) or hydralazine (Apresoline), only in the presence of negative inotropic drugs, such as beta blockers. The target systolic BP in a patient with a history of dissection is 130 mm Hg.

Surveillance Imaging
Surveillance imaging for patients with history of dissection is done at high frequency for the first 2 yrs, during which complications are most likely. A reasonable approach would be to obtain CT, MRI, or TEE at 3, 6, 12, 18, and 24 mos after the event, followed by studies q6–12mos thereafter, to ensure the dissection has healed.

INTRAMURAL HEMATOMA

In a subset of aortic dissections, no intimal flap or false lumen can be identified. In reality, these entities are often intramural hematomas, which are spontaneous hemorrhages into the aortic wall in the absence of an intimal flap or penetrating atherosclerotic ulcer (see Penetrating Atherosclerotic Ulcer). Its etiology is presumed to be due to rupture of the vasa vasorum; in some cases, a penetrating atherosclerotic ulcer may have been an inciting influence. Risk factors include age, HTN, and atherosclerosis. Symptoms are **similar to those of aortic dissection.** Imaging assessment is similar to that of aortic dissection, as is management. Treatment includes immediate surgical correction for ascending aortic hematomas. Close follow-up with serial imaging is required for those who are medically managed. Complete resolution is possible over 1–2 yrs with appropriate therapy.

PENETRATING ATHEROSCLEROTIC ULCER

An aortic intimal atheroma can develop a surface erosion or ulceration. When this erosion penetrates into the media, a penetrating atherosclerotic ulcer exists. Most of these occur in the mid- and distal descending aorta in elderly patients with multiple comorbidities. Presentation is similar to that of dissection or hematoma, with the possible addition of limb or end-organ ischemia due to atheroembolization. Unlike dissection or intramural hematoma, angiography is the gold standard for imaging, although TEE, CT, and MRI are useful. **A penetrating ulcer is rarely the cause for aortic dissection. Complications** of the penetrating ulcer include distal emboli, spontaneous aortic rupture, and aneurysm/pseudoaneurysm formation. Treatment includes early surgery for hemorrhage, recurrent chest or back pain, and enlarging (pseudo)aneurysm. Diligent control of HTN is mandatory. Close follow-up with serial imaging is required.

KEY POINTS TO REMEMBER

- Atherosclerotic aortic disease (e.g., AAA) and CAD are highly correlated.
- Aortic dissection should be considered in any patient describing acute-onset severe chest pain. If ischemia is effectively ruled out and severe chest pain is ongoing, an imaging study to rule out dissection is often indicated. Dissection can occur in the setting of inferior ischemia or injury, due to involvement of the right coronary artery.
- Any aortic dissection involving the ascending aorta requires emergent surgical repair, and some dissections that do not involve the ascending aorta also require surgical repair. All aortic dissections require urgent BP control, focusing initially on the reduction of stroke volume.
- Marfan syndrome is an autosomal-dominant (with variable expressivity) disorder that is a common cause of thoracic aortic aneurysm and aortic dissection in young to middle-aged adults.

SUGGESTED READING

Braverman AC. Aortic dissection. *Curr Opin Cardiol* 1997;12:389–390.
Braverman AC. Penetrating atherosclerotic ulcers of the aorta. *Curr Opin Cardiol* 1994;9:591–597.
Braverman AC, Harris KM. Management of aortic intramural hematoma. *Curr Opin Cardiol* 1995;10:501–504.
Kouchoukos NT, Dougenis D. Surgery of the thoracic aorta. *N Engl J Med* 1997;336:1876–1888.
Marso SP, Griffin BP, Topol EJ. *Manual of cardiovascular medicine.* Philadelphia: Lippincott Williams & Wilkins, 2000.
Pretre R, Von Segesser LK. Aortic dissection. *Lancet* 1997;349:1461–1464.

REFERENCES

1. Lederle FA, Wilson SE, Johnson GR, et al. Immediate repair compared with surveillance of small abdominal aortic aneurysms. *N Engl J Med* 2002;346:1437–1444.
2. Long-term outcomes of immediate repair compared with surveillance of small abdominal aortic aneurysms. *N Engl J Med* 2002;346:1445–1452.

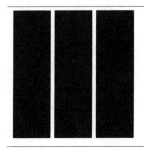

Testing and Procedures in Cardiology

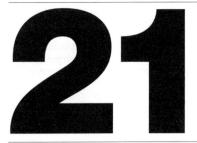

Noninvasive Cardiac Assessment for Coronary Artery Disease

Richard G. Garmany and
Peter A. Crawford

INTRODUCTION

The noninvasive assessment for CAD involves a number of different agents to challenge the cardiovascular system and a number of different forms of assessment. First, it is important to determine the indications and contraindications for testing. Next, the type of test needs to be selected. This chapter addresses these issues. Chap. 22, Imaging and Diagnostic Testing Modalities (Nuclear Imaging, Echocardiography, and Cardiac Catheterization), provides a description of the imaging procedures used for assessment of CAD.

General **indications** for **stress testing** include **diagnosing** CAD, **evaluating therapy** in patients with known disease, and **assessing risk** in patients with symptoms or a history of an acute coronary syndrome. The basic goal of all modalities is to assess prognostic indices, such as exercise capacity, myocardial function, and perfusion in response to stress. The decision to order any diagnostic test must take into account the implications of **Bayes' theorem,** which states that the pretest probability heavily influences the interpretation of the result of the test. Among patients at high risk of having CAD, false-negative results of stress tests are much more prevalent than patients with average or low risk of disease. Therefore, a negative test result in a high-risk patient is less useful at excluding CAD. Moreover, in patients at very low risk of disease, a positive result is much less likely to indicate presence of CAD. For example, in ECG stress testing, the sensitivity is 68% and specificity 77% for detection of CAD. These values were determined by comparing the results of stress ECG with angiographic data in populations of patients at moderate risk for disease. In a high-risk population in which, for example, 90% can be expected to have CAD, a positive test would carry a 96% probability of having disease on angiography. In the same group, however, *79% of those with a negative test would also have disease* and would be falsely identified as not having CAD. For this reason, an ideal patient for a noninvasive stress test has a **intermediate risk** of having coronary disease. In patients at very high pretest risk, proceeding directly to angiography is more useful. Stress testing in low-risk, asymptomatic patients is likely to produce many false positives, leading to further unnecessary invasive testing. Pretest probability can be determined by taking into consideration a patient's age, sex, and quality of symptoms, as shown in Table 21-1.

EXERCISE STRESS TESTING

Each testing method described requires a physiologic stress to be applied. **Exercise is the preferred method of stress, as it provides the most physiologic stress and yields independent prognostic information. Exercise ECG** is based on the observation that ST-segment depression occurs during induced ischemia. For most patients, it can be safely performed in an office setting and is the least expensive of all the modalities commonly used. **Complications** are rare but include arrhythmias, cardiac arrest, death (1 in 10,000), and worsening of other medical problems, and patients should be made aware of these risks as part of informed consent. In preparation for the test, digoxin, beta blockers, and other antianginal medications should be withheld for sev-

TABLE 21-1. CONSIDERATIONS FOR DETERMINING PRETEST PROBABILITY

Age (yrs)	Sex	Asymptomatic	Nonanginal chest pain	Atypical anginal symptoms	Classic anginal symptoms
30–39	Male	Very low	Low	Intermediate	Intermediate
	Female	Very low	Very low	Very low	Intermediate
40–49	Male	Low	Intermediate	Intermediate	High
	Female	Very low	Very low	Low	Intermediate
50–59	Male	Low	Intermediate	Intermediate	High
	Female	Very low	Low	Intermediate	Intermediate
60–69	Male	Low	Intermediate	Intermediate	High
	Female	Low	Intermediate	Intermediate	High

From Gibbons RJ, Balady GJ, Beasley JW, et al. ACC/AHA guidelines for exercise testing: executive summary. A report of the American College of Cardiology/American Heart Association Task Force on Practice Guidelines (Committee on Exercise Testing). *Circulation* 1997;96:345–354, with permission.

eral days if possible; no food, alcohol, or caffeine should be taken at least 4 hrs before the test. Patients should bring a list of their medications with them.

Table 21-2 lists guidelines for exercise ECG testing, and Table 21-3 highlights contraindications to exercise stress testing.

TABLE 21-2. GUIDELINES FOR EXERCISE ECG TESTING

For diagnosis of CAD

Class I: appropriate	Adult patients with an intermediate pretest probability of CAD based on gender, age, and symptoms, including those with RBBB or <1-mm ST depression at rest
IIa: probably appropriate	Patients with vasospastic angina
IIb: possibly appropriate	Patients with high pretest probability of CAD
	Patients with a low pretest probability of CAD
	Patients with <1-mm ST depression at baseline on digoxin
	Patients with LVH and <1-mm ST depression on baseline ECG
III: inappropriate	Preexcitation syndromes (WPW)
	Ventricular-paced rhythm
	>1-mm ST depression at baseline
	Complete LBBB
	Patients with established diagnosis of CAD based on past MI or angiogram

For risk assessment and prognosis in patients with symptoms or history of CAD

Class I: appropriate	Initial evaluation of patients with suspected or known stable CAD, including those with RBBB or <1-mm ST depression at rest
	Patients with known CAD with a significant clinical change
	Low-risk unstable angina patients after ruling out for MI, without angina or HF

(continued)

TABLE 21-2. CONTINUED

	Intermediate-risk unstable angina patients 2–3 days after presenting, without angina or HF
IIa: probably appropriate	Intermediate-risk unstable angina patients after ruling out for MI, without angina or HF
IIb: possibly appropriate	Preexcitation syndromes (WPW)
	Ventricular-paced rhythm
	>1-mm ST depression at baseline
	Complete LBBB
	Patients with a stable clinical course
III: inappropriate	Patients with severe comorbidity likely to limit life expectancy and/or candidacy for revascularization
	High-risk unstable angina patients
After MI	
Class I: appropriate	Before discharge for prognosis and evaluation of medical therapy (given as a submaximal study at 4–7 days)
	Early after discharge for same indications if not done before discharge (symptom-limited study at 14–21 days)
	3–6 wks after discharge to evaluate medical treatment and prognosis in patients who undergo a submaximal test before discharge
IIa: probably appropriate	After discharge for activity prescription as part of rehabilitation in patients who have undergone revascularization
IIb: possibly appropriate	Complete LBBB
	Preexcitation syndrome
	LVH
	Digoxin therapy
	>1-mm resting ST segment depression
	Electronically paced ventricular rhythm
	Periodic monitoring in asymptomatic patients during rehabilitation
III: inappropriate	Severe comorbidities likely to limit life expectancy and/or candidacy for revascularization
	Decompensated HF, arrhythmias, or other serious condition
	Patients who have already undergone cardiac catheterization (borderline lesions should be assessed with imaging)
Exercise testing in asymptomatic individuals without known CAD	
Class I: appropriate	None
IIa: probably appropriate	Asymptomatic patients with diabetes who plan a rigorous exercise program
IIb: possibly appropriate	Guide to risk-reduction therapy
	Asymptomatic patients (male: >45 yrs, female: >55 yrs) who plan to exercise, have jobs impacting public safety, peripheral vascular disease, or chronic renal insufficiency
III: inappropriate	As routine screening

HF, heart failure; LBBB, left bundle-branch block; RBBB, right bundle-branch block; WPW, Wolff-Parkinson-White syndrome.
From Gibbons RJ, Balady GJ, Bricker JT, et al. ACC/AHA 2002 guideline update for exercise testing: summary article: a report of the ACC/AHA Task Force on Practice Guidelines (Committee to Update the 1997 Exercise Testing Guidelines). *Circulation* 2002;106:1883, with permission.

TABLE 21-3. CONTRAINDICATIONS TO EXERCISE STRESS TESTING

Absolute	Relative
Recent (~4 days) STEMI	BP >200/115
Unstable angina	Moderate valvular heart disease
Ventricular arrhythmia, uncontrolled	Electrolyte abnormalities
Atrial arrhythmia, uncontrolled	Fixed-rate pacemaker
Third-degree heart block	Ventricular aneurysm
Acute CHF	Uncontrolled medical disease
Severe aortic stenosis	Chronic infectious disease
Aortic dissection	Medical disorders exacerbated by exercise
Myocarditis, pericarditis, endocarditis	Known left main or proximal LAD stenosis
Recent DVT or PE	HCM
Acute infection	Mental impairment
Patient refusal	
Acute medical disorder	
Psychosis	

DVT, deep venous thrombosis; LAD, left anterior descending coronary artery; PE, pulmonary embolism.
From Fletcher GF, Balady GJ, Amsterdam EA, et al. Exercise standards for testing and training: a statement for healthcare professionals from the American Heart Association. *Circulation* 2001;104:1694–1740, with permission.

Unlike pharmacologic testing, exercise testing provides more reliable information on symptoms, BP response, heart rate response and arrhythmias, and exercise capacity. **High-risk features** include inability to perform 6 mins of the Bruce protocol (see below), ischemia early in the test, >2-mm ST depression, sustained ST depression after cessation of exercise, ischemia at low heart rates, flattened or lowered BP response to exercise, angina that limits exercise, and serious ventricular arrhythmia.

The number of metabolic equivalents (METs) achieved is used to assess exercise capacity. One MET is approximately 3.5 mL O_2/kg/min; 2–3 METs approximates slow walking on flat ground; 4–5 METs approximates doubles tennis; 6–7 METs approximates yard work; 8–9 METs describes a slow jog; 10–11 METs describes a medium jog. Exercise protocols have been established using the treadmill, bicycle ergometer, and hand-grip. Of these, the treadmill is most frequently used in the United States. Protocols share the common features of gradually increasing workload to a peak over 10–12 mins. The **Bruce protocol** is the historical standard and has been modified for use in debilitated patients (lower workload earlier). In general, the speed and grade of incline start low, and each gradually increases in 3-min stages. One MET approximates 1 min on the Bruce protocol.

1 mm of horizontal or downsloping ST depression seen during or after exercise indicates ischemia. It does *not* indicate the site of myocardial ischemia or which vessel is involved. ST-segment elevation is rather specific for the area involved and indicates areas of severe ischemia, unless Q waves were already present in those leads; in this case, the ST elevation suggests aneurysmal change in previously infarcted regions caused by tachycardia and increased contractility of other segments. T wave inversion is not specific for ischemia. Most normal adults show an increase in systolic BP during exercise; a decrease indicates a higher probability of ischemia and grounds for terminating the test (Table 21-4). Variables other than ECG measured during the test include BP, maximal work capacity, heart rate response, and heart rate–pressure product. These can be integrated with ECG changes to improve the prognostic value of the test. The *sensitivity and specificity of exercise ECG testing are approximately 68% and 77%*, respectively. The specificity is reduced by digoxin, LVH, and resting ST-segment/

TABLE 21-4. INDICATIONS FOR EXERCISE STRESS TEST TERMINATION

Absolute

    ST elevation suspicious for acute myocardial injury

    Moderate to severe angina

    Drop in systolic BP

    Serious arrhythmias (high-grade heart block, VT, AF with RVR)

    Severe dyspnea

    CNS symptoms

    Patient request

Relative

    Pronounced (>2 mm) horizontal or downsloping ST depressions

    BP >250/115

    Less serious arrhythmias, including exercise-induced BBB

BBB, bundle-branch block; RVR, rapid ventricular response.
From Fletcher GF, Balady GJ, Amsterdam EA, et al. Exercise standards for testing and training: a statement for healthcare professionals from the American Heart Association. *Circulation* 2001;104:1694–1740, with permission.

T wave changes. Sensitivity is maximized if maximum heart rate reaches 85% of **age-predicted maximum (= 220 – age)**; if the maximum heart rate is below this and there are no ECG changes, the test is **nondiagnostic.** Results of ECG stress testing are reported as normal, abnormal, or nondiagnostic. The **Duke nomogram** allows prediction of annual mortality by incorporating ST changes, amount of anginal symptoms, and exercise capacity. It is less useful in elderly patients as well as those with positive findings on echocardiography or perfusion imaging. The **Duke score = (exercise time in mins) – (5 × the ST-segment deviation in mm) – (4 × the angina index). Angina score value** of 0 is no angina, 1 if angina occurs, and 2 if angina is the reason for stopping the test. A Duke score of ≥ +5 denotes low risk (0.25% annual mortality), –10 to +4 denotes intermediate risk (1.25% annual mortality), and <–10 denotes high risk for cardiovascular events (5% annual mortality).

PHARMACOLOGIC STRESS

Patients who are unable to exercise at sufficient intensity to achieve a target heart rate have several options for testing. The choice of which pharmacologic agent to use depends on the patient and the assessment method being used.

    Coronary vasodilators include **dipyridamole (Persantine)** and **adenosine (Adenocard)**. These agents work on the principle that when they are administered in normal coronary arteries, they produce vasodilatation and increased blood flow. In coronary arteries with stenosis that obstructs flow, the segment distal to the stenosis is maximally vasodilated chronically. Blood is preferentially shunted away from these diseased vessels when normal arteries are vasodilated. Dipyridamole acts by inhibiting adenosine reuptake. It has a much longer half-life than adenosine, and side effects include flushing, AV block, headache, nausea, and chest pain. The effect of dipyridamole may be reversed with aminophylline. Given the extremely short half-life of adenosine, it has fewer side effects than dipyridamole.

    Contraindications to these vasodilators include reactive airway disease, AV block, and allergy to aminophylline or dipyridamole. Patients must not receive caffeine or theophylline for 24–48 hrs before the test.

    These agents are especially useful in patients with left bundle-branch block, those on beta blockers, those who have a paced rhythm, poorly controlled ventricular ectopy, or

poorly controlled HTN. They are not appropriate in patients with moderate to severe COPD or asthma because of bronchospasm.

Positive inotropic agents include **dobutamine (Dobutrex)** and the less frequently used agent **arbutamine (GenESA)**, which are both similar in their effects. Dobutamine causes an increase in myocardial O_2 demand by increasing inotropy and heart rate. These agents may be reversed with beta blockers. If the heart rate response is insufficient with dobutamine alone, it may be augmented with atropine.

These agents are especially useful in patients with moderate to severe COPD or asthma but are not useful in patients with left bundle-branch block, those who are on beta blockers, or those who have a paced rhythm, poorly controlled ventricular ectopy or atrial arhythmias, or poorly controlled HTN.

Atrial pacing can be used as a last resort in patients in whom other methods are contraindicated. Given the invasive nature and poor increase in BP, this technique is rarely used.

IMAGING WITH STRESS TESTS

Most stress testing of inpatients and many stress tests in outpatients occur with some form of imaging. Although this is often not necessary, it is useful in several circumstances. Many patients are unable to exercise due to COPD, peripheral vascular disease, arthritis, or general deconditioning. In addition, ventricular function, valvular function, pulmonary artery pressures, and myocardial viability are all examples of information that imaging adds to exercise or pharmacologic stress testing. The sensitivity of the stress test is usually higher with an imaging modality. Imaging is sometimes useful to further risk-stratify patients with intermediate-risk Duke treadmill scores. The functional significance of a known borderline lesion on angiography can be assessed. Finally, some patients have certain features that render them poor candidates for ECG testing alone (Table 21-5).

Nuclear Imaging

Nuclear imaging studies provide information beyond that obtained from ECG stress testing. Uses for imaging studies include diagnosis of coronary disease in patients with a history of angina or an abnormal exercise ECG. Nuclear imaging potentially localizes the ischemic myocardium. For the diagnosis of coronary disease, the *sensitivity of nuclear imaging is 90%, and the specificity is 74%.* Additional uses include risk

TABLE 21-5. INDICATIONS FOR USE OF NUCLEAR PERFUSION IMAGING STUDY INSTEAD OF EXERCISE ECG

1. Complete left bundle-branch block (should be performed with adenosine)
2. Paced ventricular rhythm (should be performed with adenosine)
3. Conduction abnormalities, such as Wolff-Parkinson-White (may be used with exercise, adenosine, or dobutamine)
4. >1-mm ST depression at rest (may be used with exercise, adenosine, or dobutamine)
5. Inability to reach exercise level sufficient to obtain ECG results (adenosine or dobutamine)
6. Known history of CAD with a history of revascularization (may be used with exercise, adenosine, or dobutamine)

Adapted from Gibbons RJ, Abrams J, Chatterjee K, et al. ACC/AHA 2002 guideline update for the management of patients with chronic stable angina: a report of the American College of Cardiology/American Heart Association Task Force on Practice Guidelines (Committee to Update the 1999 Guidelines for the Management of Patients with Chronic Stable Angina), 2002. Available at www.acc.org/clinical/guidelines/stable/stable.pdf.

stratification in patients with an anginal history before surgery, determination of myocardial viability, and assessment of fixed coronary lesions to determine if they cause symptomatic ischemia. Imaging studies also allow assessment of medical, percutaneous, or surgical therapy for CAD. **High-risk features** include a large perfusion defect, multiple perfusion defects, LV dilatation, and high lung uptake of the tracer.

Patients with recent exposure to radiation should not undergo a nuclear imaging study. All patients should be NPO for at least 4 hrs before the test. In addition, if the stress is to be induced with dipyridamole or adenosine, patients should not receive caffeine for 12 hrs before the test and should not be taking theophylline. See Chap. 22, Imaging and Diagnostic Testing Modalities (Nuclear Imaging, Echocardiography, and Cardiac Catheterization) for details on performing nuclear imaging stress tests.

In addition to nuclear imaging in the setting of stress testing, nuclear perfusion studies can be performed in people with ongoing chest pain but with low liklihood of an ACS [see Chap. 7, Acute Coronary Syndromes (Unstable Angina/Non–ST-Segment Elevation Myocardial Infarction), and Chap. 8, Acute ST-Segment Elevation Myocardial Infarction].

Stress Echocardiography

Echocardiography using an exercise or pharmacologic stress can be useful as a screening test for coronary ischemia or to define the anatomic location of ischemia with similar indications as perfusion imaging. **Stress echocardiography** is based on the increased global contractility of the normal heart during stress. This normally leads to hyperdynamic wall motion, increased heart rate, and increased ejection fraction. Coronary ischemia during stress produces segmental wall motion abnormalities of decreased myocardial thickening and excursion. **High-risk features** include diminished ejection fraction with stress, resting diminished ejection fraction, two or more segments with wall motion abnormalities, and failure to augment contractility at low heart rate or dobutamine dose. When executing this study, a resting echocardiogram is performed first, followed by exercise or drug administration and repeat echocardiogram immediately after the stress. The two sets of images are then compared side by side. If a pharmacologic stress is required, inotropic agents, such as dobutamine, provide a more physiologic approximation of exercise than vasodilators and are more commonly used.

Stress echocardiography is best suited for patients in whom a formal structural assessment of the heart is desired and/or in the setting of the features limiting the sensitivity/specificity of ECG testing alone (Table 21-5). Of these indications, left bundle-branch block and a paced rhythm are reasons to strongly prefer nuclear imaging over echocardiography. For the other four indications, echocardiography may be used. *Sensitivity and specificity of exercise echocardiograms are 80–85% and 85–90%, respectively, whereas those for dobutamine stress are 68–98% and 80–85%, respectively.*

KEY POINTS TO REMEMBER

- Stress testing is useful in risk stratifying patients who are at intermediate risk for CAD based on history, risk factors, and physical exam.
- Exercise stress testing should be the default, unless the patient is unable to exercise or has a significantly abnormal resting ECG.
- The addition of imaging (beyond ECG recording) is not necessary unless other information is desired, or other factors exist that limit the sensitivity/specificity of ECG alone.
- If a patient is unable to walk (peripheral vascular disease, osteoarthritis, severe LV dysfunction, severe deconditioning, COPD), the choice of pharmacologic stress agent depends on the individual patient. Adenosine is a good choice for patients with tachyarrhythmias, left bundle-branch block, or a paced rhythm, whereas dobutamine is a good choice for patients with severe COPD, asthma, or AV block.
- The choice of an imaging modality also depends on the patient. Nuclear studies are more sensitive in extremely overweight patients, those with COPD, and those who cannot receive dobutamine (tachyarrhythmias, severe valvular disease). Echocardi-

ography is more appropriate in patients in whom additional information is desired, such as hemodynamic and valvular disease status. ECG alone is used in the setting of exercise in low- to intermediate-probability patients (and is the correct answer for board examinations regarding stress testing in most intermediate-risk patients).

REFERENCES AND SUGGESTED READINGS

Braunwald E, Zipes DP, Libby P. *Heart disease,* 6th ed. Philadelphia: WB Saunders. 2001:129–160, 273–324.

Fletcher GF, Balady GJ, Amsterdam EA, et al. Exercise standards for testing and training: a statement for healthcare professionals from the American Heart Association. *Circulation* 2001;104:1694–1740.

Gibbons RJ, Abrams J, Chatterjee K, et al. ACC/AHA 2002 guideline update for the management of patients with chronic stable angina: a report of the American College of Cardiology/American Heart Association Task Force on Practice Guidelines (Committee to Update the 1999 Guidelines for the Management of Patients with Chronic Stable Angina), 2002. Available at www.acc.org/clinical/guidelines/stable/stable.pdf.

Gibbons RJ, Abrams J, Chatterjee K, et al. ACC/AHA 2002 guideline update for the management of patients with chronic stable angina—summary article: a report of the American College of Cardiology/American Heart Association Task Force on Practice Guidelines (Committee on the Management of Patients With Chronic Stable Angina). *Circulation* 2003;107:149–158.

Gibbons RJ, Balady GJ, Bricker JT, et al. ACC/AHA 2002 guideline update for exercise testing: a report of the American College of Cardiology/American Heart Association Task Force on Practice Guidelines (Committee on Exercise Testing), 2002. American College of Cardiology Web site. Available at www.acc.org/clinical/guidelines/exercise/dirIndex.htm.

Gibbons RJ, Balady GJ, Bricker JT, et al. ACC/AHA 2002 guideline update for exercise testing: summary article: a report of the ACC/AHA Task Force on Practice Guidelines (Committee to Update the 1997 Exercise Testing Guidelines). *Circulation* 2002;106:1883–1892.

Lee TH, Boucher CA. Noninvasive tests in patients with stable CAD. *N Engl J Med* 2001;344(24):1840–1844.

Marso SP, Griffin BP, Topol EJ, eds. *Manual of cardiovascular medicine.* Philadelphia: Lippincott Williams & Wilkins, 2000.

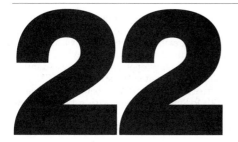

Imaging and Diagnostic Testing Modalities (Nuclear Imaging, Echocardiography, and Cardiac Catheterization)

Douglas R. Bree and
Peter A. Crawford

NUCLEAR IMAGING

Introduction

Nuclear cardiology has evolved over the past two decades to become an integral discipline in noninvasive diagnostic testing for CAD as well as LV systolic function. Use of radionuclide imaging modalities provides information in the diagnosis of CAD, assessment of myocardial viability, and risk stratification/prognosis in known CAD. Advances in radiopharmaceuticals, imaging equipment, and techniques have increased testing sensitivity and specificity. Assessment of cardiac function is also available using gated-imaging techniques. A variety of different methods to induce cardiac stress and imaging agents exist, and the clinician must be aware of differences among these options to obtain the appropriate data.

Indications

Several clinical scenarios exist in which cardiac stress testing is considered warranted (see Chap. 6, Stable Angina; Chap. 7, Acute Coronary Syndromes (Unstable Angina/Non–ST-Segment Elevation Myocardial Infarction); Chap. 8, Acute ST-Segment Elevation Myocardial Infarction; and Chap. 21, Noninvasive Cardiac Assessment for Coronary Artery Disease).

In addition to the indications for stress testing (see Chap. 21, Noninvasive Cardiac Assessment for Coronary Artery Disease), several guidelines exist for the use of **nuclear imaging.** The ACC/AHA guidelines provide specific indications for the use of radionuclide perfusion imaging rather than ECG in the following situations:

- Complete left bundle-branch block
- Electronically paced ventricular rhythm
- Preexcitation (Wolff-Parkinson-White) syndrome
- >1 mm of ST-segment depression at rest
- Inability to exercise to achieve adequate stress
- Angina and a history of revascularization

Perfusion imaging is also useful **before or after revascularization.** It is used to demonstrate ischemia and viability before revascularization (class I indication), evaluate recurrent symptoms after revascularization (class I), and occasionally to assess the significance of a lesion on which no intervention was performed.

The use of nuclear imaging is generally thought to be more beneficial than routine ECG stress tests due to improved sensitivity and specificity. Using data from multiple trials, the sensitivity and specificity for exercise ECG testing are 68% and 77%, respectively [1]. These values increase to 88% and 77% if the study is performed with single-photon emission CT (SPECT) with radionucleotide imaging [1].

Contraindications

- **Standard contraindications to stress testing:** Discussed in Chap. 6, Stable Angina, and Chap. 21, Noninvasive Cardiac Assessment for Coronary Artery Disease.

- **Contraindications to use of dipyridamole (Persantine) or adenosine (Adeno-card):** History of asthma or wheezing on exam, allergy to dipyridamole, allergy to aminophylline (which reverses bronchospasm), caffeine consumption within 12–24 hrs, high-grade AV block, ongoing theophylline (Bronkodyl, Elixophyllin, Slo-bid, Uniphyl, Slo-Phyllin, Theo-24) treatment (should be stopped 36 hrs before exam).
- **Relative contraindications to dobutamine:** Significant aortic stenosis or HCM, significant tachyarrhythmias; also less effective if recent (<12 hrs) beta blocker use.
- **Contraindications to nuclear studies [2]:** Iodine-131 therapy within 12 wks, **technetium-99m** studies within 48 hrs, indium-111 scans within 30 days, gallium-67 scans within 30 days, recent PO intake (except for water), recent caffeine consumption (4 hrs).

STRESS AGENTS

Exercise

Exercise is the **stress agent of choice,** as it provides functional and prognostic information that pharmacologic stress does not provide. Using standard exercise protocols (see Chap. 6, Stable Angina, and Chap. 21, Noninvasive Cardiac Assessment for Coronary Artery Disease), the patient is asked to signal when his or her exercise threshold is about to be reached. At this point, the radioisotope is injected, and exercise continues for an additional minute to allow adequate agent perfusion.

Dipyridamole

Dipyridamole (Persantine) inhibits the metabolism of adenosine and acts as a coronary vasodilator that selectively dilates normal arteries, leaving stenotic arteries with a relative lower flow rate. The infusion lasts for 4 mins, after which the radioisotope is injected. As mentioned in Contraindications above, dipyridamole is contraindicated in bronchospastic lung diseases and in patients who have recently taken theophylline or caffeine. The effects of dipyridamole can be reversed by aminophylline (Phyllocontin, Truphylline), 50–100 mg IV bolus.

Adenosine

Adenosine has the safety benefit of a much shorter half-life than dipyridamole. The infusion lasts for 6 mins (0.142 μg/kg/min), with radioisotope injection administered at 3 mins. Reversal of the effects is similar to dipyridamole but is rarely needed due to the short half-life of this agent. It may cause AV block.

Dobutamine

Dobutamine (Dobutrex) causes increased myocardial work by stimulation of beta-adrenergic receptors. In the setting of nuclear perfusion imaging, it is used primarily in asthmatic patients who are unable to exercise (also in patients scheduled for echocardiographic imaging). Patients previously taking beta blockers should hold dosing for 4–5 half-lives before test if feasible. Infusion is started at 5 μg/kg/min and increased in graded steps until maximal heart rate is achieved (maximum dose = 40 μg/kg/min). Additional atropine may be given to help obtain maximal heart rate. Side effects include chest pain, flushing, nausea, palpitations, dyspnea, and frequently ectopy. The effects are reversed by IV beta blockade at the study's conclusion (e.g., esmolol or metoprolol).

RADIOPHARMACEUTICALS (RADIONUCLIDES)

- Thallium-201
  - General information
    - Produced in a cyclotron.
    - Half-life = 73 hrs.
    - Acts similarly to potassium (imported to cells by Na-K-ATPase).

- Kinetics
  - Initial uptake in myocytes is approximately 85% [3] and is directly proportional to regional blood flow.
  - Extraction increases with slow flow rates and decreases with fast flow rates.
  - After initial extraction, **thallium** redistributes throughout the myocardium, with a slower rate of "washout" occurring in regions with limited perfusion.
  - Therefore, lack of uptake in a region immediately after injection demonstrates lack of regional blood flow, and lack of redistribution on delayed images demonstrates decreased myocardial viability.
- Technetium-99m (sestamibi)
  - General information
    - Produced on-site in molybdenum-99–technetium-99m generators.
    - Half-life = 6 hrs.
    - Enters myocytes by passive diffusion and binds to cell membranes (mitochondria primarily).
    - Shorter half-life allows larger doses for gated images for assessment of ventricular function [assuming a regular heart rhythm (no AF or frequent PVC)].
  - Kinetics
    - Approximately 65% extraction on first pass [3].
    - Uptake related directly to myocardial perfusion.
    - Very slow to no redistribution occurs.

IMAGING PROTOCOLS

Nuclear imaging employs radiopharmaceuticals with SPECT imaging to provide information about myocardial perfusion and ventricular function. Different protocols used for stress testing include

- Thallium stress/redistribution
  - Thallium given at stress with images, then redistribution images taken at approximately 4 hrs for rest imaging (or longer for viability).
  - Advantages: simplicity, low cost.
  - Disadvantages: increased time, no gated images for estimation of LV ejection fraction.
- Thallium stress/reinjection
  - Thallium given at stress with images, then reinjection at 4 hrs for rest imaging (or longer for viability).
  - Advantage: improved viability imaging.
  - Disadvantages: time, cost of reinjection, no gated images.
- Technetium rest/stress
  - Technetium given at rest with images, then given with stress and images taken at later time.
  - Advantages: better image quality, ability to obtain gated images, ability to perform stress without immediately acquiring images.
  - Disadvantages: poorer assessment of viability, higher cost, decreased extraction fraction during increased flow periods.
- Dual isotope
  - Thallium given at rest with images, then technetium-sestamibi given with stress and images obtained.
  - Advantages: speed of study, ability to test for viability, ability to obtain gated images.
  - Disadvantage: higher cost.
  - Despite high cost, it is nevertheless the test of choice in many centers.

TYPES OF DEFECTS

- **Fixed:** Areas without tracer uptake in both stress and rest images; can represent either scarring or hibernating myocardium. Delayed imaging or rest reinjection with thallium helps differentiate viable myocardium from scar; determined by improvement in tracer uptake.

- **Reversible:** Areas without tracer uptake on stress images that resolve in rest or delayed imaging; suggests myocardial ischemia.
- **Partially reversible:** Defects present on stress but improve on resting images, although they do not completely return to uniform uptake; typically considered to be a combination of both myocardial ischemia and scar.

Viability assessment can be made with nuclear imaging studies. If a fixed perfusion deficit is present, then reinjection of thallium with reimaging 6–24 hrs later can be performed. If the region persists in its poor uptake of thallium, the region is termed a **scar.** If fixed defect shows evidence of perfusion on reinjection images, the region is termed **hibernating** and may benefit from revascularization. This is in contrast to **stunned** myocardium, which appears perfused but exhibits diminished wall motion. Stunned myocardium usually occurs in a periinfarct territory and, with revascularization, improves function over days to weeks. Note that the gold standard for assessing the viability of myocardium is PET, but SPECT is commonly used for practical issues. **High-risk features** include a large perfusion defect, multiple perfusion defects, LV dilatation, and high lung uptake of the tracer.

ASSESSMENT OF LEFT VENTRICULAR SYSTOLIC FUNCTION

In addition to the ability to use gated imaging to assess LV systolic function in the setting of perfusion imaging, radionuclides can be used solely for the assessment of LV and RV systolic function by a test called **radionuclide ventriculogram (RVG).** **Multigated acquisition (MUGA)** uses ECG-derived gating to compare blood pool images with the cardiac cycle. The blood pool is labeled by acquiring a 2-cc sample of the patient's blood and tagging the erythrocytes with technetium-99m. An ejection fraction is calculated.

ECHOCARDIOGRAPHY

Introduction

The use of **echocardiography** in modern cardiology is widespread in the diagnosis and assessment of a multitude of indications. The resting echocardiography study provides valuable information about cardiac anatomy and specific structures (i.e., valve function, septal defects, pericardial diseases); Doppler imaging helps further assessment of hemodynamics; **stress echocardiography** provides information regarding areas of ischemia; and TEE can help assess the aorta, valvular structures, and atrial anatomy accurately. Indications for echocardiography are numerous, and the usefulness of information gained from these studies has taken an increasingly important role in the management of many cardiac conditions.

Two-Dimensional Imaging (Resolution of 30 Frames/Sec)

Standard Views

See Fig. 22-1 for an example.

- **Parasternal long axis:** Obtained with the probe positioned in the fifth intercostal space at the lower left sternal border with the probe marker pointing toward the right shoulder. This view (Fig. 22-1) gives a longitudinal perspective of the LV, with views of mitral and aortic valves along with anteroseptal and posterior wall segments (but not the apical segments).
- **Parasternal short axis:** From the parasternal long-axis view, the transducer is rotated 90 degrees so that the marker points to the left shoulder. This provides a cross-sectional view of the LV. With various degrees of angulation, views can be obtained at the level of the aortic valve, the mitral valve, and the papillary muscles.
- **Apical four-chamber view:** With the marker pointing toward the left shoulder, the transducer may now be brought to the cardiac apex. This view allows visualization of all four chambers of the heart and is useful in measuring ventricular dimensions,

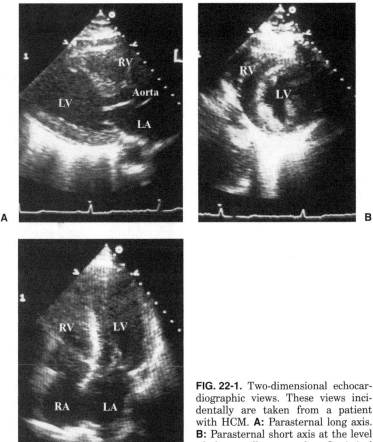

FIG. 22-1. Two-dimensional echocardiographic views. These views incidentally are taken from a patient with HCM. **A:** Parasternal long axis. **B:** Parasternal short axis at the level of the papillary muscles. **C:** Apical four-chamber view. LA, left atria; RA, right atrium.

as well as mitral inflow patterns and Doppler tissue imaging. Slight angulation cranially enables visualization of the aortic valve (the five-chamber view).

- **Apical two-chamber view:** Still at the apex, the transducer is now rotated so the marker again faces the right shoulder. This view displays the LV longitudinally but with better visualization of the apex along with the anterior and inferior walls.

Wall Segment Model

The American Society of Echocardiography classification system uses the above four standard views to help divide the LV into a uniform 16-segment reporting system. Circumferentially, the ventricle is divided into anterior, lateral, posterior, inferior, septal, and anteroseptal segments. Longitudinally, the ventricle is divided into basal, mid, and apical segments. The apical segments are divided circumferentially into four, rather than six, segments (ant, lat, inf, sep), thus giving a total of 16 segments (6 + 6 + 4 = 16).

Wall Motion Grading

The uniform system to grade each segment for wall motion is as follows: 1 = normal, 2 = hypokinetic, 3 = akinetic, 4 = dyskinetic, 5 = aneurysmal. In some centers, the average of these scores, the segmental wall motion index, is reported to help track ventricular function.

M-Mode Echocardiography (Resolution of 1000 Frames/Sec)

Although two-dimensional imaging provides a satisfying picture of the heart in real time, M-mode imaging adds helpful information to the echocardiographic study by providing a one-dimensional sampling line through the heart that shows the cardiac structures related to time. M-mode has existed longer than two-dimensional imaging. The vertical axis represents tissue depth of the image, and the horizontal axis is a representation of time. The information obtained provides objective data regarding cardiac chamber dimensions, wall thickness, fractional shortening, and valve motion. M-mode provides much higher resolution than two-dimensional in terms of time.

Doppler Echocardiography

Color-Flow Mapping

Color-flow mapping applies a color image superimposed on a two-dimensional image. The color is dependent on the **velocity** of flow and the **direction** of flow relative to the transducer. Typically, flow toward the transducer is red, and flow away is blue. Turbulent flow produces a mosaic or, in some systems, a green image (known as **aliasing**). This technique is useful in detecting valvular dysfunction (stenosis or regurgitation), as well as shunting through anatomic defects.

Spectral Doppler

This technique shows the graphic relationship between blood flow velocity and time. Similarly to M-mode, the U/S beam is projected through a single line. Color-flow mapping in two-dimensional images is performed to guide proper placement of the sampling beam. It is important that the sampling beam be positioned within 20 degrees of the direction of blood flow for results to be considered accurate. Flow velocity can be measured by **pulsed-wave (PW)** or **continuous-wave (CW)** Doppler techniques. PW Doppler sends short bursts of U/S beams at a specific frequency and is, therefore, useful to interrogate flow velocities at a discrete location in the line of measure. CW Doppler continuously sends and receives U/S information and is helpful in determining the maximal velocity at any point along the line of measure. The use of spectral Doppler is helpful in multiple regards:

- **Diastolic function:** PW measurement of mitral inflow velocity reveals E wave (early diastolic filling) and a wave (atrial contraction). Typically, E wave is $>a$ wave; E/a wave reversal suggests impaired relaxation; and if E wave is $>>a$ wave, then a restrictive filling pattern is suggested (more severe diastolic dysfunction). "Pseudonormal" pattern is a stage between impaired relaxation and restrictive filling patterns. In this setting, Valsalva maneuver often unveils E/a reversal.
- **Assessment of pulmonary artery (PA) pressure:** In the presence of tricuspid regurgitation, a CW assessment of peak flow across the valve provides an estimated RV systolic pressure when estimated right atrial pressure is added to the gradient. In the absence of pulmonary stenosis this provides an accurate estimate of PA systolic pressure using **the modified Bernoulli equation** (peak pressure gradient = $4 \times$ velocity^2).
  - An important example of an application of this method is the assessment of PA pressure. The systolic BP in the PA is assessed by using the velocity of the tricuspid regurgitant jet in the modified Bernoulli's equation, which provides the systolic pressure gradient between the right atrium and RV. Adding the right atrial pressure to this result gives the PA systolic pressure, assuming there is no gradient between the RV and PA (such as pulmonic stenosis). The right atrial pressure is estimated according to inferior vena cava (IVC) size: 0–5 mm Hg if normal-diameter IVC collapses >50% on inspiration; 5–10 mm Hg if IVC is mildly dilated and collapse normally; 10–15 mm Hg if mildly dilated IVC only partially collapses with inspiration; 15–20 mm Hg if dilated IVC does not collapse. Thus, for a velocity of 2.5 m/sec in the setting of a normal IVC, the systolic BP in the PA is 30 mm Hg.

- **Assessment of stenoses and other obstructions:** The estimation of pressure gradient across a narrowing can be made based on the velocity immediately after the obstruction, using the modified Bernoulli equation. The severity of aortic stenosis or mitral stenosis can be determined, for example (see Chap. 13, Valvular Heart Disease).
- **Cardiac output:** A CW Doppler envelope over the aortic outflow provides the velocity-time integral (VTI). The area under this envelope is directly proportional to cardiac output and can actually help estimate cardiac output if the aortic root area and heart rate are also measured.

Stress Echocardiography

Introduction
Stress echocardiography is an effective technique for the assessment of CAD, detection of viable myocardium, and localization of significant coronary artery lesions. The interpretation of stress echocardiography depends on the typical response of myocardial wall segments to become hypercontractile with increased stress. The assessment of focal wall motion abnormalities provides anatomic information suggestive of ischemia. For indications for this form of stress testing, see Chap. 21, Noninvasive Cardiac Assessment for Coronary Artery Disease.

Imaging
Before the stress portion, a resting study is performed, along with a single cardiac cycle in each of the four standard views stored digitally. The patient is stressed by dobutamine or exercise, and stress images are obtained in the four standard views. With pharmacologic stress, images are taken with each level of agent infused. With exercise stress, the images are obtained as rapidly as possible after the patient has exercised to maximal capacity. A single cardiac cycle is digitized for side-by-side comparison. The addition of echocardiographic contrast agents may be warranted to improve accuracy, particularly for patients with technically difficult studies. For image interpretation, the rest and stress images may be displayed synchronously. Full interpretation of the study requires review of the digital images and videotape. The degree of wall thickening is the parameter of interest, with each wall segment under careful scrutiny.

Stress Modalities
EXERCISE. Again, exercise is the preferred method of stress, as it reproduces physiologic conditions, provides independent prognostic information, and is sensitive if the patient can exercise to reach maximal heart rate. A standard Bruce protocol provides functional assessment of exercise tolerance and prognosis using the Duke treadmill score (see Chap. 6, Stable Angina, and Chap. 21, Noninvasive Cardiac Assessment for Coronary Artery Disease).

DOBUTAMINE. Dobutamine causes an increase in heart rate and hyperdynamic wall motion, and it is indicated for patients unable to exercise or in patients with resting wall motion abnormalities to assess viability during inotrope infusion. Images are taken at infusion rates of 10 μg/kg/min, 30 μg/kg/min, and maximal dose. For patients who have not achieved maximal heart rate with 40 μg/kg/min infusion, atropine may be given (to max. 1–2 mg IV) and/or dobutamine may be increased to 50 μg/kg/min for a brief period.

Interpretation
Image interpretation is subjective, and accurate readings are highly dependent on the skill of the reader. The images obtained in the standard four-chamber view provide assessment of all 16 segments of wall motion. The normal response to stress is an increase in contractility in all segments. A new wall motion abnormality with stress is suggestive of ischemia. A segment that is impaired at rest but worsens with stress is also suggestive of ischemia. A segment that is akinetic and shows no improvement is **scar.** A segment that is akinetic but shows improvement with stress is **viable.** A normal or impaired segment that shows little or no improvement with stress is said to have **impaired contractile reserve,** which could be due to ischemia, severe HTN, or cardiomyopathy.

Dobutamine echocardiography is also useful in **patients with underlying LV dysfunction** to assess the functional and perfusion status of myocardial segments with abnormal function. In this case, a lower dose of dobutamine is used and is slowly increased during the test. Assessment is made for improvement of the baseline wall motion abnormalities with dobutamine. If there is no improvement, then the segment is **scar.** If there is initial improvement that continues to improve, the myocardium is **viable.** If initial improvement subsequently worsens at higher doses of dobutamine (which increase demand), a **biphasic response** has been demonstrated; this indicates **viable but ischemic** tissue that would possibly benefit from revascularization.

CORONARY ARTERIOGRAPHY/ANGIOGRAPHY (CARDIAC CATHETERIZATION)

Introduction

Selective coronary arteriography is considered the gold-standard imaging technique in the evaluation of CAD. It involves the injection of iodinated contrast material directly into the coronary arteries and the heart. It is common practice in cardiology, with ever-increasing numbers of centers and cardiologists performing these studies. The data obtained from cardiac catheterization are invaluable in the management of CAD, as they provide specific information regarding severity and location of coronary lesions. The attendant risks of left-heart catheterization are significant, and adequate experience in performing the study is paramount for study accuracy and patient safety. The expanding field of interventional cardiology has seen rapid advancements in catheter-based techniques in the treatment of CAD that are beyond the scope of this chapter; therefore, what follows is a primer on the technique of diagnostic coronary arteriography. See Chap. 6, Stable Angina, Chap. 7, Acute Coronary Syndromes (Unstable Angina/Non–ST-Segment Elevation Myocardial Infarction), and Chap. 8, Acute ST-Segment Elevation Myocardial Infarction, for a description of the appropriate use of balloon angioplasty and stenting.

Indications

Acute MI

Cardiac catheterization in the setting of acute STEMI is dependent on the volume of the center performing the study and must have the urgent goal of reperfusion by primary angioplasty. For patients in an appropriate center in whom percutaneous coronary intervention (PCI) is planned, patients with new ST-segment elevations or presumably new left bundle-branch block within 12 hrs of symptom onset, coronary angiography is a class I indication as an alternative to thrombolytic therapy. In addition, for those presenting within 36 hrs of symptom onset who are in cardiogenic shock and are <75 yrs, coronary angiography is a class I indication. For patients receiving thrombolytic therapy, catheterization is considered class I for patients with persistent pain or unresolved ECG findings, but it is class III in patients who have clinically reperfused.

Acute Coronary Syndromes (Unstable Angina/Non–ST-Segment Elevation MI)

The role for early (within 48 hrs) cardiac catheterization in patients with acute coronary syndromes (NSTEMI, unstable angina) has become more widely accepted [see Chap. 7, Acute Coronary Syndromes (Unstable Angina/Non–ST-Segment Elevation Myocardial Infarction)]. **Any patient with elevated troponin, new ST-segment depression, angina with CHF or worsening mitral regurgitation, decreased LV function, hemodynamic instability, a high-risk result on stress testing, sustained VT, prior PCI within 6 mos, prior bypass surgery, or recurrent rest angina despite medical therapy merits coronary angiography within 48 hrs, if stable, and sooner if unstable** (Class I).

Chronic Stable Angina

Considered class I indication if poorly controlled on maximal medical regimen, but class III if angina is satisfactorily controlled. Additional Class I indications include high-risk results on stress testing (Duke score of –11 or lower, ejection fraction <35%, significant perfusion imaging defects and/or wall motion abnormalities), patients surviving a sudden cardiac death, and patients with sustained monomorphic VT or nonsustained polymorphic VT.

Ventricular Arrhythmia

Patients with sustained VT or sudden cardiac death without other clear causes merit a class I indication as an alternative modality to stress testing.

Relative Contraindications

Coagulopathy

In elective cases, coagulopathy should be corrected before catheterization. Recommendations include holding warfarin 3 days prior and stopping heparin 2 hrs before arterial puncture. Thrombocytopenia (platelet count <50,000) or INR >2 also substantially increases bleeding risk and should be corrected if possible.

Renal Failure

Contrast-induced nephrotoxicity poses a considerable risk for a percentage of potential catheterization candidates. The risks of this complication must be considered against the management benefit on a case-by-case basis. Risks include advanced age, underlying renal insufficiency, diabetes, and the amount of dye used. Optimization of fluid status and renal function before catheterization may help limit this possibility, but the risk of dialysis should be discussed before the study. Pre- and postprocedure IV saline is the best known renal protective agent. In addition, N-acetylcysteine (Mucomyst) is used (600 mg PO bid on the day before, the day of, and the day after catheterization) in patients with baseline renal insufficiency; a few studies have demonstrated a protective effect for patients receiving contrast for CT scans or cardiac catheterization [4,5].

Dye Allergy

Seek an adequate history of IV contrast administration, and consider significant adverse reactions. In many cases, the reaction is minor and generally well tolerated, and the patient can simply have a standard premedication regimen (see Preparation for Study).

Infection

Patients with active infections may have catheterization deferred pending resolution of the infection, if feasible. Local infection over a puncture site warrants consideration of alternative sites.

Uncontrolled HTN

Manage severe HTN before catheterization.

Decompensated Heart Failure

Optimize treatment before catheterization, **unless coronary ischemia is causative, which is a class I indication for cardiac catheterization.**

Preparation for Study

The patient should be NPO for at least 6 hrs before the procedure.

Informed Consent

Before the study, complete an open discussion with the patient and family that outlines the purposes of the test, what it involves, the risks involved with catheterization, as well as alternatives and the proposed benefits. Make specific mention of a risk for MI of approximately 0.05% and a risk of death of 0.1%. Discuss additional plans in case further intervention, by either catheter or surgery, may be necessary based on the study results.

Medications

Patients should hold anticoagulant medications, as listed in Contraindications. Withhold metformin in patients undergoing coronary arteriography, as lactic acidosis can result if renal failure occurs. Other oral hypoglycemics should also be withheld on day of test, because patient is NPO. ASA is typically given before the study, and clopidogrel (Plavix), 300 mg PO, can be given in patients about to have intervention. The continuation of heparin and glycoprotein IIb–IIIa inhibitors is patient and operator dependent. Discontinue NSAIDS to limit additional nephrotoxins.

Premedication

In patients with prior dye allergy, a regimen of steroids and histamine-blocking agents can be given before catheterization. One regimen includes prednisone, 50 mg PO q6h for four doses; famotidine (Pepcid), 20 mg PO q12h for two doses; and diphenhydramine (Benadryl), 50 mg IV on call to the catheterization lab.

IV Fluids

In patients with renal insufficiency, administering IV fluids before catheterization can help avoid any prerenal insults added to the dye load (this must be weighed against the patient's volume status). The contrast dye also can cause a large osmotic diuresis after catheterization, and pericatheterization fluids help prevent hypovolemia in all patients not in heart failure. Give special consideration to patients with poor systolic function to avoid pulmonary edema. Mucomyst can be given in the setting of underlying renal insufficiency (see Renal Failure).

Procedure

Arterial Access

Typically, the femoral artery is used for most cardiac catheterizations unless patients have contraindications to this approach, such as severe peripheral artery disease, abdominal aortic aneurysm, prior grafting in the area, or overlying infection (the radial or brachial artery can be used in these cases). The cannulation of the femoral artery should occur approximately 2–3 cm below the inguinal ligament. This helps minimize potential complications, such as retroperitoneal bleeding from a superior puncture and pseudoaneurysm or AV fistula formation from an inferior site. Once the artery is entered, use the Seldinger technique to cannulate the artery with the introducer catheter. In most diagnostic cases, a 6-Fr. (1-Fr. = 0.3 mm) system is used. For planned interventions, an 8-Fr. system is used. Alternative access sites, such as radial and brachial arteries, may be used in special circumstances.

Engaging the Vessels

Using fluoroscopic guidance, any of a wide variety of catheters is advanced to selectively engage the coronary arteries. Difficulty in engaging a native vessel or bypass graft can be countered with a variety of techniques applied by the cardiologist, including use of specialized catheters and special catheter manipulations with advancement and torque. Usually, the left main coronary artery is engaged first, and views of the left system are obtained. This is followed by the right coronary artery, internal mammary arteries, and then grafts arising from the anterior aorta, such as saphenous vein grafts and radial artery grafts, are injected and imaged.

Views

Typically, low- or isoosmolar and nonionic contrast is selected, as these have been demonstrated to be safer in ACS, chronic renal insufficiency, heart failure, or history of contrast allergy. Several views of each coronary artery are obtained to assess degrees of stenosis in multiple planes to improve diagnostic accuracy. The views are taken with varying degrees of angulation in multiple planes. The common vernacular describing the views includes left anterior oblique, right anterior oblique, and anteroposterior, each with varying degrees of cranial (beam toward feet) or caudal (beam toward head) angulation. The title of the view indicates the position of the source of the x-ray in relation to the patient. Therefore, an easy way to orient to the specific view is to remember that left anterior oblique projections display the spine on the right, and vice versa. Any lesions that are seen in one view must have a perpendicular view taken to accurately assess the degree of stenosis. A substantial amount of error can occur if a lesion is eccentric and viewed in only one plane.

Left Ventriculography

A pigtail catheter can be advanced across most native aortic valves without much difficulty to obtain important data regarding the LV. Attempts to pass a stenotic aortic valve can prove much more difficult, even for experienced cardiologists; crossing a mechanical valve is contraindicated.

- **LV end-diastolic pressure (LVEDP):** Once the ventricle has been entered and the cardiac rhythm stabilizes, the catheter may be used to monitor ventricular pressure. High LVEDP (>25 mm Hg) is associated with heart failure (both systolic and diastolic.) If the LVEDP is normal, the patient may proceed to left ventriculography.
- **Left ventriculogram:** In patients without elevated LVEDP or renal dysfunction, the injection of 30–50 cc of contrast under cineangiography can provide useful information. The images are usually obtained in the 30-degree right anterior oblique projection and provide information on regional contractility of anterior, apical, and inferior walls. It also helps assess any degree of mitral regurgitation that may be present.

Postcatheterization Care

Sheath Removal
The introducer sheath is commonly removed after completion of the procedure unless repeat catheterization for intervention is possible. After local anesthesia is given, the sheath is removed, and direct manual pressure is applied for >20 mins to provide hemostasis. Bed rest is required for a duration that depends on the size of the sheath used, as well as other parameters; requirements differ between operators, centers, and closure techniques. Observe closely for bleeding or hematoma formation.

Closure Devices
A variety of closure devices exist to help decrease bleeding complications and allow earlier ambulation.

- **Angio-Seal and VasoSeal:** These are biodegradable collagen plugs deployed at the puncture site; they require no manual pressure and allow ambulation after <1 hr.
- **Perclose:** A percutaneous suture device that closes the arterial puncture site and allows immediate ambulation.

Complications

Death
Overall risk of death during cardiac catheterization is 0.1%. The likelihood increases on several clinical variables, including emergent catheterizations, patients with left main coronary disease, and patients with advanced age.

MI
The risk of causing an MI during catheterization is 0.05%. Possible causes include disruption of previous coronary plaque, coronary dissection, and large air emboli.

Arrhythmias
There is a 0.5% chance of VF during catheterization. This complication can occur particularly during engagement and injection of the right coronary artery. Treatment includes rapid electrical cardioversion.

Emergent CABG
Address this possibility before catheterization, in case the patient is found to have critical disease or a complication from catheterization or percutaneous intervention needing emergent CABG.

Cerebrovascular Accident
The risk of cerebrovascular accident is 0.05%. This complication may occur by disruption of an aortic plaque or by injection of air though the catheter.

Vascular Complications
Multiple complications may arise at the site of arterial puncture, including **pseudoaneurysms**, large **hematomas, arteriovenous fistulas, arterial thrombosis,** and **retroperito-**

neal bleeding. Cumulatively, these events are not uncommon in the practice of cardiac catheterization, and diligent monitoring of a patient's site is important to diagnose these complications rapidly. **Use of U/S** in patients with evidence of a large groin hematoma is essential in the early diagnosis and management of these vascular problems. Consider **retroperitoneal bleeding** in a patient who complains of new back pain and experiences a drop in hemoglobin and/or BP. The appropriate study used to diagnose this bleeding is a noncontrast abdominal CT scan, and consultation with the vascular surgery service is appropriate, as is maintaining an active type and cross, discontinuing anticoagulants (only if the bleed is hemodynamically significant), and transfusing as needed.

Miscellaneous
Hypotension (vasodilation from the contrast), transient myocardial dysfunction, and osmotic diuresis–induced hypovolemia are also possible. IV fluid is usually given after the procedure to prevent some of these effects.

Infection
Infection is rare and is minimized by proper sterile technique. Prophylactic antibiotics are not routinely given for diagnostic cases.

Renal Failure
The administration of contrast dye during catheterization may cause renal dysfunction in some patients, particularly in those with preexisting renal dysfunction, dehydration, advanced age, or diabetes mellitus. To prevent this complication, patients are commonly prehydrated before the procedure, and a limited amount of contrast dye is used during the procedure. Mucomyst is also used (see Contraindications).

KEY POINTS TO REMEMBER

- Imaging tests in cardiology are important components of the assessment of CAD, ventricular function, and valvular function.
- The choice of exercise ECG, nuclear perfusion imaging, and echocardiography with stress testing depends on a number of patient characteristics, including the baseline ECG and the patient's ability to walk.
- Cardiac catheterization with coronary angiography is an extremely powerful tool, but because it is an invasive procedure, it is selected for relatively high-risk patients.
- Consult an attending cardiologist when planning cardiac catheterization, even when the indication for the test seems readily apparent. After the results of coronary angiography are obtained, the decision-making process with regard to revascularization and future medical management will benefit significantly from cardiology evaluation.

SUGGESTED READING

Bhatt DL. Left heart catheterization. In: Marso SP, Griffin BP, Topol EJ, eds. *Manual of cardiovascular medicine*. Philadelphia: Lippincott Williams & Wilkins, 2000.

Bonow RO. Identification of viable myocardium. *Circulation* 1996;94:2674–2680.

Braunwald E, Antman EM, Beasley JW, et al. ACC/AHA 2002 guideline update for the management of patients with unstable angina and non-ST-segment elevation myocardial infarction: a report of the American College of Cardiology/American Heart Association Task Force on Practice Guidelines (Committee on the Management of Patients With Unstable Angina). 2002. Available at: http://www.acc.org/clinical/guidelines/unstable/unstable.pdf.

Deedy M. Stress echocardiography. In: Marso SP, Griffin BP, Topol EJ, eds. *Manual of cardiovascular medicine*. Philadelphia: Lippincott Williams & Wilkins, 2000.

DeMaria AN, Blanchard DG. The echocardiogram. In: Alexander RW, Schlant RC, Fuster V, et al., eds. *Hurst's the heart,* 10th ed. New York: McGraw-Hill, 2000.

Gibbons RJ, Abrams J, Chatterjee K, et al. ACC/AHA 2002 guideline update for the management of patients with chronic stable angina: a report of the American College of

Cardiology/American Heart Association Task Force on Practice Guidelines (Committee to Update the 1999 Guidelines for the Management of Patients with Chronic Stable Angina). 2002. Available at http://www.acc.org/clinical/guidelines/stable/stable.pdf.

Grubb NR, Newby DE. Echocardiography. In: *Churchill's pocketbook of cardiology.* Edinburgh: Churchill Livingstone, 2000.

Lin S, Armstrong G. Transthoracic echocardiography. In: Marso SP, Griffin BP, Topol EJ, eds. *Manual of cardiovascular medicine.* Philadelphia: Lippincott Williams & Wilkins, 2000.

Patterson RE, Eisner RL, Williams BR. Nuclear cardiology. In: Alexander RW, Schlant RC, Fuster V, et al., eds. *Hurst's the heart,* 10th ed. New York: McGraw-Hill, 2000.

Ryan TJ, Antman EM, Brooks NH, et al. 1999 update: ACC/AHA guidelines for the management of patients with acute myocardial infarction: executive summary and recommendations: a report of the American College of Cardiology/American Heart Association Task Force on Practice Guidelines (Committee on Management of Acute Myocardial Infarction). *Circulation* 1999;100:1016–1030.

Scanlon PJ, Faxon DP, Audet AM, et al. ACC/AHA guidelines for coronary angiography: a report of the American College of Cardiology/American Heart Association Task Force on Practice Guidelines (Committee on Coronary Angiography). *J Am Coll Cardiol* 1999;33:1756–1824

Skiles JA. Nuclear imaging. In: Marso SP, Griffin BP, Topol EJ, eds. *Manual of cardiovascular medicine.* Philadelphia: Lippincott Williams & Wilkins, 2000.

Wackers FJT, Soufer R, Zaret BL. Nuclear cardiology. In: Braunwald E, ed. *Heart disease: a textbook of cardiovascular medicine,* 5th ed. Philadelphia: WB Saunders, 1997.

REFERENCES

1. Cole C. Exercise electrocardiographic testing. In: Marso SP, Griffin BP, Topol EJ, eds. *Manual of cardiovascular medicine.* Philadelphia: Lippincott Williams & Wilkins, 2000.

2. Nissen SE. Shortcomings of coronary angiography and their implications in clinical practice. *Cleve Clin J Med* 1999;66(8):479–485.

3. Lee TH, Boucher CA. Noninvasive tests in patients with stable coronary artery disease. *N Engl J Med* 2001;344:1840–1844.

4. Tepel M, van der Giet M, Schwarzfeld C, et al. Prevention of radiographic-contrast-agent-induced reductions in renal function by acetylcysteine. *N Engl J Med* 2000;343:180–184.

5. Shyu KG, Cheng JJ, Kuan P. Acetylcysteine protects against acute renal damage in patients with abnormal renal function undergoing a coronary procedure. *J Am Coll Cardiol* 2002;40:1383–1388.

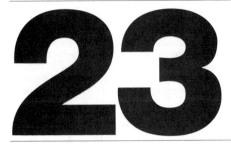

Management of Anticoagulation in Patients Requiring Surgical Procedures

Alan Zajarias

INTRODUCTION

The most common indications for anticoagulation are deep venous thrombosis (DVT)/ pulmonary embolism, AF, and the presence of a mechanical heart valves. Chronically anticoagulated patients occasionally require surgical intervention, and decisions must be made according to the management of the anticoagulation in the pre-, intra- and postop periods. Risk of thrombotic complications associated with discontinuation of anticoagulation must be weighed against the risk of bleeding complications postop. Some important considerations include

- 6% of recurrent cases of DVT are fatal, and 2% result in serious permanent disability.
- 20% of arterial emboli are fatal, and 40% result in serious permanent disability.
- In patients with DVT, incidence of bleeding in the first 5 postop days was 11%.
- 3% of major postop bleedings are fatal.

This chapter covers the management of anticoagulation in those patients with baseline indications for anticoagulation. Primary prophylaxis against DVT in the surgical setting is a distinct topic beyond the scope of this chapter.

Incidence of major bleeding in patients with prosthetic valves varies and increases with higher INRs. Bleeding rates are 1.2% per yr and 3.8% per yr in patients whose INRs were 2.5–3.5 vs 3.5–4.5, respectively.

Factors that influence anticoagulation management in these patients include several features. Patient characteristics, such as age and indication for anticoagulation, are important. Surgical determinants, such as urgency of surgery [when possible, surgery in patients receiving **PO anticoagulation (OAC)** should be elective, allowing planned anticoagulation reversal and correction of medical comorbidities to reduce complications]; area, approach, expected blood loss, type of incision, and closure; and immobilization, endothelial damage, activation of the inflammatory cascade (Virchow's triad), platelet activation, and exposure of thrombogenic material (collagen, tissue factor, sutures), make surgery a prothrombotic event. The mode of anesthesia is also an important consideration: Regional or epidural anesthesia is accompanied by risk of hematoma formation and cord compression. Of note, the administration of low-molecular-weight heparin (LMWH) is not approved by the U.S. FDA for patients receiving epidural anesthesia.

PROSTHETIC HEART VALVES

The **incidence** of embolization secondary to prosthetic heart valves differs according to multiple factors. **Valve type** plays a role, because older-generation valves (Björk-Shiley and the caged-ball Starr-Edwards valves) are more thrombogenic and require anticoagulation at higher INRs. Björk-Shiley valves in the aortic position in the absence of OAC are associated with thromboembolic events at a rate of 23% per yr. St. Jude's valves in the same position had a rate of 12.3% per yr. OAC reduces the risk of embolic thromboembolic events by 75%. Bioprosthetic valves have a higher risk of events during the first 3 mos after implantation but become endothelialized and carry a much lower risk thereafter. **Valve position** is also important: Embolic risk is higher in the mitral than in the aortic position. St. Jude's valves in the mitral position have a 22.2% per yr incidence rate of thromboembolic event without anticoagulation, whereas the same valve in the aortic position was associated with a lower incidence, 12.3% per yr. **Valve number** is important, as the greater the number of prosthetic valves, the greater the risk of embolic events. Other factors that increase the risk of thrombosis and embolic events are the presence of AF, severe LV dysfunction, prior embolic event, and the presence of a hypercoagulable state. Prosthetic valve–associated thromboembolic events were estimated to be 10% in a series published by the Mayo Clinic but were evident after a follow-up of 2 yrs [1].

Mechanisms of Valve Thrombosis

Thrombus formation within a prosthetic valve is associated with endothelial and endocardial damage during surgery. The presence of suture material (at the valvular sewing ring and site of atriotomy closure) stimulates platelet and coagulation factor activation. Prosthetic valves cause turbulent flow, which in turn damages formed blood elements, traps platelets, and favors thrombosis. Fluctuations in anticoagulant levels may increase thrombus formation (when subtherapeutic) and decrease adherence to the valvular surface once therapeutic levels are reached. Discontinuation of anticoagulation is associated with a 3.7-fold increase in risk of thromboembolic event [2].

Current Use of Anticoagulation

Current guidelines for anticoagulation of the American College of Chest Physicians (ACCP) recommend the following:

- **St. Jude Medical bi-leaflet valve, CarboMedics-Hall bi-leaflet valve, or Medtronic-Hall tilting disk in the aortic position in a patient with normal sinus rhythm and no left atrial enlargement:** INR target of 2.5 (range, 2–3). Target INR of 3.0 or addition of 80–100 mg/day of ASA is favored if the patient has AF.
- **St. Jude Medical bi-leaflet valve, CarboMedics bi-leaflet valve, or Medtronic-Hall tilting disk in the mitral position:** INR target of 3.0 (range, 2.5–3.5).
- **Patients with a prior embolic event despite adequate anticoagulation or those with a caged-ball or caged-disk valve:** Target INR of 3.0 (range, 2.5–3.5) and ASA, 80–100 mg/day.
- **Patients with bioprosthetic valves:** INR of 2.5 (2.0–3.0) for the first 3 mos postop, followed by daily ASA, 80 mg/day, if they do not have other risk factors for embolic events (AF, left atrial thrombus). If other risk factors are present, patients should remain anticoagulated for the other indication.

Periop Management of PO Anticoagulation in the Setting of Mechanical Valves

There is no overall consensus on the management of patients with prosthetic heart valves and surgery, as there is a dearth of randomized trials evaluating these questions. Nevertheless, several key articles have been published, and the ACC/AHA have published recommendations. One review article [3] reported the risk of embolism in patients with AF or valve replacements is not high enough to warrant treatment with IV heparin pre- and postop due to high complication rates. The authors recommended stopping OAC before surgery, operating when INR 1.3–1.5, and avoiding use of postop IV heparin in patients with prosthetic heart valves and no prior thrombotic events. Postop SC heparin was recommended for DVT prophylaxis in high-risk patients. Avoid elective surgery during the first month after an arterial embolic event, but if it is entertained, use preop IV heparin; postop IV heparin is indicated if the risk of bleeding is low. The ACC/AHA guidelines, as well as another review [4], recommend stratifying patients according to risk factors. Conventional anticoagulation can be undertaken in patients with low risk (low thromboembolic events in new-generation prosthetic valves, no prior embolic events). This consists of discontinuing warfarin preop. Perform surgery once INR <1.5, and resume OAC once patient is tolerating

PO intake. IV heparin is recommended for use only if INR <2.0 for >5 days. An aggressive approach is undertaken in high-risk patients. In this setting, discontinue warfarin preoperatively. Bridge with IV heparin once INR <2.0, keeping activated partial thromboplastin time at 2–2.5 times the upper limit of normal, and discontinue heparin 4 hrs preop. Resume heparin and OAC as soon as possible. Discontinue heparin once INR >2.0. A third review [5] published an observational study in patients with chronic anticoagulation (prosthetic valves, AF, or hypercoagulable state) undergoing surgical, dental, or invasive procedures in which warfarin was discontinued. They were treated with enoxaparin, 1 mg/kg q12h SC, continued until 12 hrs before the procedure and restarted once hemostasis was achieved and discontinued once a therapeutic INR was obtained. They reported three postprocedure bleeding complications; however, **it is important to stress that LMWH has not been deemed adequate and may, in fact, be inadequate for thromboembolic protection in the setting of prosthetic valves.** Many cardiologists recommend preprocedural heparin as soon as the INR falls to <2 for all patients with prosthetic heart valves and, similarly, restarting it postprocedure as soon as surgically acceptable.

ATRIAL FIBRILLATION

Risk of Embolization

LV dysfunction, age >75, HTN, previous stroke or TIA, and diabetes mellitus increase the likelihood of an embolic event in patients with AF. Patients with nonvalvular AF have a 4.5% per yr risk of systemic embolization. The risk is 0.5% per day in the first 30 days after an arterial embolic event. The risk is 12% per yr (0.032%/day) if there is a previous episode of cerebrovascular disease. OAC reduces risk of systemic embolization in patients with nonvalvular AF by 66%.

Risk of Bleeding

In patients with a previous episode of GI bleeding and age >75, OAC increases the risk of bleeding. The SPAF II trial demonstrated that major bleeding was found at 2.3% per yr in patients >75 yrs who were treated with OAC and had an INR of 2–4.5. In patients with the same characteristics but treated with 325 mg of ASA, bleeding was evidenced in 1.1% per yr. Intracranial hemorrhages were only seen in patients with INR >3.0. In SPAF III, high-risk patients (mean age, 71 yrs) with an INR of 2–3 had a rate of intracranial bleeding of 0.5% per yr [7].

Recommendations

OAC can be discontinued before surgery, letting the INR drift to <1.5 for an invasive procedure. The risk of postop bleeding outweighs the benefit of pre- and postop anticoagulation, because the incidence of embolic events in patients with AF is so small when it is calculated on a daily basis. Resume OAC once the patient tolerates PO intake and the risk of bleeding has diminished. Initiate DVT prophylaxis with LMWH or SC unfractionated heparin in high-risk patients. The cost of in-hospital anticoagulation for postop patients with chronic AF does not justify in-house anticoagulation with IV heparin and bridging to OAC if the discharge is being held by a subtherapeutic INR. **However, patients with prior thromboembolic event or LV dysfunction may warrant IV heparin pre- and postop.**

DEEP VENOUS THROMBOSIS

Risk Factors

Risk factors for DVT include increasing age, neoplasia, immobility, paralysis, stroke, previous DVT, trauma, obesity, cardiac dysfunction, intravascular catheters, inflammatory bowel disease, nephrotic syndrome, pregnancy, estrogen administration (PO contraception), antiphospholipid antibody syndrome, activated protein C resistance–factor V

Leiden mutation, and deficiency of natural anticoagulant proteins (proteins C and S, antithrombin III). The risk of recurrence depends on the presence of modifiable risk factors, circumstances precipitating the initial DVT, and the time treated with OAC. The risk of DVT recurrence at 3 mos without anticoagulation is approximately 50%. If anticoagulated for 1 mo, the risk drops to 10%, and after 3 mos, the risk is 5%. The risk of DVT in patients with recurrent DVTs from a hypercoagulable state is 15% per yr. In the first month after DVT, each day not anticoagulated has a 1% absolute increase in the risk of recurrence.

Risk Stratification

ACCP stratifies patients according to their risk of developing DVT postop. Low-risk patients include those <40 yrs undergoing minor surgery. Those at moderate risk include patients with risk factors (see Risk Factors) undergoing minor surgery, patients aged 40–60 yrs without risk factors and not undergoing major surgery, and patients <40 yrs submitted to major surgery. The high-risk group includes patients >60 yrs undergoing nonmajor surgery, patients with risk factors, or those >40 yrs undergoing major surgery. Very high-risk patients include those >40 yrs with prior DVT; patients with hypercoagulable state or cancer; patients undergoing hip or knee surgery; and those with major trauma or spinal cord injury.

Recommendations

Ideally, surgery should be delayed at least 3 mos after the DVT or until OAC treatment has been completed. One set of recommendations [3] holds the following: If the DVT occurred <1 mo ago, and surgery is needed, initiate full anticoagulation with IV heparin and discontinue 4–8 hrs preop. Restart IV heparin at the previous maintenance rate without a bolus 12 hrs postop. If the DVT occurred 1–3 mos before the surgery, no preop IV heparin is needed unless other risk factors (debilitating illness, neoplasia, immobilization) are encountered. Postop IV heparin should be used until the INR is >2.0 on warfarin (Coumadin). If the DVT occurred >3 mos before surgery, there is no need for preop heparin. Postop SC DVT prophylaxis with unfractionated heparin or LMWH should be used until INR >2.0. The ACCP guidelines contend that patients with previous DVT >3 mos ago or AF without prior cerebrovascular accident are considered low risk for thromboembolic event. Recommendations suggest letting the INR drift down preop and beginning postop DVT prophylaxis if the intervention increases risk for thromboembolism. Patients with DVT <3 mos ago, mechanical valve in mitral position, or presence of caged-ball valve are at high risk for a thromboembolic event and should receive LMWH or full-dose unfractionated heparin IV for 2 days before surgery while the INR is drifting down and should stop warfarin 48 hrs preop. Continue anticoagulation at full dose postop until INR becomes therapeutic. For gynecologic and urologic surgery, the ACCP recommends decreasing the dose of Coumadin to obtain an INR 1.3–1.5 to perform surgery. Initiate Coumadin at full dose and 5000 U of unfractionated heparin bid SC after surgery.

KEY POINTS TO REMEMBER

- Patients with prior DVT, AF, or prosthetic heart valves require attention to their anticoagulation before and after any surgical procedure.
- In general, consensus guidelines and review articles recommend risk-stratifying patients when making a decision. Low-risk patients may only require cessation of Coumadin in the 48–72 hrs before surgery and DVT prophylaxis after surgery. High-risk patients may require full heparinization as soon as Coumadin is stopped, with anticoagulation resumed as soon as is surgically acceptable.

SUGGESTED READING

Albers G, Dalen J, Laupacis A, et al. Antithrombotic therapy in atrial fibrillation. *Chest* 2001;119[Suppl 1]:194s–206s.

Ansell J, Hirsh J Dalen J, et al. Managing oral anticoagulant therapy. *Chest* 2001;119 [Suppl 1]:22s–38s.

Eckman M, Beshanksy J, Durand-Zaleski I, et al. Anticoagulation for noncardiac procedures in patients with prosthetic heart valves. Does low risk mean high cost? *JAMA* 1990;263:1513–1521.

Geerts W, Heit J, Clagett P, et al. Prevention of venous thromboembolism. *Chest* 2001; 119[Suppl 1]:176s–193s.

Hirsh J, Dalen J, Anderson D, et al. Oral anticoagulants: mechanism of action, clinical effectiveness and optimal therapeutic range. *Chest* 2001;119[Suppl 1]:8s–21s.

Jacobs L, Nusbaum N. Perioperative management and reversal of antithrombotic therapy. *Clin Geriatr Med* 2001;17:189–203.

Levine M, Raskob G, Landefeld S, et al. Hemorrhagic complication of anticoagulant treatment. *Chest* 2001;119[Suppl 1]:108s–121s.

Pengo V, Barbero F, Banzato A, et al. A comparison of a moderate with a moderate-high intensity oral anticoagulant treatment in patients with mechanical heart valves prosthesis. *Thromb Haemost* 1997;77:839–844.

Stein P, Alpert J, Bussey H, et al. Antithrombotic therapy in patients with mechanical and biological prosthetic heart valves. *Chest* 2001;119[Suppl 1]:220s–227s.

REFERENCES

1. Tinker J, Tarhan S. Discontinuing anticoagulant therapy in surgical patients with cardiac prosthesis. *JAMA* 1978;239:738–739.
2. Cannegieter SC, Rosendaal FR, Briet E. Thromboembolic and bleeding complications in patients with mechanical heart valve prostheses. *Circulation* 1994;89: 635–641.
3. Kearon C, Hirsh J. Management of anticoagulation before and after elective surgery. *N Engl J Med* 1997;336:1506–1511.
4. Tiede D, Nishimura R, Gastineau D. Modern management of prosthetic valve anticoagulation. *Mayo Clin Proc* 1998;73:665–680.
5. Spandorfer J, Lynch S, Weitz H, et al. Use of enoxaparin for the chronically anticoagulated patient before and after procedures. *Am J Cardiol* 1999;84:478–480.
6. Warfarin vs. aspirin for prevention of thromboembolism in atrial fibrillation: Stroke prevention in atrial fibrillation II study. *Lancet* 1994;343:687–691.
7. Adjusted-dose warfarin versus low intensity, fixed dose warfarin plus aspirin for high risk patients with atrial fibrillation: Stroke Prevention in Atrial Fibrillation III randomized clinical trial. *Lancet* 1996;348:633–638.

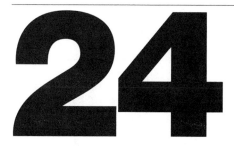

Procedures in Cardiovascular Critical Care (Intraaortic Balloon Pump, Swan-Ganz Catheterization, and Temporary Transvenous Pacemaker)

Michael O. Barry

INTRAAORTIC BALLOON PUMP

The intraaortic balloon pump (IABP) was the first hemodynamic support device developed in the 1960s. The hemodynamic support device provided improvements in the myocardial O_2 supply/demand ratio and circulatory support.

The IABP remains the most widely used mechanical cardiac support device because of its simplicity, ease of insertion, and long clinical track record.

Hemodynamic Effects of Counterpulsation

The intraaortic balloon exerts its hemodynamic effects through counterpulsation (Fig. 24-1; Table 24-1). The balloon rapidly inflates during diastole and deflates during systole. The inflation and deflation provide two specific hemodynamic effects.

The IABP rapidly expands in early diastole (i.e., just after aortic valve closure) and thus produces an increase in diastolic pressure, which translates into a marked increase in coronary perfusion pressure. The abrupt deflation of the balloon during isovolumetric contraction just before the opening of the aortic valve removes effective aortic volume. This removed volume decreases the aortic systolic pressure and, thus, resistance. The reduced aortic resistance allows for greater LV systolic ejection. The systolic deflation decreases the myocardial O_2 requirements through a reduction in afterload.

Technique

An appropriate-sized balloon is obtained based on patient size. Needle access to the common femoral artery is obtained. Through the needle, a guidewire is passed into the abdominal aorta, making sure no resistance is encountered. Placement of the wire is confirmed by fluoroscopy. A 7–9-Fr. introducer sheath is placed over the wire by the modified Seldinger technique. A small amount of contrast dye is injected through the sheath, and using cineangiography, the suitability of the ileo-femoral arterial system is assessed (severe vascular disease precludes placement of the IABP). Of note, some IABP systems allow placement over a long wire without a sheath. In emergent situations, when fluoroscopy is not available, the procedure can be done at the bedside. Confirmation by chest x-ray of IABP tip position just below the aortic arch is essential. The balloon line is connected to the pump, which injects helium, and the blood port is connected to the pressure transducer.

Troubleshooting

Late Balloon Inflation

- The balloon inflates after the aortic valve closes, thereby shortening the period of diastolic augmentation. This reduced augmentation time translates into reduced coronary perfusion.
- The waveform illustrates that the dicrotic notch occurs significantly before the balloon inflation point.

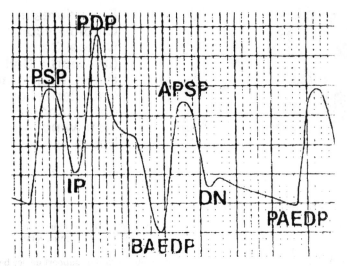

FIG. 24-1. Normal arterial waveform with intraaortic balloon pump (IABP) set at 1:2 pulsation (with every other beat, the balloon inflates and deflates). APSP, assisted peak systolic pressure; BAEDP, balloon aortic end-diastolic pressure; DN, dichrotic notch; IP, inflation point; PAEDP, patient aortic end-diastolic pressure; PDP, peak diastolic pressure; PSP, peak systolic pressure. [From Sorrentino M, Feldman T. Techniques for IABP timing, use, and discontinuance. *J Crit Illn* 1992;7(4):597–604, with permission.]

Early Balloon Deflation

- The balloon deflates before isovolumetric contraction, allowing refilling of the aorta before ventricular ejection. Therefore, the afterload reduction is lessened.
- On the waveform, the peak systolic pressure is ≤ assisted peak systolic pressure.

TABLE 24-1. INTRAAORTIC BALLOON PUMP TERMINOLOGY

Terminology (at a 1:2 pumping rate)	Effects
Peak systolic pressure	Systolic pressure without activity related to the balloon pump
Inflation point	Point on the arterial pressure tracing where balloon inflation originates; just after the dicrotic notch
Peak diastolic pressure	Augmented increase in diastolic pressure that occurs when the balloon inflation displaces aortic blood volume due to counterpulsation
Balloon aortic end-diastolic pressure	Lowest pressure in the aorta, reflecting balloon deflation
Assisted peak systolic pressure	Systolic peak that reflects the afterload reduction produced by the balloon pump
Dicrotic notch	Landmark on the downslope of the arterial pressure waveform that signals aortic valve closure and the beginning of diastole

Early Balloon Inflation

- The balloon inflates before the closure of the aortic valve, thereby increasing the afterload and, thus, increasing myocardial stress.
- The waveform illustrates the inflation point occurring before the dicrotic notch.

Late Balloon Deflation

- The balloon deflation occurs after the aortic valve is open. This causes a reduced ejection fraction and increases the myocardial work.
- The waveform illustrates that the peak systolic pressure is significantly greater than the augmented peak systolic pressure.

Indications for Intraaortic Balloon Pumps

Cardiogenic Shock

- IABPs are useful in the setting of cardiogenic shock secondary to multiple causes, some of which include acute MI, continuing ischemia, acute mitral regurgitation, VSD, myocarditis, or drug toxicity.
- Generally, the initiation of counterpulsation in shock leads to a marked rise in systemic diastolic pressure and cardiac index, along with a fall in LV filling pressure.
- Hemodynamic benefits are usually maintained for only 3–4 days unless revascularization or corrective surgery is performed.

Unstable Angina

- Addition of an IABP to a maximal medical program produces marked improvement in angina status in 95% of unstable patients.
- It has been hypothesized that counterpulsation improves unstable angina by increasing collateral flow to the ischemic area.

Prophylactic High-Risk Intervention

- IABPs have been used prophylactically during percutaneous angioplasty in patients with severe LV dysfunction or patients who have a larger territory of myocardium at risk (e.g., the anterior wall).
- Other situations in which IABPs have been used include stabilizing patients with severe aortic stenosis and in patients with severe multivessel or left main CAD requiring urgent cardiac or noncardiac surgery.
- Promising data suggest that IABPs prevent reocclusion after angioplasty.

Table 24-2 lists contraindications for IABP use.

Complications of Intraaortic Balloon Pumps

Complications of IABPs are listed in Table 24-3 and reviewed below.

TABLE 24-2. CONTRAINDICATIONS FOR INTRAAORTIC BALLOON PUMPS

Significant aortic regurgitation

Abdominal aortic aneurysm

Aortic dissection

Septicemia

Uncontrolled bleeding

Severe bilateral peripheral vascular disease

Bilateral femoral-popliteal bypass grafts for severe peripheral vascular disease

TABLE 24-3. COMPLICATIONS OF INTRAAORTIC BALLOON PUMPS

Limb ischemia	Sepsis
Arterial dissection	Balloon rupture
Cholesterol emboli	Thrombocytopenia
Cerebrovascular accident	

Limb Ischemia

- Limb ischemia is usually apparent within a few hours of insertion and is related to simple mechanical obstruction of the circulation by the balloon catheter at the insertion site.
- Removal of the balloon generally alleviates the problem. Rarely is surgical thrombectomy or vascular repair necessary.
- Loss of the limb is rare. It occurs in the setting of severe peripheral vascular disease or as the result of extensive thrombus formation.

Arterial Dissection

- Iatrogenic retrograde dissection may occur as a result of wire advancement. The IABP may then be inserted into the false lumen. This usually presents with severe back pain. There is a high incidence of aortic rupture and sudden hemodynamic collapse.
- The best defense against arterial dissection is avoidance of stiff guidewires and avoiding forcing the guidewire when resistance is encountered.

Cholesterol Embolization

Cholesterol emboli usually present with bilateral, painful, cold, mottled limbs indicative of livedo reticularis. There is also associated eosinophilia, eosinophiluria, and thrombocytopenia, as well as renal failure secondary to cholesterol emboli.

Cerebrovascular Accident

Embolic cerebrovascular accident may occur if the IABP's central lumen has been flushed vigorously in an attempt to correct damping of the central arterial pressure due to thrombus. Therefore, do not use the central lumen of the IABP as a site for obtaining arterial blood.

Sepsis

Sepsis is a rare complication if the device is placed under sterile technique and its duration of use is 3–7 days; however, if the device used >1 wk, the risk of infection increases.

Balloon Rupture

- Balloon rupture rarely occurs due to calcification in the aorta. The ruptured balloon may produce thrombus within the balloon, making percutaneous removal impossible.
- In even more rare incidences, balloon rupture has been associated with helium embolization.

RIGHT-HEART CATHETERIZATION

- The decision to place a pulmonary artery (PA) catheter (Swan-Ganz catheter) should always be preceded by a specific question regarding the patient's hemodynamics. The answer to the question should have significant bearing on the management of the patient, because placement of a PA catheter is not without risk.
- During routine right-heart catheterization, measurements of pressures and O_2 saturations in the vena cava, right atrium, RV, PA, and pulmonary capillary wedge position can be performed, and cardiac output (CO) can be quantified.
- The determination of O_2 saturation from various sections of the right-heart chambers may be used to assess the location and magnitude of an intracardiac left-to-

right shunt, which would occur with an atrial septal defect or VSD or even possibly a patent ductus arteriosus.

- When the catheter is in the correct location (zone III), the pulmonary capillary wedge pressure (PCWP) usually accurately reflects left atrial pressure. The left atrial pressure in the absence of mitral stenosis reflects LV end-diastolic pressure, which is a measurement of preload.
- Also, right-heart catheterization allows for evaluation of the severity of tricuspid or pulmonic stenosis, pulmonary HTN, and calculation of pulmonary vascular resistance (PVR).
- Table 24-4 lists risks and complications associated with right-heart catheterization.

Approaches and Catheterization Technique

- Choice of insertion site should be determined individually according to the risks and benefits of each location. Nevertheless, the left subclavian and the right internal jugular approaches probably permit easiest passage of the catheter into the PA. The femoral veins can be used but require more skill in placement and are associated with a higher risk of infection or deep venous thrombosis if left in place.
- The technique of insertion of the 7–8-Fr. introducer (also called *sheath* or *cordis*) is the same as that for any central venous access—the Seldinger technique. The PA catheter is passed through the introducer into the vein.
- The balloon is inflated when the tip of the catheter exits the sheath. Continuous pressure tracing and fluoroscopy aid with establishment of catheter tip position. When advancing the catheter, the balloon should be fully inflated. As the catheter is advanced through the tricuspid valve, the pressure tracing records a dramatic change appropriate to the higher pressures seen in the RV. This location is the greatest risk for arrhythmias; thus, proceed without delay.
- Arrival at the PA is heralded by the pressure tracing appearance of the dicrotic notch. Also, the diastolic pressure is greater than that of the RV.
- From the PA, **slowly** advance the inflated balloon catheter until a fall in the systolic pressure is noted compared with the pressure in the PA; this is the PCWP. The balloon may be deflated, and the PA tracing should reappear. The balloon should be **slowly** reinflated. If too little balloon volume is required to reach the wedge position, the catheter tip is positioned too distally, and further inflation risks rupture of the PA.
- Perform chest x-rays to confirm the position of the PA catheter. The tip should be no more than 3–5 cm from the midline. Also, ideally, the catheter tip should be in zone III of the lung, where arterial pressure exceeds venous and alveolar pressure, thereby creating a column of blood to the left atrium.

The balloon should always be maintained in the deflated position, except when making a PCWP measurement.

Hemodynamic Measurements

See Fig. 24-2.

TABLE 24-4. RISKS AND COMPLICATIONS OF RIGHT-HEART CATHETERIZATION

Air embolism	Pulmonary infarction
Endocarditis/sepsis	Right bundle-branch block (complete
PA rupture	heart block if underlying left bundle-
Bleeding	branch block)
Cardiac tamponade/perforation	Pneumonthora (if superior approach)
	Sustained ventricular arrhythmias
	Thromboembolism

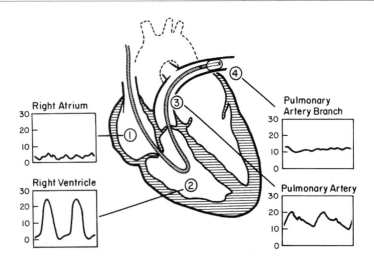

FIG. 24-2. Pressure tracing exhibited in the various chambers and positions during right-heart catheterization. (From Marino PL. *The ICU book,* 2nd ed. Philadelphia: Lippincott Williams & Wilkins, 1997:157, with permission.)

Pressure Measurement and Waveforms

- Once the catheter has been positioned in the desired cardiac chamber, it is connected directly through a fluid-filled tubing to a pressure transducer. This transducer transforms a pressure signal into an electrical signal. See Table 24-5 for normal hemodynamic values.
- Errors in pressure measurements can result from several sources, such as inaccurate zero referencing of the manometer.

Right Atrial Tracing

- Right atrial systole follows the P wave on the ECG and produces the *a* wave of the right atrial pressure tracing. With relaxation, there is a decline in the pressure, known as the *x* descent.

TABLE 24-5. NORMAL HEMODYNAMIC VALUES

Cardiac index (L/min/m^2)	2.6–4.2
PCWP (mm Hg)	6–12
PA (mm Hg)	16–30/3–12
Mean	10–16
RV (mm Hg)	16–30/0–8
Right atrium (mm Hg)	0–8
SVR (dynes/sec/cm^{-5})	700–1600
PVR (dynes/sec/cm^{-5})	20–130

PCWP, pulmonary capillary wedge pressure; PVR, pulmonary vascular resistance; SVR, systemic vascular resistance.

- Filling of the right atrium from the venous circulation and retrograde movement of the tricuspid valve annulus during RV systole produces the v wave. When the tricuspid valve opens, blood from the right atrium empties into the RV, thus causing a decline in the right atrial pressure, producing the y descent.
- Typically, the peak a wave is higher than the peak v wave pressure.

Right Ventricular Tracing
Atrial systole produces a small a wave. RV systole follows the QRS complex, which gives rise to a rapidly increasing systolic pressure waveform. With ventricular relaxation, the pressure waveform declines and reaches a nadir.

Pulmonary Artery Tracing
The normal PA pressure consists of a systolic wave that coincides with RV systole. The decline in the pressure wave is usually interrupted by the **dicrotic notch,** which corresponds to the pulmonic valve closure. The nadir of the decline represents the end-diastolic pressure (see Fig. 24-2).

Pulmonary Capillary Wedge Tracing

- The pressure waveform obtained is a transmitted left atrial pressure. The tracing is similar to the right atrial waveform. There are a wave, x descent, v wave, and y descents; these correspond with left atrial systole, relaxation, filling, and emptying, respectively.
- Typically, the v wave is greater than the a wave.

Cardiac Output

- Recall that the CO is defined as liters of output/min, whereas the cardiac index is the magnitude of CO proportional to the body surface area.
- The two commonly used methods of measuring CO are the Fick method and the thermodilution technique.

FICK METHOD

- The Fick method of CO measurement is based on the hypothesis that the consumption of oxygen ($\dot{V}O_2$) by an organ is the product of the blood flow to that organ and the regional arteriovenous concentration difference of the substance.
- **CO (L/min) = O_2 consumption (mL/min)/arteriovenous O_2 difference (AVO$_2$) across the lungs (mL/L).**
- To measure CO in humans, this principle is applied to the lungs. By measuring the amounts of O_2 extracted from inspired air and the $A\dot{V}O_2$ across the lungs, one can calculate the pulmonary blood flow. Because pulmonary blood flow is equal to systemic blood flow, in the absence of a significant shunt, it can be extrapolated as CO.
- In many labs, the O_2 consumption is estimated from a nomogram. Determining $A\dot{V}O_2$ differences across the lungs requires blood from the PA and pulmonary vein to be analyzed for O_2 content. Because the O_2 content of the pulmonary venous blood is similar to the systemic arterial blood (in the absence of a right-to-left inter-atrial shunt), these values may be interchanged.
- **The Fick method is most accurate for patients with a low CO and least accurate in patients with a high CO or significant shunts.**

THERMODILUTION TECHNIQUE

- To determine CO, a known amount of indicator is injected into the circulation and allowed to mix completely in the blood, then its concentration is measured over time (Fig. 24-3). A time-concentration curve is generated, and the area under the curve, as calculated by minicomputers, corresponds to the CO.
- The indicator most often used is cold saline. A balloon-tipped, flow-direct catheter with a thermistor at the tip is used. The distal tip with the thermistor is advanced to the PA, and the proximal port is within the right atrium. Next, 5–10 cc of iced

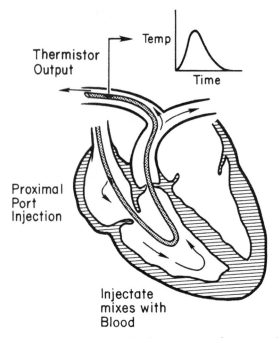

FIG. 24-3. The thermodilution technique for determining cardiac output. (From Marino PL. *The ICU book,* 2nd ed. Philadelphia: Lippincott Williams & Wilkins, 1997:179, with permission.)

fluid is injected through the proximal port, and the temperature change at the distal thermistor is recorded as time. This allows for a thermodilution curve to be formulated and converted into CO.

- The thermodilution technique is inexpensive, easy to perform, and does not require arterial sampling; **however, certain conditions may render the results unreliable, such as tricuspid regurgitation, pulmonic regurgitation, or intracardiac shunts.**

Vascular Resistance

- The resistance of a vascular bed is calculated by dividing the pressure gradient across the bed by the flow through it.

$$\text{Sytemic vascular resistance (SVR)} = \frac{\text{Mean systemic arterial pressure} - \text{Mean right atrial pressure}}{\text{Systemic blood flow (CO)}}$$

- Increased SVR is usually present in patients with systemic HTN. It also may be seen in patients with low COs who have compensatory vasoconstriction.
- Reduced SVR is seen with inappropriately increased CO (e.g., sepsis, AV fistulas, anemia, fever, thyrotoxicosis).

$$\text{PVR} = \frac{\text{Mean PA pressure} - \text{Mean PCWP}}{\text{Pulmonary blood flow (CO)}}$$

- Elevated PVR is seen in pulmonary diseases, Eisenmenger syndrome, or a significant left-sided valvular lesion or wall motion defect.
- Table 24-6 lists etiology-dependent hemodynamics in shock.

TABLE 24-6. SHOCK: ETIOLOGY-DEPENDENT HEMODYNAMICS

Etiology of shock	PCWP	RAP	CO	SVR
Cardiogenic	High	High	Low	High
Septic	Low	Low	High/normal	Low
Pulmonary embolism/pulmonary HTN	Normal	High	Low	High/ normal
Hypovolemic	Low	Low	Low	High

CO, cardiac output; PCWP, pulmonary capillary wedge pressure; RAP, right arterial pressure; SVR, systemic vascular resistance.

Shunt Calculation

- The magnitude and direction of any shunt can be calculated by oximetry using the following equation:

$$\frac{Q_p}{Q_s} = \frac{SaO_2 - M\bar{v}O_2}{P\bar{v}O_2 - PaO_2}$$

- $M\bar{v}O_2$ is usually equal to the PaO_2, unless there is a shunt and/or congenital anomaly. In this case, $M\bar{v}O_2$ is calculated as follows:

$$M\bar{v}O_2 = \frac{3 \times SVCO_2 + IVCO_2}{4}$$

- The $P\bar{v}O_2$ can be drawn from the catheter tip in the wedge position (carefully!), although a true $P\bar{v}O_2$ is drawn from the left atrium.
- Qp/Qs of >1 suggests a net left-to-right shunt; <1 is right to left.

TEMPORARY TRANSVENOUS PACING

Initially, temporary cardiac pacing was solely used to increase heart rate, although improvements in understanding of electrophysiology and pacing electrodes have meant that temporary cardiac pacing can by used as a technique in control of brady- and tachyarrhythmias.

Basic Anatomy and Physiology of the Conduction System

- The normal heart beat arises from the sinoatrial (SA) node, located in the right atrium near its junction with the superior vena cava. The blood supply to the SA node is predominantly via the SA nodal artery, a branch of the right coronary artery in approximately 60% of people and the left circumflex coronary artery in approximately 40% of people.
- The AV node is located posteriorly in the right atrium, adjacent to the tricuspid annulus. The AV node blood supply arises from the distal right coronary artery in 90% of people and the left circumflex coronary artery in 10% of people.
- There is a delay within the AV node allowing for atrial contraction, then it travels through the His bundle to the Purkinje system and the ventricular myocardium.
- Both the SA node and AV node are richly innervated by the autonomic nervous system.
- The relative balance between the parasympathetic and sympathetic nervous system accounts for the resting autonomic tone. Increased parasympathetic output (i.e., increased vagal tone) can result in clinically significant bradycardia.
- Table 24-7 lists common vagal stimuli.

TABLE 24-7. COMMON VAGAL STIMULI

Intubation	Urination or defecation
Suctioning	Vomiting
Increased ICP	Sleeping
Markedly increased BP	

Diagnostic Evaluation

- Bradyarrhythmias can be caused by intrinsic disease of the conduction system or by extrinsic factors acting on the conduction system (Table 24-8).
- Bradyarrhythmias occur in 4–5% of patients with acute MI. Sinus node dysfunction (which may present as bradycardia, sinus pauses, or sinus arrest) is most common, with an inferior MI from occlusion of the right coronary artery.
- Varying degrees of AV block can also be seen with an acute MI (see Chap. 8, Acute ST-Segment Elevation Myocardial Infarction). In the case of an **inferior MI,** the site of block is usually at the AV node, due to occlusion of the AV nodal artery, a branch of the right coronary artery. This results in first-degree heart block, second-degree (Mobitz I) heart block, or, rarely, third-degree heart block. These are usually transient or at least not life threatening. The Bezold-Jarisch reflex is the mechanism.
- AV block caused by an **anterior MI** due to occlusion of the left anterior descending artery usually occurs below the AV node. This infranodal block results in symptomatic and often irreversible Mobitz II block or third-degree AV block.

TABLE 24-8. EXTRINSIC AND INTRINSIC CAUSES OF CONDUCTION DISEASE

Extrinsic causes

  Medications

    Beta blockers; calcium channel blockers; digoxin; class IA, IC, and III antiarrhythmics

  Acute MI

  Hyperkalemia

  Hypothyroidism

  Infectious causes

    Endocarditis, Lyme disease AV block, sepsis

  Autonomic excess

    Increased vagal output or carotid hypersensitivity

  Surgical trauma

    Aortic or mitral valve rings

Intrinsic causes

  Degenerative idiopathic disease

  CAD

  Cardiomyopathy

  Hypertensive heart disease

  Myocarditis

  Collagen vascular disease

  Infiltrative diseases

    Amyloid, sarcoid, neoplasm, hemochromatosis, radiation treatment

Temporary Treatment for Bradycardia

- Medical treatment with atropine, epinephrine, or dopamine is useful in emergency situations requiring immediate intervention until pacing can be initiated.
- Transcutaneous pacing, first introduced by Zoll in 1952, is the oldest form of pacing. Pacing is achieved by stimulation through electrodes placed on the chest wall. Limitations of this procedure include pain with impulse delivery. Also of importance, there is **limited ability of the electrical impulse to capture the ventricle** due to heavy interference caused by the skeletal muscles and chest wall.
- **Epicardial pacing** is frequently encountered in patients after cardiac surgery. Typically, the leads are placed on the epicardium during surgery and can be readily removed at any time. Epicardial pacing wires serve dual diagnostic and therapeutic functions: They record atrial and/or ventricular electrical activity. Therefore, these dual wires allow easier differentiation between ventricular and supraventricular arrhythmias.
- Epicardial pacing can also be used to terminate certain atrial and ventricular tachyarrhythmias by overdrive pacing. This overdrive pacing is done by pulse generators capable of pacing above the tachycardia rate to "overdrive" the heart.

Technique

- A pacing catheter is inserted into the heart, directly stimulating the RV. A percutaneous entry site is chosen, typically the right internal jugular vein or the femoral vein. **The left-sided central veins should be left uncontaminated, because if a permanent pacer will be required, they are the preferred sites of access and should be free of hardware.**
- The modified Seldinger technique allows placement of a 6-Fr. introducer sheath.
- A bipolar pacing lead is introduced into the RV under the aid of a balloon-tipped catheter, which allows easy floatation of the pacing wire to the apex of the RV. Special J-shaped wires are also available to allow atrial stimulation in dual-chamber temporary pacing. Situations that require atrial and ventricular activity include aortic stenosis, mitral stenosis, and obstructive myopathies. Nevertheless, single-chamber ventricular pacing is by far the most common approach.
- Guidance systems to assure proper placement of the bipolar pacing lead include fluoroscopy (most common), catheter-tip electrogram, or ECG-rhythm strip during pacemaker stimulation.
- A prosthetic tricuspid valve is a relative contraindication to placement of a transvenous pacer. Also, the femoral vein should not be used if the patient has an inferior vena cava filter.

Indications for Temporary Pacing

Some common indications for temporary pacemaker insertion within the context of acute MI include complete heart block or Mobitz type II AV block, as well as digoxin toxicity. Indications outside of acute MI include complete heart block caused by structural heart disease and symptomatic bradycardia with sinus pauses >3–4 secs (Table 24-9). **Medications,** such as beta blockers, nondihydropyridine calcium channel blockers, and digoxin toxicity, are common causes for third-degree heart block. See Chap. 5, Cardiovascular Emergencies, and Chap. 14, Bradycardia and Permanent Pacemakers, for further descriptions of treatment.

Troubleshooting with Temporary Transvenous Pacemakers

- Table 24-10 lists complications of temporary transvenous pacemakers.
- Once the introducer sheath has been established in a good position, it is sutured in place at the skin surface. The lead is attached to a pacing generator after confirmation of placement by fluoroscopy.
- The pacing generator sensitivity may be set on demand (synchronous) mode or fixed (asynchronous) mode. In demand mode, the lead "senses" the heart's intrinsic electrical activity, and in the absence of conduction, the pulse generator delivers an

TABLE 24-9. COMMON INDICATIONS FOR TRANSVENOUS TEMPORARY PACING

Condition	Setting
Third-degree AV block	Symptomatic congenital complete heart block
	Symptomatic acquired complete heart block
	Postop symptomatic complete heart block
Second-degree AV block	Symptomatic Mobitz I or II AV block
Acute MI	Symptomatic bradycardia
	High-grade AV block (trifascicular block)
	Complete AV block
Sinus node dysfunction	Symptomatic bradyarrhythmias
Tachycardia prevention treatment	Bradycardia-dependent arrhythmias
	Long QT syndrome with ventricular arrhythmias

impulse at a preset adjustable voltage. This impulse initiates depolarization and contraction of the ventricles.

- Fixed or asynchronous mode delivers a set amount of impulses per time, regardless of the underlying native conduction. This fixed pacing mode is rarely used, as this may precipitate ventricular arrhythmias via an R on T phenomenon.
- A pacing threshold must be established; this is defined as the least amount of current (in mA) necessary to depolarize or capture the ventricle. The threshold gives the operator an idea of the proximity of the pacing lead to the ventricular wall. Therefore, the lower the threshold, the closer the pacing wire is to the ventricle. The optimal pacing threshold is <1 mA. The voltage delivered by the pulse generator is usually set at least 2 mA above the pacing threshold.
- Pacing failure may be as simple as the disconnection of a loose wire, but the most common cause is failure of the lead to initiate sufficient voltage to pace the ventricle (i.e., failure of the ventricle to capture).
- Failure to capture is illustrated on the rhythm strip as pacer spikes that do not initiate capture (i.e., there is no ventricular depolarization). This is most likely due to displacement of the lead, which means the pacing threshold will have increased beyond the voltage delivered by the pulse generator. The generator voltage should be increased immediately until appropriate pacing is seen, and the lead should be repositioned.
- The set **rate** depends on the clinical scenario. Usually, it is set at 40–50 bpm as a back-up to the intrinsic heart rate, unless the CO is very low. In this setting, AV pacing may be required. For tachyarrhythmia prevention, pacing is usually set at ~100 bpm until the underlying predisposition is corrected.
- Other reasons for failure to pace include fracture of the lead or an overly sensitive pacing generator that detects impulses traveling from the chest muscles that inhibit the pulse generator. This can be corrected by reducing the sensitivity of the pulse generator.

TABLE 24-10. COMPLICATIONS OF TEMPORARY TRANSVENOUS PACEMAKERS

Pneumothorax	Ventricular ectopy/nonsustained VT
Myocardial perforation	Thromboembolism
Bleeding	Infection

- Diaphragmatic pacing is a complication associated with a high preset voltage; as a result, the phrenic nerve is stimulated through the wall of the RV. It also may indicate a perforation of the RV wall, with the lead stimulating the diaphragm directly. Beware of a patient hiccupping at a rate identical to the pacer rate.
- The pacer threshold should be checked twice daily; if the threshold is >2 mA, the patient should be restricted to bed rest, and repositioning of the lead should be considered.

KEY POINTS TO REMEMBER

- After central venous line placement, right-heart catheterization, temporary transvenous pacemaker implantation, and IABP placement are the most commonly used procedures in the cardiac ICU.
- Careful decision with regard to necessity and site of insertion must be made. Coagulopathy and/or thrombocytopenia should be corrected.
- These procedures always require the assistance of those trained in the procedure to promote avoidance of complications and rapid appropriate action in the setting of a complication.

REFERENCES AND SUGGESTED READINGS

Gore JM. *Handbook of hemodynamic monitoring*. Boston: Little, Brown and Co., 1985.

Gregoratos G, Cheitlin MD, Gonill A, et al. ACC/AHA guidelines for implantation of cardiac pacemakers and antiarrhythmia devices: executives summary. A report of the American College of Cardiology/American Heart Association task force on practice guidelines (committee on pacemaker implantation). *Circulation* 1998;97:1325–1335.

Grossman W. *Cardiac catheterization and angiography*, 4th ed. Philadelphia: Lea & Febiger, 1996:113–125.

Kaushik V, Leon A, Forrester J, et al. Bradyarrhythmias, temporary and permanent pacing. *Crit Care Med* 2000;28(10):N121–N128.

Keenan J. Cardiology update. Temporary cardiac pacing. *Nurs Stand* 1995;9(20):50–51.

Lumia FJ, Rios JC. Temporary transvenous pacemaker therapy: an analysis of complications. *Chest* 1973;64:604–608.

Marino P. *The ICU book*, 2nd ed. Philadelphia: Lippincott Williams & Wilkins, 1997.

Mueller HS. Role of intra-aortic counterpulsation in cardiogenic shock and acute myocardial infarction. *Cardiology* 1994;84:168.

O'Rourke MF, Sammel N, Chang VP. Arterial counterpulsation in severe heart failure complication acute myocardial infarction. *Br Heart J* 1979;41:308.

Putterman C. The Swan-Ganz catheter: a decade of hemodynamic monitoring. *J Crit Care* 1989;4:127.

Sasayama S, Osakada G, Takahash M, et al. Effects of intraaortic balloon counterpulsation on regional myocardial function during acute coronary occlusion in the dog. *Am J Cardiol* 1979;43:59.

Topol E. *Textbook of cardiovascular medicine*. Philadelphia: Lippincott–Raven Publishers, 1998:1957–1969.

Zoll PM. Resuscitation of the heart in ventricular standstill by external electric stimulation. *N Engl J Med* 1952:247:768–781.

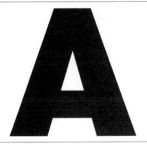

Preop Cardiac Assessment

Michael E. Lazarus

The most widely used algorithm for preop assessment of cardiac risk was updated in 2002 by the AHA (Fig. A-1). The following eight-step approach accompanies this algorithm.

1. What is the urgency of the surgery? If the surgery is emergent or urgent, your time would best be spent concentrating on periop medical management and surveillance.
2. Has the patient undergone coronary revascularization within the past 5 yrs? If so, and the patient is asymptomatic, no further workup is needed.
3. Has the patient undergone a coronary evaluation within the last 2 yrs? If so, repeat testing may be redundant.
4. Does the patient have an unstable coronary syndrome or major clinical predictors? In the setting of unstable coronary disease, decompensated CHF, symptomatic arrhythmias, or severe valvular heart disease, patients most often will benefit from cardiac catheterization.
5. Does the patient have intermediate predictors of risk? These include history of MI, angina pectoris, compensated or prior CHF, and diabetes mellitus. Consideration of functional capacity and the level of surgery-specific risk allow you to identify those patients most likely to benefit from noninvasive cardiac testing. To evaluate surgery-specific cardiac risk, consider the type of procedure (e.g., vascular procedures are more likely to be associated with underlying CAD than nonvascular surgery) and the degree of hemodynamic stress associated with surgery-specific procedures (certain procedures are more likely than others to result in prolonged periop alterations in heart rate and BP, fluid shifts, pain, bleeding, clotting tendencies, oxygenation, and neurohumoral activation).
6. Patients with intermediate clinical predictors of risk who have moderate to excellent functional capacity can generally undergo an intermediate risk operation with little likelihood of periop cardiac complications. Further testing is often required in patients who have poor functional capacity and/or are undergoing high-risk surgery.
7. Noncardiac surgery is generally safe in patients with no high or intermediate risk factors and who have moderate or excellent functional capacity (>4 metabolic equivalents).
8. Results of noninvasive testing guide further cardiac management, be it medical or invasive.

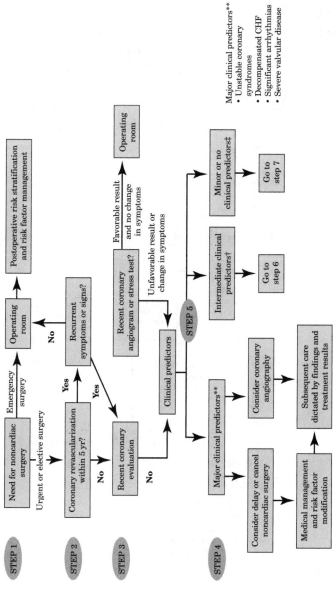

FIG. A-1. Stepwise approach to preop cardiac assessment. *Subsequent care may include cancellation or delay of surgery, coronary revascularization followed by noncardiac surgery, or intensified care. METs, metabolic equivalents. (From Eagle KA, Berger PB, Calkins H, et al. ACC/AHA guideline update for perioperative cardiovascular evaluation for noncardiac surgery: executive summary: a report of the American College of Cardiology/American Heart Association Task Force on Practice Guidelines (Committee to Update the 1996 Guidelines on Perioperative Cardiovascular Evaluation for Noncardiac Surgery. *Circulation* 2002;105:1257–1267.) *(continued)*

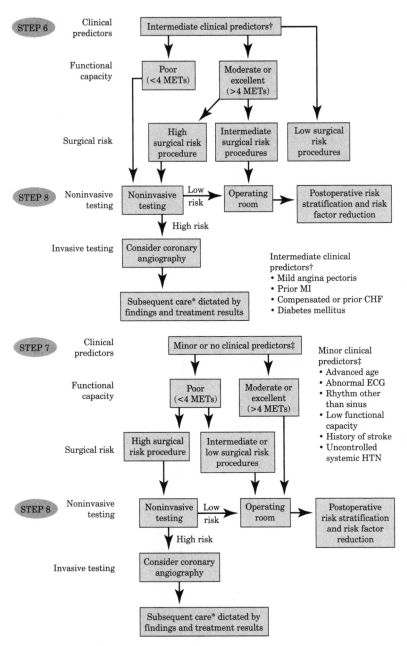

FIG. A-1. Continued.

Index

Page numbers followed by *t* indicate tables; numbers followed by *f* indicate figures.